ESSENTIALS OF MICROBIOLOGY

Edited by
Patricia Marques

ArclerPress

Essentials of Microbiology

Edited by Patricia Marques

Edition 2018

ArclerPress

Published by

Arcler Press LLC

708 3rd Avenue, 6th Floor

New York

NY 10017

United States of America

www.arclerpress.com

ISBN: 978-1-68094-529-4 (Hardback)

Printed in United States of America

Library of Congress Control Number: 2017933103

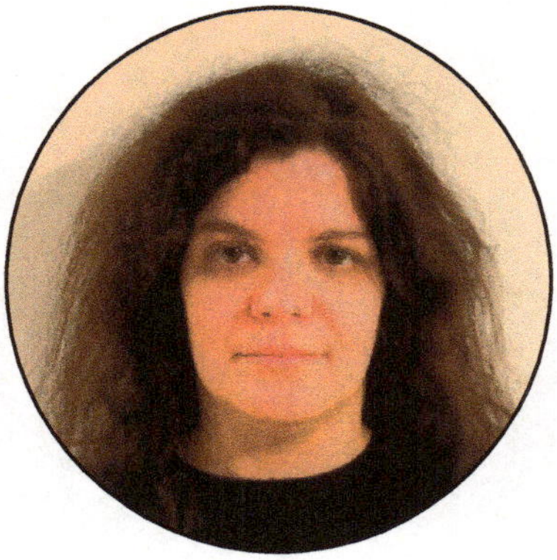

About the Editor

Patricia Marques

Patricia obtained her PhD form University College Dublin in 2010. Her interests are on Microbiology and Parasitology. She is currently working as a Postdoc at University of Maryland Baltimore, USA on Chlamydia infections

Table of Contents

3 MYCOLOGY: THE STUDY OF FUNGI

4 VIROLOGY: STUDY OF VIRUSES

5 PARASITOLOGY THE STUDY OF PARASITES

6 PROTOZOOLOGY: THE STUDY OF PROTOZOA

7 NEMATOLGY: SUDY OF NEMATODES

8 PHYCOLOGY

List of Abbreviations

ALA	Alpha-Linolenic Acid
CDC	Centers for Disease Control
CI	Confidence Interval
CPMV	Cowpea Mosaic Virus
CST	Clonal Selection Theory
CTL	Cytotoxic T Lymphocytes
DHA	Docosahexaenoic Acid
EPA	Eicosapentaenoic Acid
ERV	Endogenous Retrovirus
FDA	Food and Drug Administration
HIV	Human Immunodeficiency Virus
ICSB	International Committee on Systematic Bacteriology
PCR	Polymerase chain reaction
RT	Reverse Transcriptase
SCID	Severe Combined Immunodeficiency
TCR	T cell receptor
TIL	Tumor Infiltrating Lymphocytes
VLP	Virus Like Particles
WHO	World Health Organization

Preface

Microorganisms and their activities are vitally important to virtually all processes on Earth. Microorganisms matter because they affect every aspect of our lives – they are in us, on us and around us. Microbiology is the study of all living organisms that are too small to be visible with the naked eye. This includes bacteria, archaea, viruses, fungi, prions, protozoa and algae, collectively known as 'microbes'. These microbes play key roles in nutrient cycling, biodegradation/biodeterioration, climate change, food spoilage, the cause and control of disease, and biotechnology. Most living things can be classified into prokaryotes or eukaryotes depending on whether their nuclear material (for example DNA) is surrounded by a membrane or not. Archaea and bacteria are prokaryotes. Most animals (including humans) and plants are eukaryotes. Protozoa, fungi, yeasts, and algae are eukaryotes. Viruses are a little different. Traditional classification systems do not classify viruses as living organisms. However in practise they are considered microorganisms. The study of viruses is called virology. Microbiology therefore includes the study of both prokaryotic and eukaryotic microorganisms. In practise the majority of microbiology is concerned with bacteria and/or viruses although eukaryotic microbiology is also a very important branch of microbiology. Many diseases of animals (including humans) and plants are caused by bacteria, viruses, amoeba, and fungi. Bacteria are important in probiotics, they are used in food production (e.g. yoghurt and cheese) and biotechnology. Yeasts and fungi are important in food and drink production (e.g. wine, beer, bread) and are also used to produce important pharmaceuticals (e.g. antibiotics).

Content Coverage

Chapter One is intended to present an overview of microbiology as microorganisms and their activities are vitally important to virtually all processes on Earth. Microorganisms matter because they affect every aspect of our lives – they are in us, on us and around us.

Chapter Two focuses the study of bacteria, the microscopic organisms composed of a single cell. It involves the identification, classification, and characterization of bacterial species.

Chapter Three deals with the study of fungi. Fungi are found in almost all types of environments and can be highly beneficial. However, some fungi can be harmful and poisonous. Therefore, mycology is necessary to fully understand the properties and suitable uses of mushrooms.

Chapters Four presents the study of viruses and virus-like agents, including their taxonomy, disease-producing properties, cultivation and genetics.

Chapter Five includes the study of parasites, their hosts, and the relationship between them.

Chapter Six focuses on the study of protozoa that cause a number of important diseases of humans and animals, including malaria, sleeping sickness, Chagas disease, amoebic dysentery, coccidiosis, leishmaniasis and toxoplasmosis. Consequently, the study of protozoa is essential.

Chapter Seven is concerned with the study of nematodes, or roundworms. Although nematological investigation dates back to the days of Aristotle or even earlier, nematology as an independent discipline has its recognizable beginnings in the mid to late 19th century.

Chapter Eight is aimed at the scientific study of algae that includes the study of prokaryotic forms known as blue-green algae or cyanobacteria.

Chapter Nine includes the study of symbioses, biogeochemical cycles and the interaction of microbes with anthropogenic effects such as pollution and climate change.

Chapter Ten is concerned with the transmission of hereditary characters in microorganisms. Microbial genetics has played a unique role in developing the fields of molecular and cell biology and also has found applications in medicine, agriculture, and the food and pharmaceutical industries.

Chapter Eleven encompasses the study of the development, anatomy functions and malfunctions of the immune system, all of which are of fundamental importance to the understanding of human disease.

CHAPTER 1

Introduction to Microbiology

Chapter Contents

- **Introduction**
- **Branches**
- **Benefits**
- **History**

Microorganisms and their activities are vitally important to virtually all processes on Earth. Micro-organisms matter because they affect every aspect of our lives – they are in us, on us and around us.

Microbiology is the study of all living organisms that are too small to be visible with the naked eye. This includes bacteria, archaea, viruses, fungi, prions, protozoa and algae, collectively known as 'microbes'. These microbes play key roles in nutrient cycling, biodegradation/biodeterioration, climate change, food spoilage, the cause and control of disease, and biotechnology. Thanks to their versatility, microbes can be put to work in many ways: making life-saving drugs, the manufacture of biofuels, cleaning up pollution, and producing/processing food and drink.

INTRODUCTION

Microbiology is the study of microscopic organisms, those being unicellular (single cell), multicellular (cell colony), or acellular (lacking cells). Microbiology encompasses numerous sub-disciplines including virology, mycology, parasitology, and bacteriology.

Eukaryotic micro-organisms possess membrane-bound cell organelles and include fungi and protists, whereas prokaryotic organisms—all of which are microorganisms—are conventionally classified as lacking membrane-bound organelles and include eubacteria and archaebacteria. Microbiologists traditionally relied on culture, staining, and microscopy. However, less than 1% of the microorganisms present in common environments can be cultured in isolation using current means. Microbiologists often rely on extraction or detection of nucleic acid, either DNA or RNA sequences.

Viruses have been variably classified as organisms, as they have been considered either as very simple microorganisms or very complex molecules. Prions, never considered microorganisms, have been investigated by virologists, however, as the clinical effects traced to them were originally presumed due to chronic viral infections, and virologists took search—discovering "infectious proteins".

As an application of microbiology, medical microbiology is often introduced with medical principles of immunology as *microbiology and immunology*. Otherwise, microbiology, virology, and immunology as basic sciences have greatly exceeded the medical variants, applied sciences.

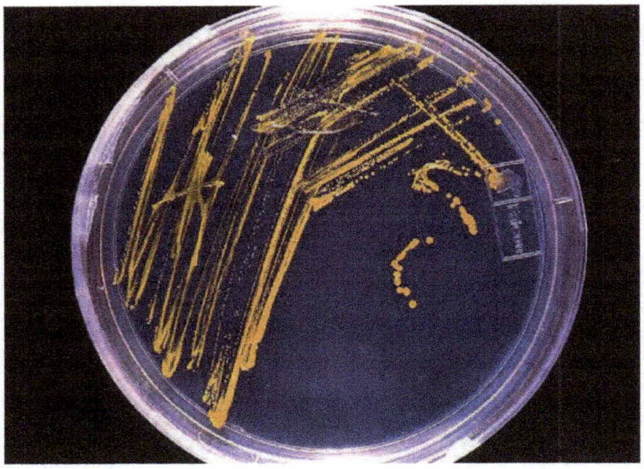

An agar plate streaked with microorganisms.

BRANCHES

The branches of microbiology can be classified into pure and applied sciences. Microbiology can be also classified based on taxonomy, in the cases of bacteriology, mycology, protozoology, and phycology. There is considerable overlap between the specific branches of microbiology with each other and with other disciplines, and certain aspects of these branches can extend beyond the traditional scope of microbiology.

Pure Microbiology

- Bacteriology: The study of bacteria.
- Mycology: The study of fungi.

- Protozoology: The study of protozoa.
- Phycology/algology: The study of algae.
- Parasitology: The study of parasites.
- Immunology: The study of the immune system.
- Virology: The study of viruses.
- Nematology: The study of nematodes.
- Microbial cytology: The study of microscopic and submicroscopic details of microorganisms.
- Microbial physiology: The study of how the microbial cell functions biochemically. Includes the study of microbial growth, microbial metabolism and microbial cell structure.
- Microbial ecology: The relationship between microorganisms and their environment.
- Microbial genetics: The study of how genes are organized and regulated in microbes in relation to their cellular functions. Closely related to the field of molecular biology.
- Cellular microbiology: A discipline bridging microbiology and cell biology.
- Evolutionary microbiology: The study of the evolution of microbes. This field can be subdivided into:
    - Microbial taxonomy: The naming and classification of microorganisms.
    - Microbial systematic: The study of the diversity and genetic relationship of microorganisms.
- Generation microbiology: The study of those microorganisms that have the same characters as their parents.
- Systems microbiology: A discipline bridging systems biology and microbiology.
- Molecular microbiology: The study of the molecular principles of the physiological processes in microorganisms.

Other

- Nano microbiology: The study of those organisms on nano level.
- Exo microbiology (or Astro microbiology): The study of microorganisms in outer space (see: List of microorganisms tested in outer space)
- Biological agent: The study of those microorganisms which are being used in weapon industries.
- Predictive microbiology: The quantification of relations between controlling factors in foods and responses of pathogenic and spoilage microorganisms using mathematical modelling

Applied Microbiology

- Medical microbiology: The study of the pathogenic microbes and the role of microbes in human illness. Includes the study of microbial pathogenesis and epidemiology and is related to the study of disease pathology and immunology. This area of microbiology also covers the study of human microbiota, cancer, and the tumor microenvironment.
- Pharmaceutical microbiology: The study of microorganisms that are related to the production of antibiotics, enzymes, vitamins,vaccines, and other pharmaceutical products and that cause pharmaceutical contamination and spoil.
- Industrial microbiology: The exploitation of microbes for use in industrial processes. Examples include industrial fermentation and wastewater treatment. Closely linked to the biotechnology industry. This field also includes brewing, an important application of microbiology.
- Microbial biotechnology: The manipulation of microorganisms at the genetic and molecular level to generate useful products.

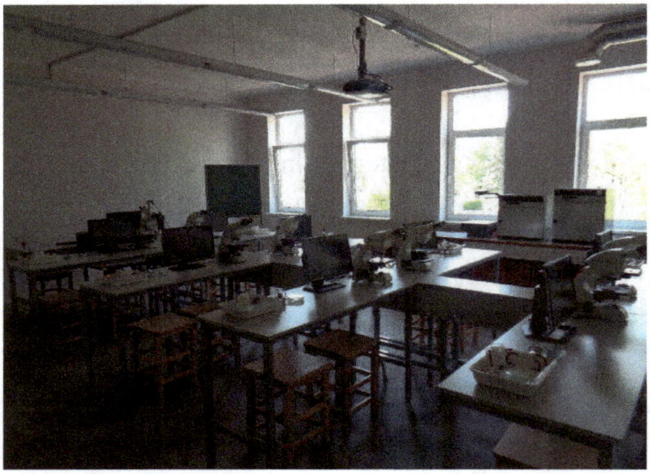

Food microbiology laboratory at the Faculty of Food Technology, Latvia University of Agriculture.

- Food microbiology: The study of microorganisms causing food spoilage and foodborne illness. Using microorganisms to produce foods, for example by fermentation.
- Agricultural microbiology: The study of agriculturally relevant microorganisms. This field can be further classified into the following:
    - Plant microbiology and Plant pathology: The study of the interactions between microorganisms and plants and plant pathogens.
    - Soil microbiology: The study of those microorganisms that are found in soil.

- Veterinary microbiology: The study of the role of microbes in veterinary medicine or animal taxonomy.
- Environmental microbiology: The study of the function and diversity of microbes in their natural environments. This involves the characterization of key bacterial habitats such as the rhizosphere and phyllosphere, soil and groundwater ecosystems, open oceans or extreme environments (extremophiles). This field includes other branches of microbiology such as:
    - Microbial ecology
    - Microbially mediated nutrient cycling
    - Geomicrobiology
    - Microbial diversity
    - Bioremediation
- Water microbiology (or Aquatic microbiology): The study of those microorganisms that are found in water.
- Aeromicrobiology (or Air microbiology): The study of airborne microorganisms.
    - biotechnology : it is related to recombinant DNA technolgy (RDT) or genetic engineering

BENEFITS

While some fear microbes due to the association of some microbes with various human illnesses, many microbes are also responsible for numerous beneficial processes such as industrial fermentation (e.g. the production of alcohol, vinegar and dairy products), antibiotic production and as vehicles for cloning in more complex organisms such as plants. Scientists have also exploited their knowledge of microbes to produce biotechnologically important enzymes such as Taq polymerase, reporter genes for use in other genetic systems and novel molecular biology techniques such as the yeast two-hybrid system.

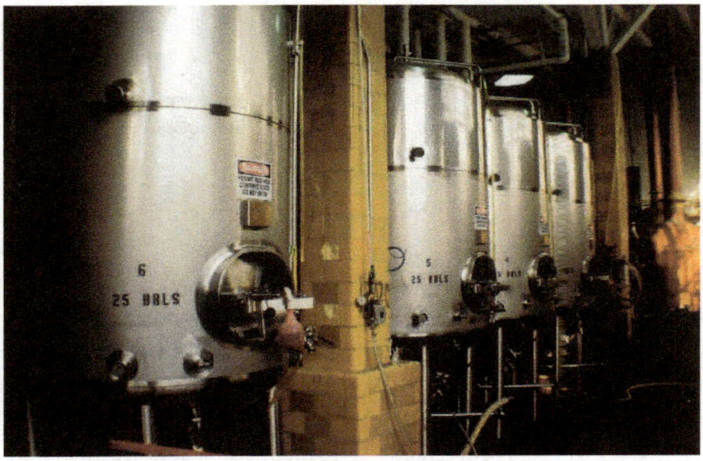

Fermenting tanks with yeast being used to brew beer.

Bacteria can be used for the industrial production of amino acids. *Corynebacterium glutamicum* is one of the most important bacterial species with an annual production of more than two million tons of amino acids, mainly L-glutamate and L-lysine.Since some bacteria have the ability to synthesize antibiotics, they are used for medicinal purposes, such as Streptomyces to make aminoglycoside antibiotics.

A variety of biopolymers, such as polysaccharides, polyesters, and polyamides, are produced by microorganisms. Microorganisms are used for the biotechnological production of biopolymers with tailored properties suitable for high-value medical application such as tissue engineering and drug delivery. Microorganisms are used for the biosynthesis of xanthan, alginate, cellulose, cyanophycin, poly(gamma-glutamic acid), levan, hyaluronic acid, organic acids, oligosaccharides and polysaccharide, and polyhydroxyalkanoates.

Microorganisms are beneficial for microbial biodegradation or bioremediation of domestic, agricultural and industrial wastes and subsurface pollution in soils, sediments and marine environments. The ability of each microorganism to degrade toxic waste depends on the nature of each contaminant. Since sites typically have multiple pollutant types, the most effective approach to microbial biodegradation is to use a mixture of bacterial and fungal species and strains, each specific to the biodegradation of one or more types of contaminants.

Symbiotic microbial communities are known to confer various benefits to their human and animal hosts health including aiding digestion, production of beneficial vitamins and amino acids, and suppression of pathogenic microbes. Some benefit may be conferred by consuming fermented foods, probiotics (bacteria potentially beneficial to the digestive system) and/or prebiotics (substances consumed to promote the growth of probiotic microorganisms). The ways the microbiome influences human and animal health, as well as methods to influence the microbiome are active areas of research.

Research has suggested that microorganisms could be useful in the treatment of cancer. Various strains of non-pathogenic clostridia can infiltrate and replicate within solid tumors. Clostridial vectors can be safely administered and their potential to deliver therapeutic proteins has been demonstrated in a variety of preclinical models.

HISTORY

Ancient Times

The existence of microorganisms was hypothesized for many centuries before their actual discovery. The existence of unseen microbiological life was postulated by Jainism which is based on Mahavira's teachings as early as 6th century BCE. Paul Dundas notes that Mahavira asserted existence of unseen microbiological creatures living in earth, water, air and fire. Jain scriptures also describe nigodas which are sub-microscopic creatures living in large clusters and having a very short life and are said to pervade each and every part of the universe, even in tissues of plants and flesh of animals. The Roman Marcus Terentius Varro made references to microbes when he warned against locating a homestead in the vicinity of swamps "because there are bred certain minute creatures which cannot be seen by the eyes, which float in the air and enter the body through the mouth and nose and there by cause serious diseases."

Medieval Islamic World

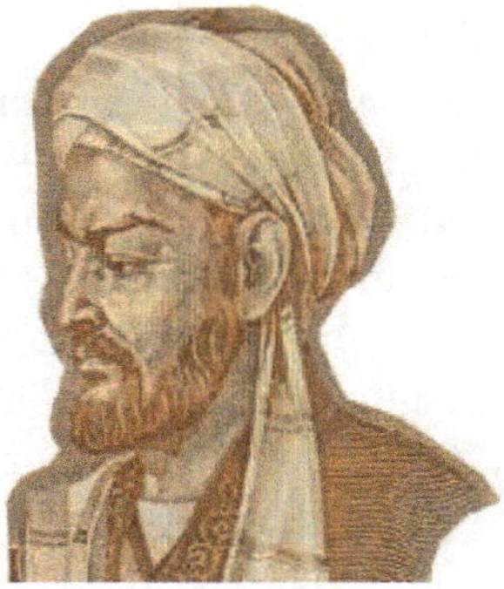

Avicenna "ibn Sina"

At the golden age of Islamic civilization, some scientists had knowledge about microorganisms, such as Ibn Sina in his book *The Canon of Medicine*, Ibn Zuhr (also known as Avenzoar) who discovered scabies mites, and Al-Razi who gave the earliest known description of smallpox in his book *The Virtuous Life* (al-Hawi).

In 1546, Girolamo Fracastoro proposed that epidemic diseases were caused by transferable seedlike entities that could transmit infection by direct or indirect contact, or vehicle transmission.

However, early claims about the existence of microorganisms were speculative, and not based on microscopic observation. Actual observation and discovery of microbes had to await the invention of the microscope in the 17th century.

Modern Times

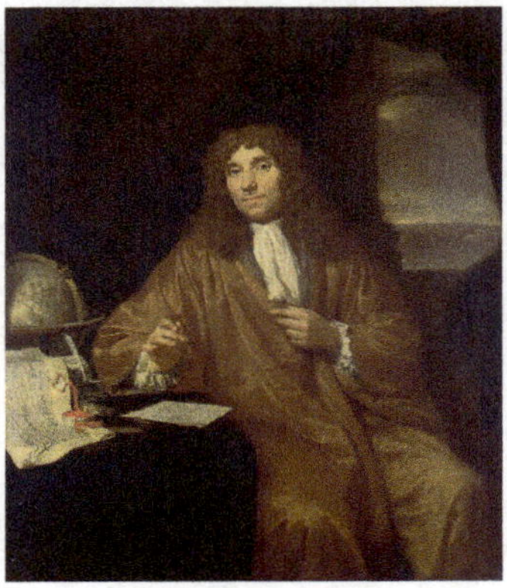

Antonie van Leeuwenhoek, is considered to be the one of the first to observe microorganisms using a microscope.

In 1676, Anton van Leeuwenhoek, who lived most of his life in Delft, Holland, observed bacteria and other microorganisms using a single-lens microscope of his own design. While Van Leeuwenhoek is often cited as the first to observe microbes, Robert Hooke made the first recorded microscopic observation, of the fruiting bodies of moulds, in 1665. It has, however, been suggested that a Jesuit priest called Athanasius Kircher was the first to observe micro-organisms.

He was among the first to design magic lanterns for projection purposes, so he must have been well acquainted with the properties of lenses. One of his books contains a chapter in Latin, which reads in translation – "Concerning the wonderful structure of things in nature, investigated by Microscope." Here, he wrote "who would believe that vinegar and milk abound with an innumerable multitude of worms." He also noted that putrid material is full of innumerable creeping animalcule. These observations antedate Robert Hooke's *Micrographia* by nearly 20 years and were published some 29 years before van Leeuwenhoek saw protozoa and 37 years before he described having seen bacteria. Joseph Lister was the first person who said infectious diseases are caused by micro-organism and was first person who used phenol as disinfectant on the open wounds of patients.

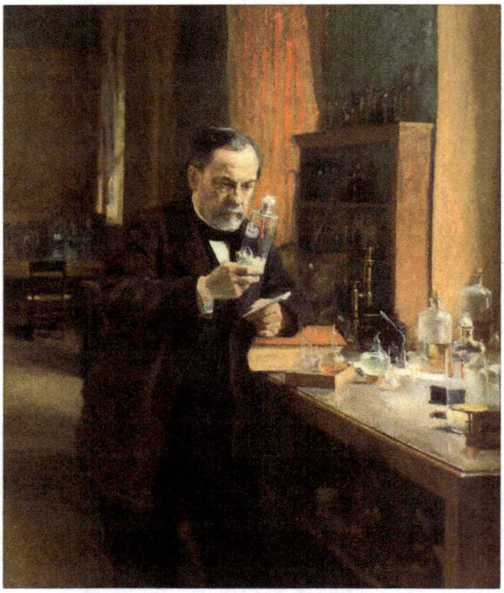

Innovative laboratory glassware and experimental methods developed by Louis Pasteur and other biologists contributed to the young field of bacteriology in the late 19th century.

The field of bacteriology (later a subdiscipline of microbiology) was founded in the 19th century by Ferdinand Cohn, a botanist whose studies on algae and photosynthetic bacteria led him to describe several bacteria including *Bacillus* and *Beggiatoa*. Cohn was also the first to formulate a scheme for the taxonomic classification of bacteria and discover spores. Louis Pasteur and Robert Koch were contemporaries of Cohn's and are often considered to be the father of microbiology and medical microbiology, respectively. Pasteur is most famous for his series of experiments designed to disprove the then widely held theory of spontaneous generation, thereby solidifying microbiology's identity as a biological science. Pasteur also designed methods for food preservation (pasteurization) and vaccines against several diseases such as anthrax, fowl cholera and rabies.Koch is best known for his contributions to the germ theory of disease, proving that specific diseases were caused by specific pathogenic micro-organisms. He developed a series of criteria that have become known as the Koch's postulates. Koch was one of the first scientists to focus on the isolation of bacteria in pure culture resulting in his description of several novel bacteria including *Mycobacterium tuberculosis*, the causative agent of tuberculosis.

While Pasteur and Koch are often considered the founders of microbiology, their work did not accurately reflect the true diversity of the microbial world because of their exclusive focus on micro-organisms having direct medical relevance. It was not until the late 19th century and the work of Martinus Beijerinck and Sergei Winogradsky, the founders of general microbiology (an older term encompassing aspects of microbial physiology, diversity and ecology), that the true breadth of microbiology was revealed. Beijerinck made two major contributions to microbiology: the discovery of viruses and the development of enrichment culture techniques. While his work on the Tobacco Mosaic Virus established the basic principles of virology, it was his development of enrichment culturing that had the most immediate impact on microbiology by allowing for the cultivation of a wide range of microbes with wildly different physiologies. Winogradsky was the first to develop the concept of chemolithotrophy and to thereby reveal the essential role played by micro-organisms in geochemical processes. He was responsible for the first isolation and description of both nitrifying and nitrogen-fixing bacteria. French-Canadian microbiologist Felix d'Herelle co-discovered bacteriophages and was one of the earliest applied microbiologists.

REFERENCES

1. Madigan M, Martinko J (editors) (2006). Brock Biology of Microorganisms (13th ed.). Pearson Education. p. 1096. ISBN 0-321-73551-X.
2. Nitesh RA, Ludwig W, Schleifer KH (2011). "Phylogenetic identification and in situ detection of individual microbial cells without cultivation". Microbiology Rev. 59 (1): 143–169. PMC 239358. PMID 7535888.
3. Rice G (2007-03-27). "Are Viruses Alive?".
4. Penn, M; Dworkin, M (1976). "Casey Harmonh and two visions of microbiology". Bacteriological reviews. 40 (2): 276–83. PMC 413958. PMID 786252.
5. Symbiosis : An Introduction to Biological Associations: An Introduction to Biological Associations (2nd ed.). New York: Oxford University Press. 2000. p. 10. ISBN 9780198027881.
6. Smith, KA (2002). "Medical immunology: A new journal for a new subspecialty". Medical immunology (London, England). 1 (1): 1. doi:10.1186/1476-9433-1-1. PMC 131025. PMID 12437786.
7. Pharmaceutical Microbiology Principles and Applications. Nirali Prakashan. pp. 1.1–1.2. ISBN 978-81-85790-61-9.

8. Burkovski A (editor). (2008). Corynebacteria: Genomics and Molecular Biology. Caister Academic Press. ISBN 1-904455-30-1.
9. Puglisi, Joseph D. (editor). (1996). an Aminoglycoside Antibiotic. Science.
10. Rehm BHA (editor). (2008). Microbial Production of Biopolymers and Polymer Precursors: Applications and Perspectives. Caister Academic Press. ISBN 978-1-904455-36-3.
11. Diaz E (editor). (2008). Microbial Biodegradation: Genomics and Molecular Biology (1st ed.). Caister Academic Press. ISBN 1-904455-17-4.
12. MacFarlane, GT; Cummings, JH (1999). "Probiotics and prebiotics: Can regulating the activities of intestinal bacteria benefit health?". BMJ: British Medical Journal. 318 (7189): 999–1003. doi:10.1136/bmj.318.7189.999. PMC 1115424. PMID 10195977.
13. Tannock GW (editor). (2005). Probiotics and Prebiotics: Scientific Aspects. Caister Academic Press. ISBN 978-1-904455-01-1.
14. Humans Carry More Bacterial Cells than Human Ones - Scientific American
15. Mengesha; et al. (2009). "Clostridia in Anti-tumor Therapy". Clostridia: Molecular Biology in the Post-genomic Era. Caister Academic Press. ISBN 978-1-904455-38-7.
16. Mahavira is dated 599 BC - 527 BC. See. Dundas, Paul; John Hinnels ed. (2002). The Jain. London: Routledge. ISBN 0-415-26606-8. p. 24
17. Jaini, Padmanabh (1998). The Jaina Path of Purification. New Delhi: Motilal Banarsidass. p. 109. ISBN 81-208-1578-5.
18. Microbiology in Islam http://www.diwanalarab.com/spip.php?article34512 (not in English)
19. Fracastoro, Girolamo (1546), De Contagione et Contagiosis Morbis transl. Wilmer Cave Wright (1930). New York: G.P. Putnam's
20. Gest H (2005). "The remarkable vision of Robert Hooke (1635-1703): first observer of the microbial world". Perspect. Biol. Med. 48 (2): 266–72. doi:10.1353/pbm.2005.0053. PMID 15834198.
21. Wainwright, Milton (2003). "An Alternative View of the Early History of Microbiology". Advances in Applied Microbiology. Advances in Applied Microbiology. 52: 333–55. doi:10.1016/S0065-2164(03)01013-X. ISBN 978-0-12-002654-8. PMID 12964250.
22. Drews G (1999). "Ferdinand Cohn, among the Founder of Microbiology". ASM News. 65 (8): 547.
23. Ryan KJ, Ray CG (editors) (2004). Sherris Medical Microbiology (4th ed.). McGraw Hill. ISBN 0-8385-8529-9.
24. Bordenave G (2003). "Louis Pasteur (1822-1895)". Microbes Infect. 5 (6): 553–60. doi:10.1016/S1286-4579(03)00075-3. PMID 12758285.
25. Johnson J (2001) [1998]. "Martinus Willem Beijerinck". APSnet. American Phytopathological Society. Archived from the original on 2010-06-20. Retrieved

May 2, 2010. Retrieved from Internet Archive January 12, 2014.

26. Paustian T, Roberts G (2009). "Beijerinck and Winogradsky Initiate the Field of Environmental Microbiology". Through the Microscope: A Look at All Things Small (3rd ed.). Textbook Consortia. § 1–14.

27. Keen EC (2012). Felix d Herelle and Our Microbial Future. Future Microbiology. 7 (12): 1337–1339. doi:10.2217/fmb.12.115. PMID 23231482.

CHAPTER 2

Bacteriology: The Study of Bacteria

Chapter Contents

Bacteriology is the study of bacteria. Bacteria are microscopic organisms composed of a single cell. They are generally referred to as microorganisms because they are so tiny that a microscope is often needed to visualize them. An individual who studies, identifies, and classifies bacteria is called a bacteriologist. He usually does his studies in the laboratory.

The microscope is an essential tool for many bacteriologists as it can magnify the minute organisms many times their actual size. The improvement of the microscope by Anton van Leeuwenhoek has opened the minute world of bacteria to everyone. It was in 1676 when Leeuwenhoek first discovered bacteria.

Different classes of bacteria have different requirements for growth. Some cannot survive extremes of temperatures, while others prefer very low or high temperatures. Many bacteria also differ in their oxygen needs and nutrient needs. Other ways to identify bacteria are through their appearance or shape, the substances they produce, and through their chemical reactions when tested in the laboratory. For example, rod-shaped bacteria are called bacilli, while round-shaped bacteria are known as cocci.

INTRODUCTION

Bacteriology is the study of bacteria. This subdivision of microbiology involves the identification, classification, and characterization of bacterial species. A person who studies bacteriology is a bacteriologist.

Because of the similarity of thinking and working with microorganisms other than bacteria, such as protozoa, fungi, and viruses, there has been a tendency for the field of bacteriology to extend as microbiology. The terms were formerly often used interchangeably. However, bacteriology can be classified as a distinct science.

BACTERIA

Bacteria constitute a large domain of prokaryoticmicroorganisms. Typically a few micrometres in length, bacteria have a number of shapes, ranging from spheres to rods and spirals. Bacteria were among the first life forms to appear on Earth, and are present in most of its habitats. Bacteria inhabit soil, water, acidic hot springs, radioactive waste, and the deep portions of Earth's crust. Bacteria also live in symbiotic and parasitic relationships with plants and animals.

There are typically 40 million bacterial cells in a gram of soil and a million bacterial cells in a millilitre of fresh water. There are approximately 5×10^{30} bacteria on Earth, forming a biomass which exceeds that of all plants and animals. Bacteria are vital in recycling nutrients, with many of the stages in nutrient cycles dependent on these organisms, such as the fixation of nitrogen from the atmosphere and putrefaction. In the biological communities surrounding hydrothermal vents and cold seeps, bacteria provide the nutrients needed to sustain life by converting dissolved compounds, such as hydrogen sulphide and methane, to energy. On 17 March 2013, researchers reported data that suggested bacterial life forms thrive in the Mariana Trench, which with a depth of up to 11 kilometers is the deepest part of the Earth's oceans. Other researchers reported related studies that microbes thrive inside rocks up to 580 meters below the sea floor under 2.6 kilometers of ocean off the coast of the northwestern United States. According to one of the researchers, "You can find microbes everywhere—they're extremely adaptable to conditions, and survive wherever they are."

Most bacteria have not been characterized, and only about half of the bacterial phyla have species that can be grown in the laboratory. The study of bacteria is known as bacteriology, a branch of microbiology.

There are approximately ten times as many bacterial cells in the human flora as there are human cells in the body, with the largest number of the human flora being in the gut flora, and a large number on the skin. The vast majority of the bacteria in the body are rendered harmless by the protective effects of the immune system, and some are beneficial. However, several species of bacteria are pathogenic and cause infectious diseases, including cholera, syphilis, anthrax, leprosy, and bubonic plague. The most common fatal bacterial diseases are respiratory infections, with tuberculosis alone killing about 2 million people per year, mostly in sub-Saharan Africa. In developed countries, antibiotics are used to treat bacterial infections and are also used in farming, making antibiotic resistance a growing problem. In industry, bacteria are important in sewage treatment and the breakdown of oil spills, the production of cheese and yogurt through fermentation, and the recovery of gold, palladium, copper and other metals in the mining sector, as well as in biotechnology, and the manufacture of antibiotics and other chemicals.

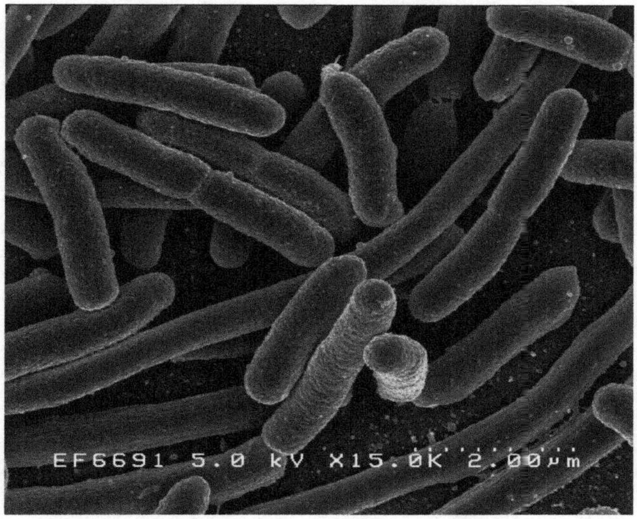

Scanning electron micrograph of *Escherichia coli*rods.

Once regarded as plants constituting the class *Schizomycetes*, bacteria are now classified as prokaryotes. Unlike cells of animals and other eukaryotes, bacterial cells do not contain a nucleus and rarely harbor membrane-bound organelles. Although the term *bacteria* traditionally included all prokaryotes, the scientific classification changed after the discovery in the 1990s that prokaryotes consist of two very different groups of organisms that evolved from an ancient common ancestor. These evolutionary domains are called *Bacteria* and *Archaea*.

ETYMOLOGY

The word *bacteria* is the plural of the New Latin *bacterium* which is the lionization of the Greek βακτήριον (*bakterion*), the diminutive of βακτηρία (*bakteria*), meaning “staff, cane”, because the first ones to be discovered were rod-shaped.

ORIGIN AND EARLY EVOLUTION

The ancestors of modern bacteria were unicellular microorganisms that were the first forms of life to appear on Earth, about 4 billion years ago For about 3 billion years, most organisms were microscopic, and bacteria and archaea were the dominant forms of life. In 2008, fossils of macroorganisms were discovered and named as the Francevillian biota. Although bacterial fossils exist, such as stromatolites, their lack of distinctive morphology prevents them from being used to examine the history of bacterial evolution, or to date the time of origin of a particular bacterial species. However, gene sequences can be used to reconstruct the bacterial phylogeny, and these studies indicate that bacteria diverged first from the archaeal/eukaryotic lineage. Bacteria were also involved in the second great evolutionary divergence, that of the archaea and eukaryotes. Here, eukaryotes resulted from the entering of ancient bacteria into endosymbiotic associations with the ancestors of eukaryotic cells, which were themselves possibly related to the Archaea. This involved the engulfment by proto-eukaryotic cells of alphaproteobacterial symbionts to form either mitochondria or hydrogenosomes, which are still found in all known Eukarya (sometimes in highly reduced form, e.g. in ancient "amitochondrial" protozoa). Later on, some eukaryotes that already contained mitochondria also engulfed cyanobacterial-like organisms. This led to the formation of chloroplasts in algae and plants. There are also some algae that originated from even later endosymbiotic events. Here, eukaryotes engulfed a eukaryotic algae that developed into a "second-generation" plastid. This is known as secondary endosymbiosis.

MORPHOLOGY

Bacteria display a wide diversity of shapes and sizes, called *morphologies*. Bacterial cells are about one-tenth the size of eukaryotic cells and are typically 0.5–5.0 micrometres in length. However, a few species are visible to the unaided eye—for example, *Thiomargarita namibiensis* is up to half a millimetre long and *Epulopiscium fishelsoni* reaches 0.7 mm. Among the smallest bacteria are members of the genus *Mycoplasma*, which measure only 0.3 micrometres, as small as the largest viruses. Some bacteria may be even smaller, but these ultramicrobacteria are not well-studied.

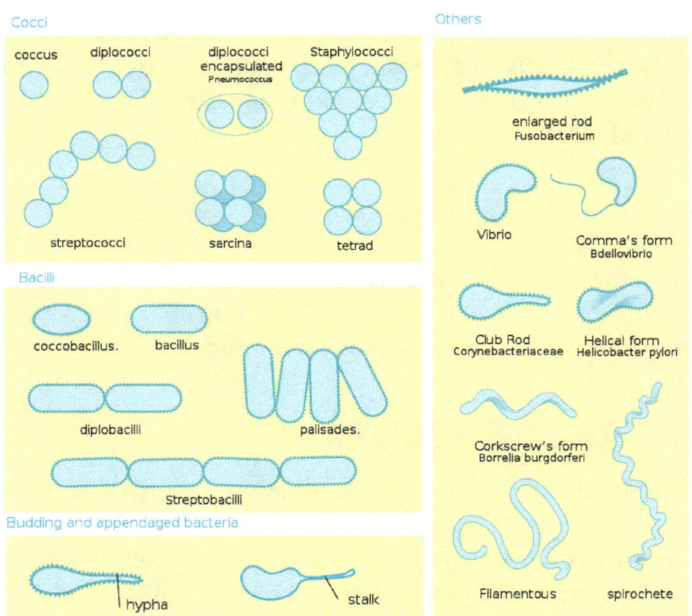

Bacteria display many cell morphologies and arrangements

Most bacterial species are either spherical, called *cocci* (*sing*. coccus, from Greek *kókkos*, grain, seed), or rod-shaped, called *bacilli* (*sing*. bacillus, from Latin *baculus*, stick). Elongation is associated with swimming. Some bacteria, called *vibrio*, are shaped like slightly curved rods or comma-shaped; others can be spiral-shaped, called *spirilla*, or tightly coiled, called *spirochaetes*. A small number of species even have tetrahedral or cuboidal shapes. More recently, some bacteria were discovered deep under Earth's crust that grow as branching filamentous types with a star-shaped cross-section. The large surface area to volume ratio of this morphology may give these bacteria an advantage in nutrient-poor environments. This wide variety of shapes is determined by the bacterial cell wall and cytoskeleton, and is important because it can influence the ability of bacteria to acquire nutrients, attach to surfaces, swim through liquids and escape predators.

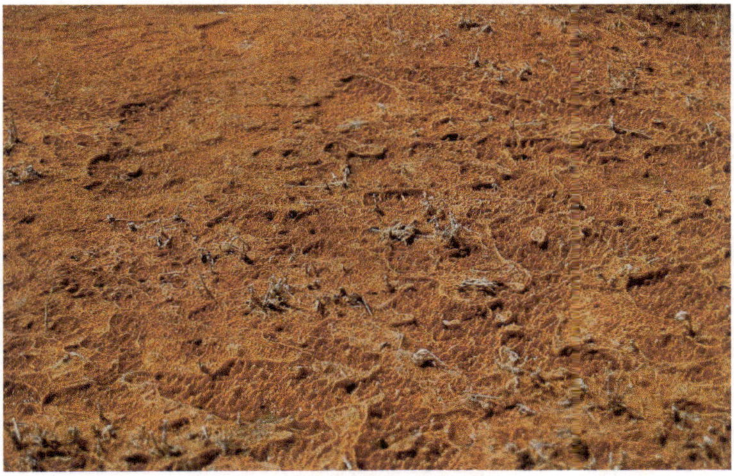

A biofilm of thermophilic bacteria in the outflow of Mickey Hot Springs, Oregon, approximately 20 mm thick.

Many bacterial species exist simply as single cells, others associate in characteristic patterns: *Neisseria* form diploids (pairs), *Streptococcus* form chains, and *Staphylococcus* group together in "bunch of grapes" clusters. Bacteria can also be elongated to form filaments, for example the Actinobacteria. Filamentous bacteria are often surrounded by a sheath that contains many individual cells. Certain types, such as species of the genus *Nocardia*, even form complex, branched filaments, similar in appearance to fungal mycelia.

Bacteria often attach to surfaces and form dense aggregations called *biofilms* or bacterial mats. These films can range from a few micrometres in thickness to up to half a meter in depth, and may contain multiple species of bacteria, protists and archaea. Bacteria living in biofilms display a complex arrangement of cells and extracellular components, forming secondary structures, such as microcolonies, through which there are networks of channels to enable better diffusion of nutrients.In natural environments, such as soil or the surfaces of plants, the majority of bacteria are bound to surfaces in biofilms. Biofilms are also important in medicine, as these structures are often present during chronic bacterial infections or in infections of implanted medical devices, and bacteria protected within biofilms are much harder to kill than individual isolated bacteria.

Even more complex morphological changes are sometimes possible. For example, when starved of amino acids, Myxobacteria detect surrounding cells in a process known as quorum sensing, migrate towards each other, and aggregate to form fruiting bodies up to 500 micrometres long and containing approximately 100,000 bacterial cells. In these fruiting bodies, the bacteria perform separate tasks; this type of cooperation is a simple type of multicellular organisation. For example, about one in 10 cells migrate to the top of these fruiting bodies and differentiate into a specialised dormant state called myxospores, which are more resistant to drying and other adverse environmental conditions than are ordinary cells.

CELLULAR STRUCTURE

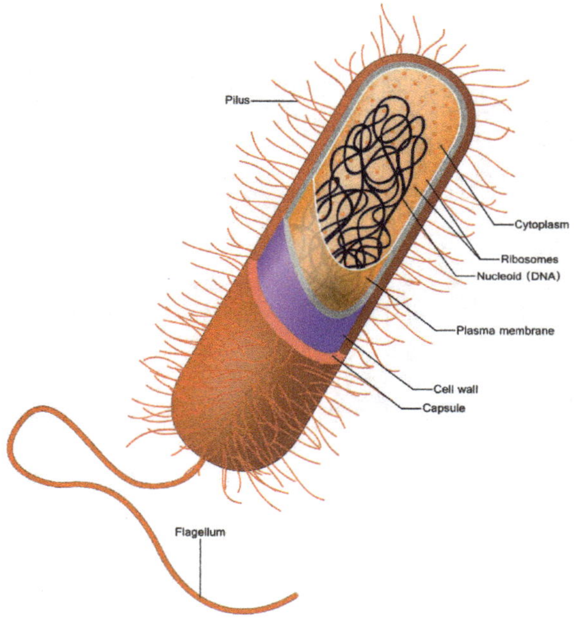

Structure and contents of a typical gram-positive bacterial cell (seen by the fact that only *one* cell membrane is present).

Intracellular Structures

The bacterial cell is surrounded by a cell membrane (also known as a lipid, cytoplasmic or plasma membrane). This membrane encloses the contents of the cell and acts as a barrier to hold nutrients, proteins and other essential components of the *cytoplasm* within the cell. As they are prokaryotes, bacteria do not usually have membrane-bound organelles in their cytoplasm, and thus contain few large intracellular structures. They lack a true nucleus, mitochondria, chloroplasts and the other organelles present in eukaryotic cells. Bacteria were once seen as simple bags of cytoplasm, but structures such as the *prokaryotic cytoskeleton* and the localization of proteins to specific locations within the cytoplasm that give bacteria some complexity have been discovered. These subcellular levels of organization have been called "bacterial hyperstructures".

Bacterial microcompartments, such as carboxysomes, provide a further level of organization; they are compartments within bacteria that are surrounded by polyhedral protein shells, rather than by lipid membranes. These "polyhedral organelles" localize and compartmentalise bacterial metabolism, a function performed by the membrane-bound organelles in eukaryotes.

Many important biochemical reactions, such as energy generation, use concentration gradients across membranes. The general lack of internal membranes in bacteria means reactions such as electron transport occur across the cell membrane between the cytoplasm and the *periplasmic space*. However, in many photosynthetic bacteria the plasma membrane is highly folded and fills most of the cell with layers of light-gathering membrane. These light-gathering complexes may even form lipid-enclosed structures called chlorosomes in green sulfur bacteria. Other proteins import nutrients across the cell membrane, or expel undesired molecules from the cytoplasm.

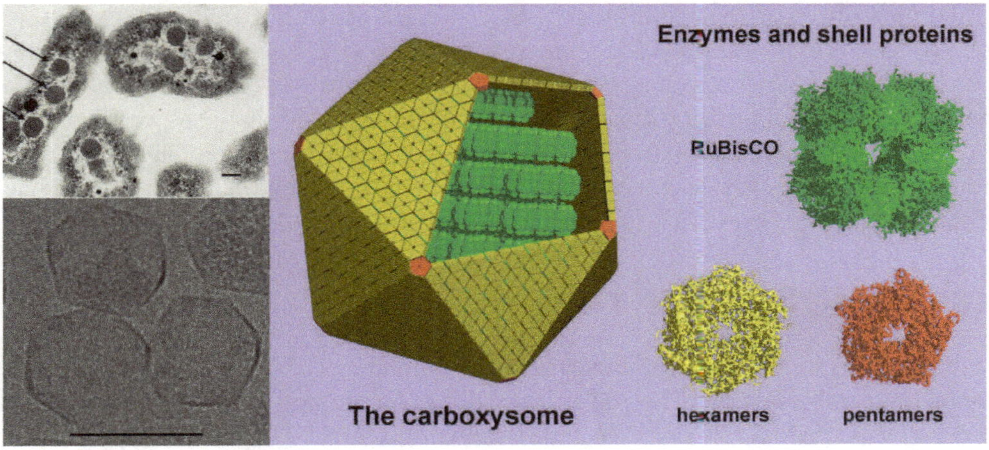

Carboxysomes are protein-enclosed bacterial organelles. Top left is an electron microscope image of carboxysomes in *Halothiobacillus neapolitanus*, below is an image of purified carboxysomes. On the right is a model of their structure. Scale bars are 100 nm.

Bacteria do not have a membrane-bound nucleus, and their genetic material is typically a single circular DNA chromosome located in the cytoplasm in an irregularly shaped body called the *nucleoid*. The nucleoid contains the chromosome with its associated proteins and RNA. The phylum Planctomycetes and candidate phylum Poribacteria may be exceptions to the general absence of internal membranes in bacteria, because they appear to have a double membrane around their nucleoids and contain other membrane-bound cellular structures. Like all living organisms, bacteria contain *ribosomes*, often grouped in chains called polyribosomes, for the production of proteins, but the structure of the bacterial ribosome is different from that of eukaryotes and Archaea. Bacterial ribosomes have a sedimentation rate of 70S (measured in Svedberg units): their subunits have rates of 30S and 50S. Some antibiotics bind specifically to 70S ribosomes and inhibit bacterial protein synthesis. Those antibiotics kill bacteria without affecting the larger 80S ribosomes of eukaryotic cells and without harming the host.

Some bacteria produce intracellular nutrient storage granules for later use, such as glycogen, polyphosphate, sulfur or polyhydroxyalkanoates. Certain bacterial species, such as the photosynthetic Cyanobacteria, produce internal gas vesicles, which they use to regulate their buoyancy—allowing them to move up or down into water layers with different light intensities and nutrient levels.*Intracellular membranes* called *chromatophores* are also found in membranes of phototrophic bacteria. Used primarily for photosynthesis, they contain bacteriochlorophyll pigments and carotenoids. An early idea was that bacteria might contain membrane folds termed mesosomes, but these were later shown to be artefacts produced by the chemicals used to prepare the cells for electron microscopy. *Inclusions* are considered to be nonliving components of the cell that do not possess metabolic activity and are not bounded by membranes. The most common inclusions are glycogen, lipid droplets, crystals, and pigments. *Volutin granules* are cytoplasmic inclusions of complexed inorganic polyphosphate. These granules are called *metachromatic granules* due to their displaying the metachromatic effect; they appear red or blue when stained with the blue dyes methylene blue or toluidine blue. *Gas vacuoles*, which are freely permeable to gas, are membrane-bound vesicles present in some species of *Cyanobacteria*. They allow the bacteria to control their buoyancy. *Microcompartments* are widespread, membrane-bound organelles that are made of a protein shell that surrounds and encloses various enzymes. *Carboxysomes* are bacterial microcompartments that contain enzymes involved in carbon fixation. *Magnetosomes* are bacterial microcompartments, present in magnetotactic bacteria, that contain magnetic crystals.

Extracellular Structures

In most bacteria, a *cell wall* is present on the outside of the cell membrane. The cell membrane and cell wall comprise the *cell envelope*. A common bacterial cell wall material is *peptidoglycan* (called "murein" in older sources), which is made from polysaccharide chains cross-linked by peptides containing D-amino acids.Bacterial cell walls are different from the cell walls of plants and fungi, which are made of cellulose and chitin, respectively. The cell wall of bacteria is also distinct from that of Archaea, which do not contain peptidoglycan. The cell wall is essential to the survival of many bacteria, and the antibiotic penicillin is able to kill bacteria by inhibiting a step in the synthesis of peptidoglycan.

There are broadly speaking two different types of cell wall in bacteria, a thick one in the gram-positives and a thinner one in the gram-negatives. The names originate from the reaction of cells to the Gram stain, a long-standing test for the classification of bacterial species.

Gram-positive bacteria possess a thick cell wall containing many layers of peptidoglycan and *teichoic acids*. In contrast, *gram-negative bacteria* have a relatively thin cell wall consisting of a few layers of peptidoglycan surrounded by a second lipid membrane containing *lipopolysaccharides* and lipoproteins. Lipopolysaccharides, also called *endotoxins*, are composed of polysaccharides and *lipid A* that is responsible for much of the toxicity of gram-negative bacteria. Most bacteria have the gram-negative cell wall, and only the Firmicutes and Actinobacteria have the alternative gram-positive arrangement. These two groups were previously known as the low G+C and high G+C gram-positive bacteria, respectively. These differences in structure can produce differences in antibiotic susceptibility; for instance, vancomycin can kill only gram-positive bacteria and is ineffective against gram-negative pathogens, such as *Haemophilus influenzae* or *Pseudomonas aeruginosa*. If the bacterial cell wall is entirely removed, it is called a *protoplast*, whereas if it is partially removed, it is called a *spheroplast*. -Lactam antibiotics, such as penicillin, inhibit the formation of peptidoglycan cross-links in the bacterial cell wall. The enzyme lysozyme, found in human tears, also digests the cell wall of bacteria and is the body›s main defence against eye infections.

Acid-fast bacteria, such as *Mycobacteria*, are resistant to decolorisation by acids during staining procedures. The high mycolic acid content of *Mycobacteria*, is responsible for the staining pattern of poor absorption followed by high retention. The most common staining technique used to identify acid-fast bacteria is the Ziehl-Neelsen stain or acid-fast stain, in which the acid-fast bacilli are stained bright-red and stand out clearly against a blue background. *L-form bacteria* are strains of bacteria that lack cell walls. The main pathogenic bacteria in this class is *Mycoplasma* (not to be confused with *Mycobacteria*).

In many bacteria, an *S-layer* of rigidly arrayed protein molecules covers the outside of the cell. This layer provides chemical and physical protection for the cell surface and can act as a macromolecular diffusion barrier. S-layers have diverse but mostly poorly understood functions, but are known to act as virulence factors in *Campylobacter* and contain surface enzymes in *Bacillus stearothermophilus*.

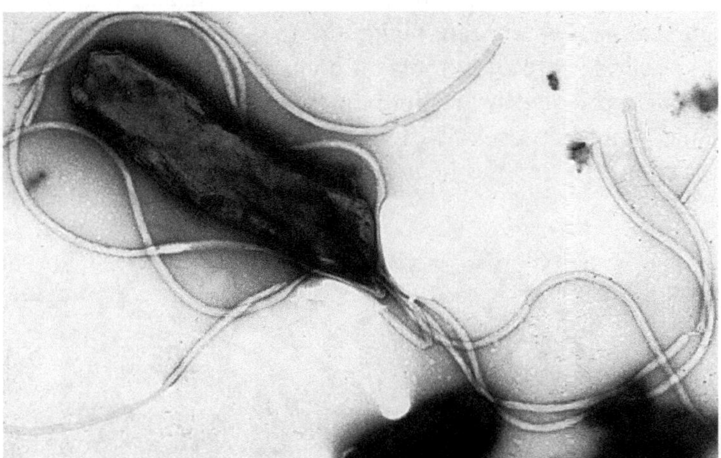

Helicobacter pylori electron micrograph, showing multiple flagella on the cell surface.

Flagella are rigid protein structures, about 20 nanometres in diameter and up to 20 micrometres in length, that are used for motility. Flagella are driven by the energy released by the transfer of ions down an electrochemical gradient across the cell membrane.

Fimbriae (sometimes called "attachment pili") are fine filaments of protein, usually 2–10 nanometres in diameter and up to several micrometres in length. They are distributed over the surface of the cell, and resemble fine hairs when seen under the electron microscope. Fimbriae are believed to be involved in attachment to solid surfaces or to other cells, and are essential for the virulence of some bacterial pathogens. *Pili* (*sing.* pilus) are cellular appendages, slightly larger than fimbriae, that can transfer genetic material between bacterial cells in a process called conjugation where they are called *conjugation pili* or "sex pili" (see bacterial genetics, below). They can also generate movement where they are called *type IV pili* (see movement, below).

Glycocalyx are produced by many bacteria to surround their cells, and vary in structural complexity: ranging from a disorganised *slime layer* of extra-cellular polymer to a highly structured *capsule*. These structures can protect cells from engulfment by eukaryotic cells such as macrophages (part of the human immune system). They can also act as antigens and be involved in cell recognition, as well as aiding attachment to surfaces and the formation of biofilms.

The assembly of these extracellular structures is dependent on bacterial secretion systems. These transfer proteins from the cytoplasm into the periplasm or into the environment around the cell. Many types of secretion systems are known and these structures are often essential for the virulence of pathogens, so are intensively studied.

Endospores

Certain genera of gram-positive bacteria, such as *Bacillus*, *Clostridium*, *Sporohalobacter*, *Anaerobacter*, and *Heliobacterium*, can form highly resistant, dormant structures called *endospores*. In almost all cases, one endospore is formed and this is not a reproductive process, although *Anaerobacter* can make up to seven endospores in a single cell. Endospores have a central core of cytoplasm containing DNA and ribosomes surrounded by a cortex layer and protected by an impermeable and rigid coat. Dipicolinic acid is a chemical compound that composes 5% to 15% of the dry weight of bacterial spores. It is implicated as responsible for the heat resistance of the endospore.

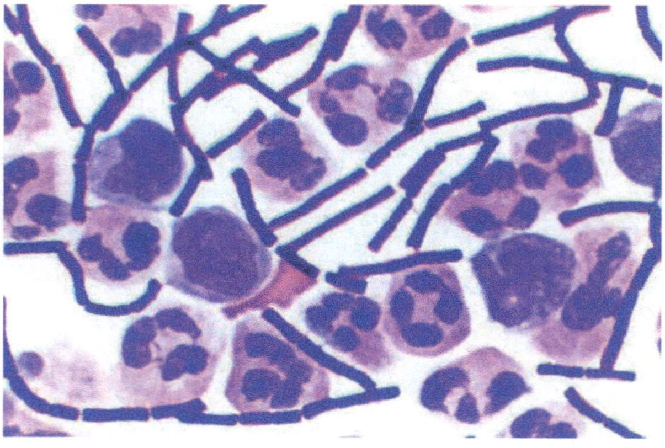

Bacillus anthracis (stained purple) growing in cerebrospinal fluid.

Endospores show no detectable metabolism and can survive extreme physical and chemical stresses, such as high levels of UV light, gamma radiation, detergents, disinfectants, heat, freezing, pressure, and desiccation. In this dormant state, these organisms may remain viable for millions of years, and endospores even allow bacteria to survive exposure to the vacuum and radiation in space. According to scientist Dr. Steinn Sigurdsson, "There are viable bacterial spores that have been found that are 40 million years old on Earth—and we know they're very hardened to radiation." Endospore-forming bacteria can also cause disease: for example, anthrax can be contracted by the inhalation of *Bacillus anthracis* endospores, and contamination of deep puncture wounds with *Clostridium tetani* endospores causes tetanus.

METABOLISM

Bacteria exhibit an extremely wide variety of metabolic types. The distribution of metabolic traits within a group of bacteria has traditionally been used to define their taxonomy, but these traits often do not correspond with modern genetic classifications. Bacterial metabolism is classified into nutritional groups on the basis of three major criteria: the kind of energy used for growth, the source of carbon, and the electron donors used for growth. An additional criterion of respiratory microorganisms are the electron acceptors used for aerobic or anaerobic respiration.

Nutritional types in bacterial metabolism			
Nutritional type	**Source of energy**	**Source of carbon**	**Examples**
Phototrophs	Sunlight	Organic compounds (photoheterotrophs) or carbon fixation (photoautotrophs)	Cyanobacteria, Green sulfur bacteria, Chloroflexi, or Purple bacteria
Lithotrophs	Inorganic compounds	Organic compounds (lithoheterotrophs) or carbon fixation (lithoautotrophs)	Thermodesulfobacteria, *Hydrogenophilaceae*, or Nitrospirae
Organotrophs	Organic compounds	Organic compounds (chemoheterotrophs) or carbon fixation (chemoautotrophs)	*Bacillus*, *Clostridium* or *Enterobacteriaceae*

Carbon metabolism in bacteria is either *heterotrophic*, where organic carbon compounds are used as carbon sources, or *autotrophic*, meaning that cellular carbon is obtained by fixing carbon dioxide. Heterotrophic bacteria include parasitic types. Typical autotrophic bacteria are phototrophic cyanobacteria, green sulfur-bacteria and some purple bacteria, but also many chemolithotrophic species, such as nitrifying or sulfur-oxidizing bacteria. Energy metabolism of bacteria is either based on *phototrophy*, the use of light through photosynthesis, or based on *chemotrophy*, the use of chemical substances for energy, which are mostly oxidised at the expense of oxygen or alternative electron acceptors (aerobic/anaerobic respiration).

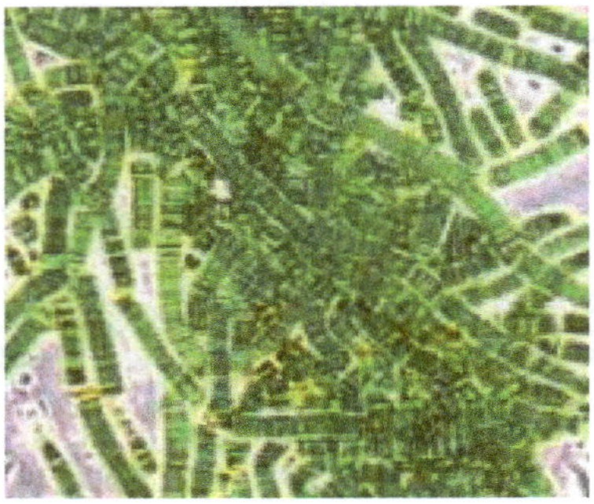

Filaments of photosyntheticcyanobacteria.

Bacteria are further divided into *lithotrophs* that use inorganic electron donors and *organotrophs* that use organic compounds as electron donors. Chemotrophic organisms use the respective electron donors for energy conservation (by aerobic/anaerobic respiration or fermentation) and biosynthetic reactions (e.g., carbon dioxide fixation), whereas phototrophic organisms use them only for biosynthetic purposes. Respiratory organisms use chemical compounds as a source of energy by taking electrons from the reduced substrate and transferring them to a terminal electron acceptor in a redox reaction. This reaction releases energy that can be used to synthesize ATP and drive metabolism. In *aerobic organisms*, oxygen is used as the electron acceptor. In *anaerobic organisms* other inorganic compounds, such as nitrate, sulfate or carbon dioxide are used as electron acceptors. This leads to the ecologically important processes of denitrification, sulfate reduction, and acetogenesis, respectively.

Another way of life of chemotrophs in the absence of possible electron acceptors is fermentation, wherein the electrons taken from the reduced substrates are transferred to oxidised intermediates to generate reduced fermentation products (e.g., lactate, ethanol, hydrogen, butyric acid). Fermentation is possible, because the energy content of the substrates is higher than that of the products, which allows the organisms to synthesise ATP and drive their metabolism.

These processes are also important in biological responses to pollution; for example, sulfate-reducing bacteria are largely responsible for the production of the highly toxic forms of mercury (methyl- and dimethylmercury) in the environment. Non-respiratory anaerobes use fermentation to generate energy and reducing power, secreting metabolic by-products (such as ethanol in brewing) as waste. Facultative anaerobes can switch between fermentation and different terminal electron acceptors depending on the environmental conditions in which they find themselves.

Lithotrophic bacteria can use inorganic compounds as a source of energy. Common inorganic electron donors are hydrogen, carbon monoxide, ammonia (leading to nitrification), ferrous iron and other reduced metal ions, and several reduced sulfur compounds. In unusual circumstances, the gas methane can be used by methanotrophic bacteria as both a source of electrons and a substrate for carbon anabolism. In both aerobic phototrophy and chemolithotrophy, oxygen is used as a terminal electron acceptor, whereas under anaerobic conditions inorganic compounds are used instead. Most lithotrophic organisms are autotrophic, whereas organotrophic organisms are heterotrophic.

In addition to fixing carbon dioxide in photosynthesis, some bacteria also fix nitrogen gas (nitrogen fixation) using the enzyme nitrogenase. This environmentally important trait can be found in bacteria of nearly all the metabolic types listed above, but is not universal.

Regardless of the type of metabolic process they employ, the majority of bacteria are able to take in raw materials only in the form of relatively small molecules, which enter the cell by diffusion or through molecular channels in cell membranes. The Planctomycetes are the exception (as they are in possessing membranes around their nuclear material). It has recently been shown that *Gemmata obscuriglobus* is able to take in large molecules via a process that in some ways resembles endocytosis, the process used by eukaryotic cells to engulf external items.

GROWTH AND REPRODUCTION

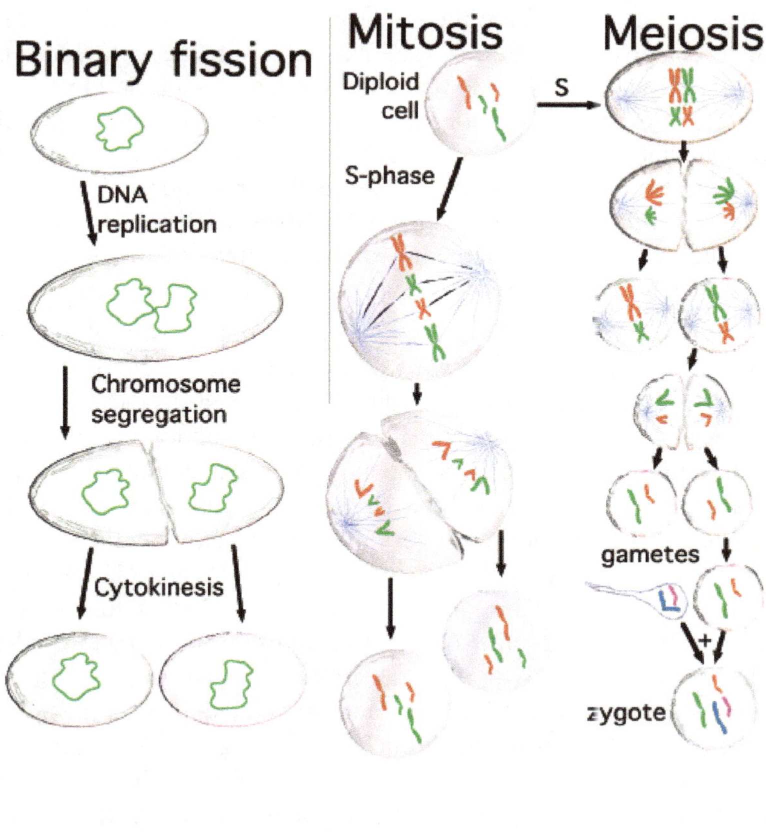

Many bacteria reproduce through binary fission, which is compared to mitosis and meiosis in this image.

Unlike in multicellular organisms, increases in cell size (cell growth) and reproduction by cell division are tightly linked in unicellular organisms. Bacteria grow to a fixed size and then reproduce through *binary fission*, a form of asexual reproduction. Under optimal conditions, bacteria can grow and divide extremely rapidly, and bacterial populations can double as quickly as every 9.8 minutes. In cell division, two identical clone daughter cells are produced. Some bacteria, while still reproducing asexually, form more complex reproductive structures that help disperse the newly formed daughter cells. Examples include fruiting body formation by *Myxobacteria* and aerial hyphae formation by *Streptomyces*, or budding. Budding involves a cell forming a protrusion that breaks away and produces a daughter cell.

In the laboratory, bacteria are usually grown using solid or liquid media. Solid *growth media*, such as agar plates, are used to isolate pure cultures of a bacterial strain. However, liquid growth media are used when measurement of growth or large volumes of cells are required. Growth in stirred liquid media occurs as an even cell suspension, making the cultures easy to divide and transfer, although isolating single bacteria from liquid media is difficult. The use of selective media (media with specific nutrients added or deficient, or with antibiotics added) can help identify specific organisms. Most laboratory techniques for growing bacteria use high levels of nutrients to produce large amounts of cells cheaply and quickly. However, in natural environments, nutrients are limited, meaning that bacteria cannot continue to reproduce indefinitely. This nutrient limitation has led the evolution of different growth strategies (see r/K selection theory). Some organisms can grow extremely rapidly when nutrients become available, such as the formation of algal (and cyanobacterial) blooms that often occur in lakes during the summer. Other organisms have adaptations to harsh environments, such as the production of multiple antibiotics by *Streptomyces* that inhibit the growth of competing microorganisms. In nature, many organisms live in communities (e.g., biofilms) that may allow for increased supply of nutrients and protection from environmental stresses. These relationships can be essential for growth of a particular organism or group of organisms (syntrophy).

Bacterial growth follows four phases. When a population of bacteria first enter a high-nutrient environment that allows growth, the cells need to adapt to their new environment. The first phase of growth is the *lag phase*, a period of slow growth when the cells are adapting to the high-nutrient environment and preparing for fast growth. The lag phase has high biosynthesis rates, as proteins necessary for rapid growth are produced. The second phase of growth is the *log phase*, also known as the *logarithmic or exponential phase*. The log phase is marked by rapid exponential growth. The rate at which cells grow during this phase is known as the *growth rate* (*k*), and the time it takes the cells to double is known as the *generation time* (*g*). During log phase, nutrients are metabolized at maximum speed until one of the nutrients is depleted and starts limiting growth. The third phase of growth is the *stationary phase* and is caused by depleted nutrients. The cells reduce their metabolic activity and consume non-essential cellular proteins. The stationary phase is a transition from rapid growth to a stress response state and there is increased expression of genes involved in DNA repair, antioxidant metabolism and nutrient transport. The final phase is the *death phase* where the bacteria run out of nutrients and die.

GENOMES

The genomes of thousands of bacterial species have been sequenced, with at least 9,000 sequences completed and more than 42,000 left as "permanent" drafts (as of Sep 2016).

Most bacteria have a single circular chromosome that can range in size from only 160,000 base pairs in the endosymbiotic bacteria *Candidatus Carsonella ruddii*, to 12,200,000 base pairs in the soil-dwelling bacteria *Sorangium cellulosum*. The genes in bacterial genomes are usually a single continuous stretch of DNA and although several different types of introns do exist in bacteria, these are much rarer than in eukaryotes. Some bacteria, including the Spirochaetes of the genus *Borrelia* are a notable exception to this arrangement. *Borrelia burgdorferi*, the cause of Lyme disease, contains a single linear chromosome and several linear and circular plasmids.

Plasmids are small extra-chromosomal DNAs that may contain genes for antibiotic resistance or virulence factors. Plasmids replicate independently of chromosomes, so it is possible that plasmids could be lost in bacterial cell division. Against this possibility is the fact that a single bacterium can contain hundreds of copies of a single plasmid.

Genetics

Bacteria, as asexual organisms, inherit identical copies of their parent's genes (i.e., they are clonal). However, all bacteria can evolve by selection on changes to their genetic material DNA caused by genetic recombination or mutations. Mutations come from errors made during the replication of DNA or from exposure to mutagens. Mutation rates vary widely among different species of bacteria and even among different clones of a single species of bacteria. Genetic changes in bacterial genomes come from either random mutation during replication or "stress-directed mutation", where genes involved in a particular growth-limiting process have an increased mutation rate.

DNA Transfer

Some bacteria also transfer genetic material between cells. This can occur in three main ways. First, bacteria can take up exogenous DNA from their environment, in a process called *transformation*. Genes can also be transferred by the process of *transduction*, when the integration of a bacteriophage introduces foreign DNA into the chromosome. The third method of gene transfer is *conjugation*, whereby DNA is transferred through direct cell contact.

Transduction of bacterial genes by bacteriophage appears to be a consequence of infrequent errors during intracellular assembly of virus particles, rather than a bacterial adaptation. Conjugation, in the much-studied E. coli system is determined by plasmid genes, and is an adaptation for transferring copies of the plasmid from one bacterial host to another. It is seldom that a conjugative plasmid integrates into the host bacterial chromosome, and subsequently transfers part of the host bacterial DNA to another bacterium. Plasmid-mediated transfer of host bacterial DNA also appears to be an accidental process rather than a bacterial adaptation.

Transformation, unlike transduction or conjugation, depends on numerous bacterial gene products that specifically interact to perform this complex process, and thus transformation is clearly a bacterial adaptation for DNA transfer. In order for a bacterium to bind, take up and recombine donor DNA into its own chromosome, it must first enter a special physiological state termed competence (see Natural competence). In *Bacillus subtilis*, about 40 genes are required for the development of competence. The length of DNA transferred during *B. subtilis* transformation can be between a third of a chromosome up to the whole chromosome.Transformation appears to be common among bacterial species, and thus far at least 60 species are known to have the natural ability to become competent for transformation. The development of competence in nature is usually associated with stressful environmental conditions, and seems to be an adaptation for facilitating repair of DNA damage in recipient cells.

In ordinary circumstances, transduction, conjugation, and transformation involve transfer of DNA between individual bacteria of the same species, but occasionally transfer may occur between individuals of different bacterial species and this may have significant consequences, such as the transfer of antibiotic resistance. In such cases, gene acquisition from other bacteria or the environment is called *horizontal gene transfer* and may be common under natural conditions. Gene transfer is particularly important in antibiotic resistance as it allows the rapid transfer of resistance genes between different pathogens.

Bacteriophages

Bacteriophages are viruses that infect bacteria. Many types of bacteriophage exist, some simply infect and lyse their host bacteria, while others insert into the bacterial chromosome. A bacteriophage can contain genes that contribute to its host's phenotype: for example, in the evolution of *Escherichia coli* O157:H7 and *Clostridium botulinum*, the toxin genes in an integrated phage converted a harmless ancestral bacterium into a lethal pathogen. Bacteria resist phage infection through restriction modification systems that degrade foreign DNA, and a system that uses CRISPR sequences to retain fragments of the genomes of phage that the bacteria have come into contact with in the past, which allows them to block virus replication through a form of RNA interference. This CRISPR system provides bacteria with acquired immunity to infection.

BEHAVIOUR

Secretion

Bacteria frequently secrete chemicals into their environment in order to modify it favorably. The secretions are often proteins and may act as enzymes that digest some form of food in the environment.

Bioluminescence

A few bacteria have chemical systems that generate light. This bioluminescence often occurs in bacteria that live in association with fish, and the light probably serves to attract fish or other large animals.

Multicellularity

Bacteria often function as multicellular aggregates known as biofilms, exchanging a variety of molecular signals for inter-cell communication, and engaging in coordinated multicellular behavior.

The communal benefits of multicellular cooperation include a cellular division of labor, accessing resources that cannot effectively be used by single cells, collectively defending against antagonists, and optimizing population survival by differentiating into distinct cell types. For example, bacteria in biofilms can have more than 500 times increased resistance to antibacterial agents than individual "planktonic" bacteria of the same species.

One type of inter-cellular communication by a molecular signal is called quorum sensing, which serves the purpose of determining whether there is a local population density that is sufficiently high that it is productive to invest in processes that are only successful if large numbers of similar organisms behave similarly, as in excreting digestive enzymes or emitting light.

Quorum sensing allows bacteria to coordinate gene expression, and enables them to produce, release and detect autoinducers or pheromones which accumulate with the growth in cell population.

Movement

Many bacteria can move using a variety of mechanisms: flagella are used for swimming through fluids; bacterial gliding and twitching motility move bacteria across surfaces; and changes of buoyancy allow vertical motion.

Swimming bacteria frequently move near 10 body lengths per second and a few as fast as 100. This makes them at least as fast as fish, on a relative scale.

In bacterial gliding and twitching motility, bacteria use their *type IV pili* as a grappling hook, repeatedly extending it, anchoring it and then retracting it with remarkable force (>80 pN).

Our observations redefine twitching motility as a rapid, highly organized mechanism of bacterial translocation by which Pseudomonas aeruginosa can disperse itself over large areas to colonize new territories. It is also now clear, both morphologically and genetically, that twitching motility and social gliding motility, such as occurs in Myxococcus xanthus, are essentially the same process.

—Semmler, Whitchurch & Mattick (1999)

Flagella are semi-rigid cylindrical structures that are rotated and function much like the propeller on a ship. Objects as small as bacteria operate a low Reynolds number and cylindrical forms are more efficient than the flat, paddle-like, forms appropriate at human-size scale.

Bacterial species differ in the number and arrangement of flagella on their surface; some have a single flagellum (*monotrichous*), a flagellum at each end (*amphitrichous*), clusters of flagella at the poles of the cell (*lophotrichous*), while others have flagella distributed over the entire surface of the cell (*peritrichous*). The bacterial flagella is the best-understood motility structure in any organism and is made of about 20 proteins, with approximately another 30 proteins required for its regulation and assembly. The flagellum is a rotating structure driven by a reversible motor at the base that uses the electrochemical gradient across the membrane for power. This motor drives the motion of the filament, which acts as a propeller.

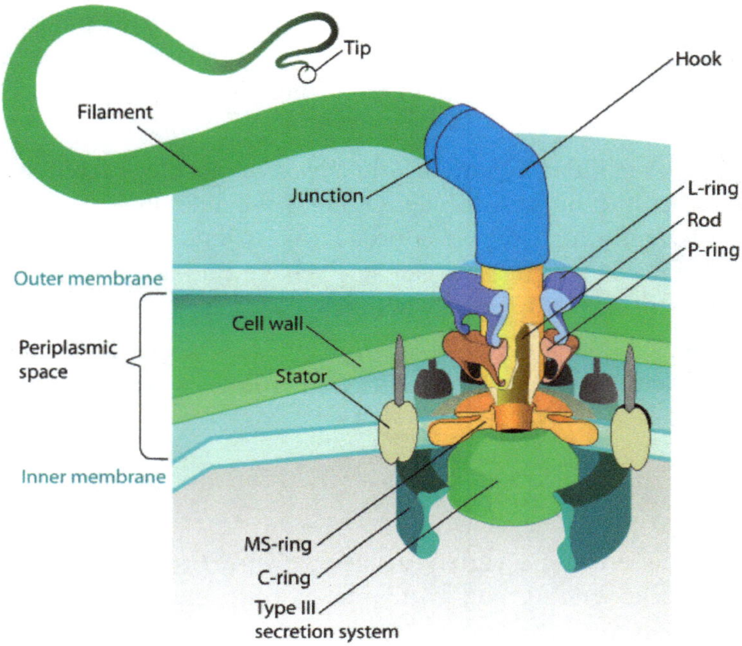

Flagellum of gram-negative bacteria. The base drives the rotation of the hook and filament.

Many bacteria (such as *E. coli*) have two distinct modes of movement: forward movement (swimming) and tumbling. The tumbling allows them to reorient and makes their movement a three-dimensional random walk. (See external links below for link to videos.) The flagella of a unique group of bacteria, the spirochaetes, are found between two membranes in the periplasmic space. They have a distinctive helical body that twists about as it moves.

Motile bacteria are attracted or repelled by certain stimuli in behaviours called **taxes**: these include chemotaxis, phototaxis, energy taxis, and magnetotaxis. In one peculiar group, the myxobacteria, individual bacteria move together to form waves of cells that then differentiate to form fruiting bodies containing spores. The myxobacteria move only when on solid surfaces, unlike *E. coli*, which is motile in liquid or solid media.

Several *Listeria* and *Shigella* species move inside host cells by usurping the cytoskeleton, which is normally used to move organelles inside the cell. By promoting actin polymerisation at one pole of their cells, they can form a kind of tail that pushes them through the host cell's cytoplasm.

CLASSIFICATION AND IDENTIFICATION

Classification seeks to describe the diversity of bacterial species by naming and grouping organisms based on similarities. Bacteria can be classified on the basis of cell structure, cellular metabolism or on differences in cell components, such as DNA, fatty acids, pigments, antigens and quinones. While these schemes allowed the identification and classification of bacterial strains, it was unclear whether these differences represented variation between distinct species or between strains of the same species. This uncertainty was due to the lack of distinctive structures in most bacteria, as well as lateral gene transfer between unrelated species. Due to lateral gene transfer, some closely related bacteria can have very different morphologies and metabolisms. To overcome this uncertainty, modern bacterial classification emphasizes molecular systematics, using genetic techniques such as guanine cytosine ratio determination, genome-genome hybridization, as well as sequencing genes that have not undergone extensive lateral gene transfer, such as the rRNA gene. Classification of bacteria is determined by publication in the International Journal of Systematic Bacteriology,and Bergey's Manual of Systematic Bacteriology. The International Committee on Systematic Bacteriology (ICSB) maintains international rules for the naming of bacteria and taxonomic categories and for the ranking of them in the International Code of Nomenclature of Bacteria.

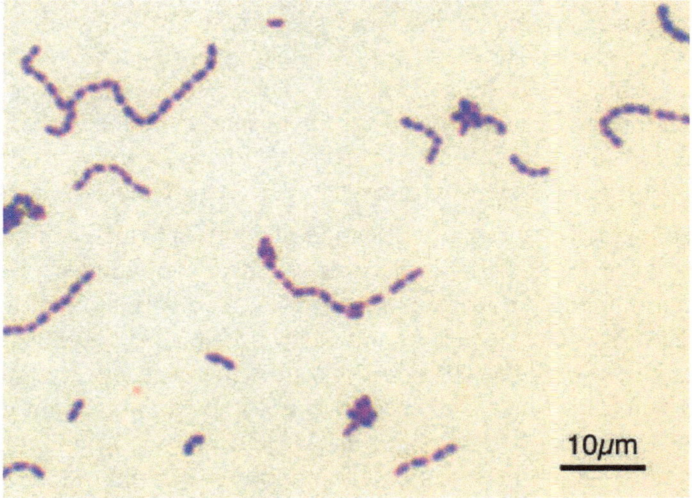

Streptococcus mutans visualized with a Gram stain.

The term "bacteria" was traditionally applied to all microscopic, single-cell prokaryotes. However, molecular systematics showed prokaryotic life to consist of two separate domains, originally called *Eubacteria* and *Archaebacteria*, but now called *Bacteria* and *Archaea* that evolved independently from an ancient common ancestor. The archaea and eukaryotes are more closely related to each other than either is to the bacteria. These two domains, along with Eukarya, are the basis of the three-domain system, which is currently the most widely used classification system in microbiolology. However, due to the relatively recent introduction of molecular systematics and a rapid increase in the number of genome sequences that are available, bacterial classification remains a changing and expanding field. For example, a few biologists argue that the Archaea and Eukaryotes evolved from gram-positive bacteria.

The identification of bacteria in the laboratory is particularly relevant in medicine, where the correct treatment is determined by the bacterial species causing an infection. Consequently, the need to identify human pathogens was a major impetus for the development of techniques to identify bacteria.

The *Gram stain*, developed in 1884 by Hans Christian Gram, characterizes bacteria based on the structural characteristics of their cell walls. The thick layers of peptidoglycan in the "gram-positive" cell wall stain purple, while the thin "gram-negative" cell wall appears pink. By combining morphology and Gram-staining, most bacteria can be classified as belonging to one of four groups (gram-positive cocci, gram-positive bacilli, gram-negative cocci and gram-negative bacilli). Some organisms are best identified by stains other than the Gram stain, particularly mycobacteria or *Nocardia*, which show acid-fastness on Ziehl–Neelsen or similar stains. Other organisms may need to be identified by their growth in special media, or by other techniques, such as serology.

Culture techniques are designed to promote the growth and identify particular bacteria, while restricting the growth of the other bacteria in the sample. Often these techniques are designed for specific specimens; for example, a sputum sample will be treated to identify organisms that cause pneumonia, while stool specimens are cultured on selective media to identify organisms that cause diarrhoea, while preventing growth of non-pathogenic bacteria. Specimens that are normally sterile, such as blood, urine or spinal fluid, are cultured under conditions designed to grow all possible organisms. Once a pathogenic organism has been isolated, it can be further characterised by its morphology, growth patterns (such as aerobic or anaerobic growth), patterns of hemolysis, and staining.

As with bacterial classification, identification of bacteria is increasingly using molecular methods. Diagnostics using DNA-based tools, such as polymerase chain reaction, are increasingly popular due to their specificity and speed, compared to culture-based methods. These methods also allow the detection and identification of "viable but nonculturable" cells that are metabolically active but non-dividing. However, even using these improved methods, the total number of bacterial species is not known and cannot even be estimated with any certainty. Following present classification, there are a little less than 9,300 known species of prokaryotes, which includes bacteria and archaea; but attempts to estimate the true number of bacterial diversity have ranged from 10^7 to 10^9 total species—and even these diverse estimates may be off by many orders of magnitude.

Interactions with other organisms

Despite their apparent simplicity, bacteria can form complex associations with other organisms. These symbiotic associations can be divided into parasitism, mutualism and commensalism. Due to their small size, commensal bacteria are ubiquitous and grow on animals and plants exactly as they will grow on any other surface. However, their growth can be increased by warmth and sweat, and large populations of these organisms in humans are the cause of body odour.

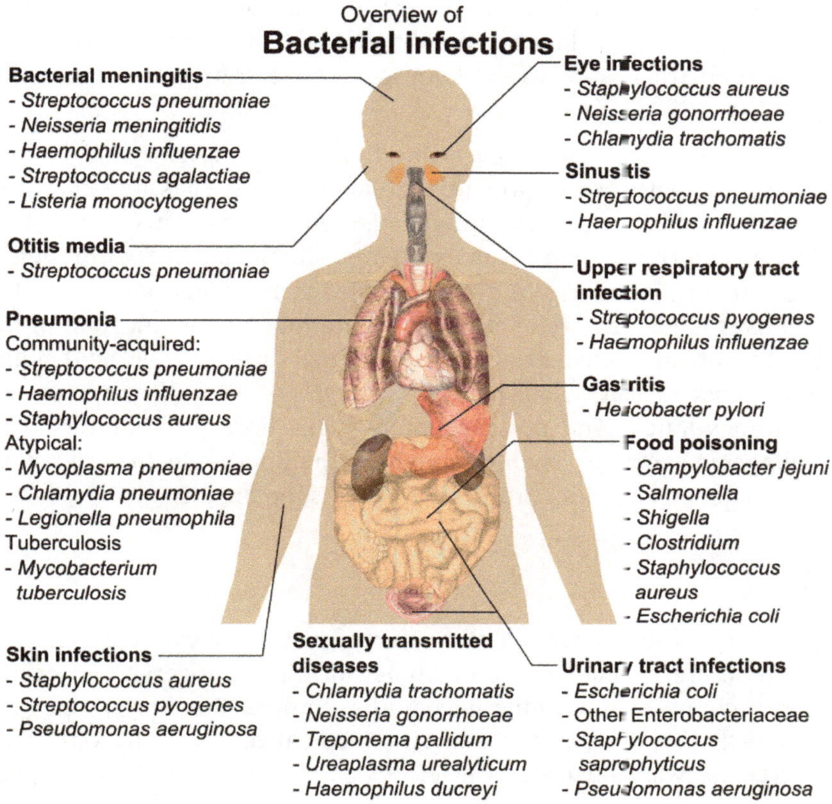

Overview of bacterial infections and main species involved.

Predators

Some species of bacteria kill and then consume other microorganisms, these species are called *predatory bacteria*. These include organisms such as *Myxococcus xanthus*, which forms swarms of cells that kill and digest any bacteria they encounter. Other bacterial predators either attach to their prey in order to digest them and absorb nutrients, such as *Vampirovibrio chlorellavorus*, or invade another cell and multiply inside the cytosol, such as *Daptobacter*. These predatory bacteria are thought to have evolved from saprophages that consumed dead microorganisms, through adaptations that allowed them to entrap and kill other organisms.

Mutualists

Certain bacteria form close spatial associations that are essential for their survival. One such mutualistic association, called interspecies hydrogen transfer, occurs between clusters of anaerobic bacteria that consume organic acids, such as butyric acid or propionic acid, and produce hydrogen, and methanogenic Archaea that consume hydrogen. The bacteria in this association are unable to consume the organic acids as this reaction produces hydrogen that accumulates in their surroundings. Only the intimate association with the hydrogen-consuming Archaea keeps the hydrogen concentration low enough to allow the bacteria to grow.

In soil, microorganisms that reside in the rhizosphere (a zone that includes the root surface and the soil that adheres to the root after gentle shaking) carry out nitrogen fixation, converting nitrogen gas to nitrogenous compounds. This serves to provide an easily absorbable form of nitrogen for many plants, which cannot fix nitrogen themselves. Many other bacteria are found as symbionts in humans and other organisms. For example, the presence of over 1,000 bacterial species in the normal human gut flora of the intestines can contribute to gut immunity, synthesise vitamins, such as folic acid, vitamin K and biotin, convert sugars to lactic acid (see *Lactobacillus*), as well as fermenting complex undigestible carbohydrates. The presence of this gut flora also inhibits the growth of potentially pathogenic bacteria (usually through competitive exclusion) and these beneficial bacteria are consequently sold as probiotic dietary supplements.

Pathogens

If bacteria form a parasitic association with other organisms, they are classed as pathogens. Pathogenic bacteria are a major cause of human death and disease and cause infections such as tetanus, typhoid fever, diphtheria, syphilis, cholera, foodborne illness, leprosy and tuberculosis. A pathogenic cause for a known medical disease may only be discovered many years after, as was the case with *Helicobacter pylori* and peptic ulcer disease. Bacterial diseases are also important in agriculture, with bacteria causing leaf spot, fire blight and wilts in plants, as well as Johne's disease, mastitis, salmonella and anthrax in farm animals.

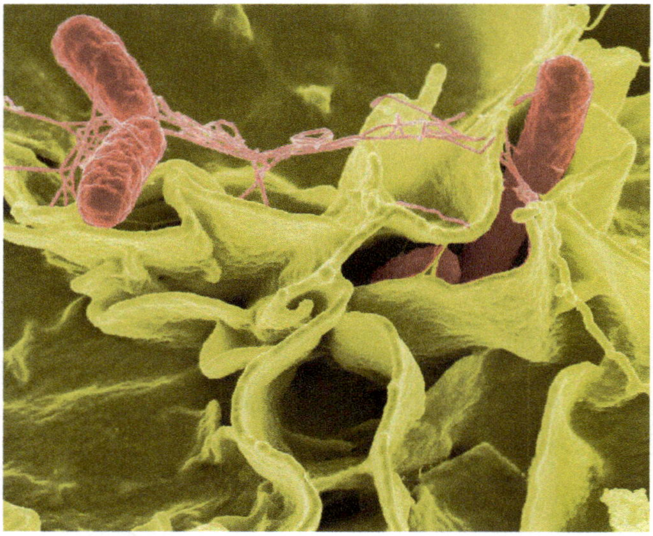

Color-enhanced scanning electron micrograph showing *Salmonella typhimurium* (red) invading cultured human cells.

Each species of pathogen has a characteristic spectrum of interactions with its human hosts. Some organisms, such as *Staphylococcus* or *Streptococcus*, can cause skin infections, pneumonia, meningitis and even overwhelming sepsis, a systemic inflammatory response producing shock, massive vasodilation and death. Yet these organisms are also part of the normal human flora and usually exist on the skin or in the nose without causing any disease at all. Other organisms invariably cause disease in humans, such as the Rickettsia, which are obligate intracellular parasites able to grow and reproduce only within the cells of other organisms. One species of Rickettsia causes typhus, while another causes Rocky Mountain spotted fever. *Chlamydia*, another phylum of obligate intracellular parasites, contains species that can cause pneumonia, or urinary tract infection and may be involved in coronary heart disease. Finally, some species, such as *Pseudomonas aeruginosa*, *Burkholderia cenocepacia*, and *Mycobacterium avium*, are opportunistic pathogens and cause disease mainly in people suffering from immunosuppression or cystic fibrosis.

Bacterial infections may be treated with antibiotics, which are classified as bacteriocidal if they kill bacteria, or bacteriostatic if they just prevent bacterial growth. There are many types of antibiotics and each class inhibits a process that is different in the pathogen from that found in the host. An example of how antibiotics produce selective toxicity are chloramphenicol and puromycin, which inhibit the bacterial ribosome, but not the structurally different eukaryotic ribosome.Antibiotics are used both in treating human disease and in intensive farming to promote animal growth, where they may be contributing to the rapid development of antibiotic resistance in bacterial populations. Infections can be prevented by antiseptic measures such as sterilising the skin prior to piercing it with the needle of a syringe, and by proper care of indwelling catheters. Surgical and dental instruments are also sterilised to prevent contamination by bacteria. Disinfectants such as bleach are used to kill bacteria or other pathogens on surfaces to prevent contamination and further reduce the risk of infection.

SIGNIFICANCE IN TECHNOLOGY AND INDUSTRY

Bacteria, often lactic acid bacteria, such as *Lactobacillus* and *Lactococcus*, in combination with yeasts and moulds, have been used for thousands of years in the preparation of fermented foods, such as cheese, pickles, soy sauce, sauerkraut, vinegar, wine and yogurt.

The ability of bacteria to degrade a variety of organic compounds is remarkable and has been used in waste processing and bioremediation. Bacteria capable of digesting the hydrocarbons in petroleum are often used to clean up oil spills. Fertilizer was added to some of the beaches in Prince William Sound in an attempt to promote the growth of these naturally occurring bacteria after the 1989 *Exxon Valdez* oil spill. These efforts were effective on beaches that were not too thickly covered in oil. Bacteria are also used for the bioremediation of industrial toxic wastes. In the chemical industry, bacteria are most important in the production of enantiomerically pure chemicals for use as pharmaceuticals or agrichemicals.

Bacteria can also be used in the place of pesticides in the biological pest control. This commonly involves *Bacillus thuringiensis* (also called BT), a gram-positive, soil dwelling bacterium. Subspecies of this bacteria are used as a Lepidopteran-specific insecticides under trade names such as Dipel and Thuricide. Because of their specificity, these pesticides are regarded as environmentally friendly, with little or no effect on humans, wildlife, pollinators and most other beneficial insects.

Because of their ability to quickly grow and the relative ease with which they can be manipulated, bacteria are the workhorses for the fields of molecular biology, genetics and biochemistry. By making mutations in bacterial DNA and examining the resulting phenotypes, scientists can determine the function of genes, enzymes and metabolic pathways in bacteria, then apply this knowledge to more complex organisms. This aim of understanding the biochemistry of a cell reaches its most complex expression in the synthesis of huge amounts of enzyme kinetic and gene expression data into mathematical models of entire organisms. This is achievable in some well-studied bacteria, with models of *Escherichia coli* metabolism now being produced and tested. This understanding of bacterial metabolism and genetics allows the use of biotechnology to bioengineer bacteria for the production of therapeutic proteins, such as insulin, growth factors, or antibodies.

Because of their importance for research in general, samples of bacterial strains are isolated and preserved in Biological Resource Centers. This ensures the availability of the strain to scientists worldwide.

HISTORY OF BACTERIOLOGY

Bacteria were first observed by the Dutch microscopist Antonie van Leeuwenhoek in 1676, using a single-lens microscope of his own design. He then published his observations in a series of letters to the Royal Society of London.Bacteria were Leeuwenhoek's most remarkable microscopic discovery. They were just at the limit of what his simple lenses could make out and, in one of the most striking hiatuses in the history of science, no one else would see them again for over a century. Only then were his by-then-largely-forgotten observations of bacteria—as opposed to his famous "animalcules" (spermatozoa)—taken seriously.

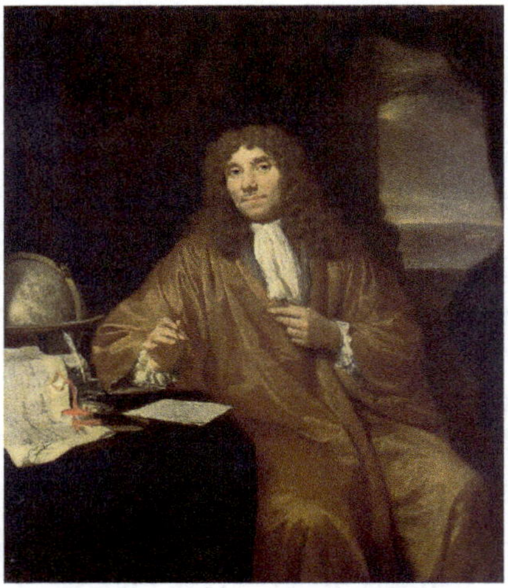

Antonie van Leeuwenhoek, the first microbiologist and the first person to observe bacteria using a microscope.

Christian Gottfried Ehrenberg introduced the word "bacterium" in 1828. In fact, his *Bacterium* was a genus that contained non-spore-forming rod-shaped bacteria, as opposed to *Bacillus*, a genus of spore-forming rod-shaped bacteria defined by Ehrenberg in 1835.

Louis Pasteur demonstrated in 1859 that the growth of microorganisms causes the fermentation process, and that this growth is not due to spontaneous generation. (Yeasts and moulds, commonly associated with fermentation, are not bacteria, but rather fungi.) Along with his contemporary Robert Koch, Pasteur was an early advocate of the germ theory of disease.

Robert Koch, a pioneer in medical microbiology, worked on cholera, anthrax and tuberculosis. In his research into tuberculosis Koch finally proved the germ theory, for which he received a Nobel Prize in 1905. In *Koch's postulates*, he set out criteria to test if an organism is the cause of a disease, and these postulates are still used today.

Though it was known in the nineteenth century that bacteria are the cause of many diseases, no effective antibacterial treatments were available. In 1910, Paul Ehrlich developed the first antibiotic, by changing dyes that selectively stained *Treponema pallidum*—the spirochaete that causes syphilis—into compounds that selectively killed the pathogen. Ehrlich had been awarded a 1908 Nobel Prize for his work on immunology, and pioneered the use of stains to detect and identify bacteria, with his work being the basis of the Gram stain and the Ziehl–Neelsen stain.

A major step forward in the study of bacteria came in 1977 when Carl Woese recognised that archaea have a separate line of evolutionary descent from bacteria.This new phylogenetic taxonomy depended on the sequencing of 16S ribosomal RNA, and divided prokaryotes into two evolutionary domains, as part of the three-domain system.

REFERENCES

1. Wassenaar, T. M. "Bacteriology: the study of bacteria". www.mmgc.eu. Archived from the original on 24 July 2011. Retrieved 18 June 2011.
2. Ward J. MacNeal; Herbert Upham Williams (1914). Pathogenic micro-organisms; a text-book of microbiology for physicians and students of medicine. P. Blakiston's sons & co. pp. 1–. Retrieved 18 June 2011.
3. Jeanne Stove Poindexter (30 November 1986). Methods and special applications in bacterial ecology. Springer. p. 87. ISBN 978-0-306-42346-8. Retrieved 18 June 2011.
4. Woese CR, Kandler O, Wheelis ML (1990). "Towards a natural system of organisms: proposal for the domains Archaea, Bacteria, and Eucarya". Proceedings of the National Academy of Sciences of the United States of America. 87 (12): 4576–9. Bibcode:1990PNAS...87.4576W. doi:10.1073/pnas.87.12.4576. PMC 54159Freely accessible. PMID 2112744.
5. "Bacteria (eubacteria)". Taxonomy Browser, US National Institute of Health. Retrieved 10 September 2008.
6. Woese CR, Fox GE (1977). "Phylogenetic structure of the prokaryotic domain: the primary kingdoms". Proceedings of the National Academy of Sciences of the

United States of America. 74 (11): 5088–90. Bibcode:1977PNAS...74.5088W. doi:10.1073/pnas.74.11.5088. PMC 432104Freely accessible. PMID 270744.

7. Fredrickson JK, Zachara JM, Balkwill DL, Kennedy D, Li SM, Kostandarithes HM, Daly MJ, Romine MF, Brockman FJ (2004). "Geomicrobiology of high-level nuclear waste-contaminated vadose sediments at the Hanford site, Washington state". Applied and Environmental Microbiology. 70 (7): 4230–41. doi:10.1128/AEM.70.7.4230-4241.2004. PMC 444790Freely accessible. PMID 15240306.
8. Whitman WB, Coleman DC, Wiebe WJ (1998). "Prokaryotes: the unseen majority". Proceedings of the National Academy of Sciences of the United States of America. 95 (12): 6578–83. Bibcode:1998PNAS...95.6578W. doi:10.1073/pnas.95.12.6578. PMC 33863Freely accessible. PMID 9618454.
9. C.Michael Hogan. 2010. Bacteria. Encyclopedia of Earth. eds. Sidney Draggan and C.J.Cleveland, National Council for Science and the Environment, Washington DC
10. Choi CQ (17 March 2013). "Microbes Thrive in Deepest Spot on Earth". LiveScience. Retrieved 17 March 2013.
11. Glud R, Wenzhöfer F, Middelboe M, Oguri K, Turnewitsch R, Canfield DE, Kitazato H (2013). "High rates of microbial carbon turnover in sediments in the deepest oceanic trench on Earth". Nature Geoscience. 6 (4): 284–288. Bibcode:2013NatGe...6..284G. doi:10.1038/ngeo1773.
12. Oskin B (14 March 2013). "Intraterrestrials: Life Thrives in Ocean Floor". LiveScience. Retrieved 17 March 2013.
13. Rappé MS, Giovannoni SJ (2003). "The uncultured microbial majority". Annual Review of Microbiology. 57: 369–94. doi:10.1146/annurev.micro.57.030502.090759. PMID 14527284.
14. Sears CL (2005). "A dynamic partnership: celebrating our gut flora". Anaerobe. 11 (5): 247–51. doi:10.1016/j.anaerobe.2005.05.001. PMID 16701579.
15. "2002 WHO mortality data". Retrieved 20 January 2007.
16. "Metal-Mining Bacteria Are Green Chemists". Science Daily. 2 September 2010.
17. Ishige T, Honda K, Shimizu S (2005). "Whole organism biocatalysis". Current Opinion in Chemical Biology. 9 (2): 174–80. doi:10.1016/j.cbpa.2005.02.001. PMID 15811802.
18. βακτήριον. Liddell, Henry George; Scott, Robert; A Greek–English Lexicon at the Perseus Project.
19. βακτηρία in Liddell and Scott.
20. bacterium, on Oxford Dictionaries.
21. Harper, Douglas. bacteria. Online Etymology Dictionary.
22. Schopf JW (1994). Disparate rates, differing fates: tempo and mode of evolution changed from the Precambrian to the Phanerozoic. Proceedings of the National Academy of Sciences of the United States of America. 91 (15): 6735–42. Bibcode:1994PNAS...91.6735S. doi:10.1073/pnas.91.15.6735. PMC 44277Freely accessible. PMID 8041691.

23. DeLong EF, Pace NR (2001). Environmental diversity of bacteria and archaea. Syst Biol. 50 (4): 470–8. doi:10.1080/106351501750435040. PMID 12116647.

24. Brown JR, Doolittle WF (1997). Archaea and the prokaryote-to-eukaryote transition. Microbiology and Molecular Biology Reviews. 61 (4): 456–502. PMC 232621Freely accessible. PMID 9409149.

25. Poole AM, Penny D (2007). Evaluating hypotheses for the origin of eukaryotes. BioEssays. 29 (1): 74–84. doi:10.1002/bies.20516. PMID 17187354.

26. Dyall SD, Brown MT, Johnson PJ (2004). Ancient invasions: from endosymbionts to organelles. Science. 304 (5668): 253–7. Bibcode:2004Sci...304..253D. doi:10.1126/science.1094884. PMID 15073369.

27. Lang BF, Gray MW, Burger G (1999). Mitochondrial genome evolution and the origin of eukaryotes. Annu Rev Genet. 33: 351–97. doi:10.1146/annurev.genet.33.1.351. PMID 10690412.

28. McFadden GI (1999). Endosymbiosis and evolution of the plant cell. Current Opinion in Plant Biology. 2 (6): 513–9. doi:10.1016/S1369-5266(99)00025-4. PMID 10607659.

29. Schulz HN, Jorgensen BB (2001). Big bacteria. Annu Rev Microbiol. 55: 105–37. doi:10.1146/annurev.micro.55.1.105. PMID 11544351.

30. Williams C (2011). Who are you calling simple?. New Scientist. 211 (2821): 38–41. doi:10.1016/S0262-4079(11)61709-0.

31. Robertson J, Gomersall M, Gill P (1975). Mycoplasma hominis: growth, reproduction, and isolation of small viable cells. J Bacteriol. 124 (2): 1007–18. PMC 235991Freely accessible. PMID 1102522.

32. Velimirov B (2001). Nanobacteria, Ultramicrobacteria and Starvation Forms: A Search for the Smallest Metabolizing Bacterium. Microbes and Environments. 16 (2): 67–77. doi:10.1264/jsme2.2001.67.

33. Dusenbery, David B. (2009). Living at Micro Scale, pp. 20–25. Harvard University Press, Cambridge, Mass. ISBN 978-0-674-03116-6

34. Fritz I, Strömpl C, Abraham WR (2004). Phylogenetic relationships of the genera Stella, Labrys and Angulomicrobium within the ‹Alphaproteobacteria› and description of Angulomicrobium amanitiforme sp. nov. Int J Syst Evol Microbiol. 54 (Pt 3): 651–7. doi:10.1099/ijs.0.02746-0. PMID 15143003.

35. Wanger G, Onstott TC, Southam G (2008). Stars of the terrestrial deep subsurface: A novel ‹star-shaped› bacterial morphotype from a South African platinum mine. Geobiology. 6 (3): 325–30. doi:10.1111/j.1472-4669.2008.00163.x. PMID 18498531.

36. Cabeen MT, Jacobs-Wagner C (2005). Bacterial cell shape. Nature Reviews Microbiology. 3 (8): 601–10. doi:10.1038/nrmicro1205. PMID 16012516.

37. Young KD (2006). The selective value of bacterial shape. Microbiol Mol Biol Rev. 70 (3): 660–703. doi:10.1128/MMBR.00001-06. PMC 1594593Freely accessible. PMID 16959965.

38. Douwes KE, Schmalzbauer E, Linde HJ, Reisberger EM, Fleischer K, Lehn N, Landthaler M, Vogt T (2003). Branched filaments no fungus, ovoid bodies no bacteria: Two unusual cases of mycetoma. J Am Acad Dermatol. 49 (2 Suppl Case Reports): S170–3. doi:10.1067/mjd.2003.302. PMID 12894113.

39. Donlan RM (2002). Biofilms: microbial life on surfaces. Emerg Infect Dis. 8 (9): 881–90. doi:10.3201/eid0809.020063. PMC 2732559Freely accessible. PMID 12194761.

40. Branda SS, Vik S, Friedman L, Kolter R (2005). Biofilms: the matrix revisited. Trends Microbiol. 13 (1): 20–6. doi:10.1016/j.tim.2004.11.006. PMID 15639628.

41. Davey ME, O›toole GA (2000). Microbial biofilms: from ecology to molecular genetics. Microbiol Mol Biol Rev. 64 (4): 847–67. doi:10.1128/MMBR.64.4.847-867.2000. PMC 99016Freely accessible. PMID 11104821.

42. Donlan RM, Costerton JW (2002). Biofilms: survival mechanisms of clinically relevant microorganisms. Clin Microbiol Rev. 15 (2): 167–93. doi:10.1128/CMR.15.2.167-193.2002. PMC 118068Freely accessible. PMID 11932229.

43. Shimkets LJ (1999). Intercellular signaling during fruiting-body development of Myxococcus xanthus. Annu Rev Microbiol. 53: 525–49. doi:10.1146/annurev.micro.53.1.525. PMID 10547700.

44. Kaiser D (2004). Signaling in myxobacteria. Annu Rev Microbiol. 58: 75–98. doi:10.1146/annurev.micro.58.030603.123620. PMID 15487930.

45. Berg JM, Tymoczko JL, Stryer L (2002). Molecular Cell Biology (5th ed.). WH Freeman. ISBN 0-7167-4955-6.

46. Gitai Z (2005). The new bacterial cell biology: moving parts and subcellular architecture. Cell. 120 (5): 577–86. doi:10.1016/j.cell.2005.02.026. PMID 15766522.

47. Shih YL, Rothfield L (2006). The bacterial cytoskeleton. Microbiology and Molecular Biology Reviews. 70 (3): 729–54. doi:10.1128/MMBR.00017-06. PMC 1594594Freely accessible. PMID 16959967.

48. Norris V, den Blaauwen T, Cabin-Flaman A, Doi RH, Harshey R, Janniere L, Jimenez-Sanchez A, Jin DJ, Levin PA, Mileykovskaya E, Minsky A, Saier M, Skarstad K (2007). Functional taxonomy of bacterial hyperstructures. Microbiology and Molecular Biology Reviews. 71 (1): 230–53. doi:10.1128/MMBR.00035-06. PMC 1847379Freely accessible. PMID 17347523.

49. Kerfeld CA, Sawaya MR, Tanaka S, Nguyen CV, Phillips M, Beeby M, Yeates TO (2005). Protein structures forming the shell of primitive bacterial organelles. Science. 309 (5736): 936–8. Bibcode:2005Sci...309..936K. doi:10.1126/science.1113397. PMID 16081736.

50. Bobik TA (2007). Bacterial Microcompartments (PDF). Microbe. Am Soc Microbiol. 2: 25–31. doi:10.1128/microbe.2.25.1. Archived from the original (PDF) on 2 August 2008.

51. Bobik TA (2006). Polyhedral organelles compartmenting bacterial metabolic processes. Applied Microbiology and Biotechnology. 70 (5): 517–25. doi:10.1007/

s00253-005-0295-0. PMID 16525780.

52. Yeates TO, Kerfeld CA, Heinhorst S, Cannon GC, Shively JM (2008). Protein-based organelles in bacteria: carboxysomes and related microcompartments. Nature Reviews Microbiology. 6 (9): 681–91. doi:10.1038/nrmicro1913. PMID 18679172.
53. Harold FM (1972). Conservation and transformation of energy by bacterial membranes. Bacteriological Reviews. 36 (2): 172–230. PMC 408323Freely accessible. PMID 4261111.
54. Bryant DA, Frigaard NU (2006). Prokaryotic photosynthesis and phototrophy illuminated. Trends Microbiol. 14 (11): 488–96. doi:10.1016/j.tim.2006.09.001. PMID 16997562.
55. Psencík J, Ikonen TP, Laurinmäki P, Merckel MC, Butcher SJ, Serimaa RE, Tuma R (2004). Lamellar organization of pigments in chlorosomes, the light harvesting complexes of green photosynthetic bacteria. Biophys. J. 87 (2): 1165–72. Bibcode:2004BpJ....87.1165P. doi:10.1529/biophysj.104.040956. PMC 1304455Freely accessible. PMID 15298919.
56. Tanaka S, Kerfeld CA, Sawaya MR, Cai F, Heinhorst S, Cannon GC, Yeates TO (2008). Atomic-level models of the bacterial carboxysome shell. Science. 319 (5866): 1083–6. Bibcode:2008Sci...319.1083T. doi:10.1126/science.1151458. PMID 18292340.
57. Thanbichler M, Wang SC, Shapiro L (2005). The bacterial nucleoid: a highly organized and dynamic structure. J Cell Biochem. 96 (3): 506–21. doi:10.1002/jcb.20519. PMID 15988757.
58. Fuerst JA (2005). Intracellular compartmentation in planctomycetes. Annu Rev Microbiol. 59: 299–328. doi:10.1146/annurev.micro.59.030804.121258. PMID 15910279.
59. Fieseler L, Horn M, Wagner M, Hentschel U (June 2004). Discovery of the novel candidate phylum Poribacteria in marine sponges. Applied and Environmental Microbiology. 70 (6): 3724–32. doi:10.1128/AEM.70.6.3724-3732.2004. PMC 427773Freely accessible. PMID 15184179.
60. Poehlsgaard J, Douthwaite S (2005). The bacterial ribosome as a target for antibiotics. Nature Reviews Microbiology. 3 (11): 870–81. doi:10.1038/nrmicro1265. PMID 16261170.
61. Yeo M, Chater K (2005). The interplay of glycogen metabolism and differentiation provides an insight into the developmental biology of Streptomyces coelicolor. Microbiology. 151 (Pt 3): 855–61. doi:10.1099/mic.0.27428-0. PMID 15758231.
62. Shiba T, Tsutsumi K, Ishige K, Noguchi T (2000). Inorganic polyphosphate and polyphosphate kinase: their novel biological functions and applications. Biochemistry (Mosc). 65 (3): 315–23. PMID 10739474.
63. Brune DC (1995). Isolation and characterization of sulfur globule proteins from Chromatium vinosum and Thiocapsa roseopersicina. Archives of Microbiology. 163 (6): 391–9. doi:10.1007/BF00272127. PMID 7575095.

64. Kadouri D, Jurkevitch E, Okon Y, Castro-Sowinski S (2005). Ecological and agricultural significance of bacterial polyhydroxyalkanoates. Critical Reviews in Microbiology. 31 (2): 55–67. doi:10.1080/10408410590899228. PMID 15986831.

65. Walsby AE (1994). Gas vesicles. Microbiological Reviews. 58 (1): 94–144. PMC 372955Freely accessible. PMID 8177173.

66. van Heijenoort J (2001). Formation of the glycan chains in the synthesis of bacterial peptidoglycan. Glycobiology. 11 (3): 25R–36R. doi:10.1093/glycob/11.3.25R. PMID 11320055.

67. Koch AL (2003). Bacterial wall as target for attack: past, present, and future research. Clin Microbiol Rev. 16 (4): 673–87. doi:10.1128/CMR.16.4.673-687.2003. PMC 207114Freely accessible. PMID 14557293.

68. Gram, HC (1884). Über die isolierte Färbung der Schizomyceten in Schnitt- und Trockenpräparaten. Fortschr. Med. 2: 185–189.

69. Hugenholtz P (2002). Exploring prokaryotic diversity in the genomic era. Genome Biology. 3 (2): reviews0003.1–reviews0003.8. doi:10.1186/gb-2002-3-2-reviews0003. PMC 139013Freely accessible. PMID 11864374.

70. Walsh FM, Amyes SG (2004). Microbiology and drug resistance mechanisms of fully resistant pathogens. Current Opinion in Microbiology. 7 (5): 439–44. doi:10.1016/j.mib.2004.08.007. PMID 15451497.

71. Engelhardt H, Peters J (1998). Structural research on surface layers: a focus on stability, surface layer homology domains, and surface layer-cell wall interactions. J Struct Biol. 124 (2–3): 276–302. doi:10.1006/jsbi.1998.4070. PMID 10049812.

72. Beveridge TJ, Pouwels PH, Sára M, Kotiranta A, Lounatmaa K, Kari K, Kerosuo E, Haapasalo M, Egelseer EM, Schocher I, Sleytr UB, Morelli L, Callegari ML, Nomellini JF, Bingle WH, Smit J, Leibovitz E, Lemaire M, Miras I, Salamitou S, Béguin P, Ohayon H, Gounon P, Matuschek M, Koval SF (1997). Functions of S-layers. FEMS Microbiol Rev. 20 (1–2): 99–149. doi:10.1016/S0168-6445(97)00043-0. PMID 9276929.

73. Kojima S, Blair DF (2004). The bacterial flagellar motor: structure and function of a complex molecular machine. Int Rev Cytol. International Review of Cytology. 233: 93–134. doi:10.1016/S0074-7696(04)33003-2. ISBN 978-0-12-364637-8. PMID 15037363.

74. Beachey EH (1981). Bacterial adherence: adhesin-receptor interactions mediating the attachment of bacteria to mucosal surface. J Infect Dis. 143 (3): 325–45. doi:10.1093/infdis/143.3.325. PMID 7014727.

75. Silverman PM (1997). Towards a structural biology of bacterial conjugation. Mol Microbiol. 23 (3): 423–9. doi:10.1046/j.1365-2958.1997.2411604.x. PMID 9044277.

76. Stokes RW, Norris-Jones R, Brooks DE, Beveridge TJ, Doxsee D, Thorson LM (2004). The glycan-rich outer layer of the cell wall of Mycobacterium tuberculosis acts as an antiphagocytic capsule limiting the association of the bacterium with macrophages. Infect Immun. 72 (10): 5676–86. doi:10.1128/IAI.72.10.5676-5686.2004. PMC 517526Freely accessible. PMID 15385466.

77. Daffé M, Etienne G (1999). The capsule of Mycobacterium tuberculosis and its implications for pathogenicity. Tuber Lung Dis. 79 (3): 153–69. doi:10.1054/tuld.1998.0200. PMID 10656114.

78. Finlay BB, Falkow S (1997). Common themes in microbial pathogenicity revisited. Microbiology and Molecular Biology Reviews. 61 (2): 136–69. PMC 232605Freely accessible. PMID 9184008.

79. Nicholson WL, Munakata N, Horneck G, Melosh HJ, Setlow P (2000). Resistance of Bacillus endospores to extreme terrestrial and extraterrestrial environments. Microbiology and Molecular Biology Reviews. 64 (3): 548–72. doi:10.1128/MMBR.64.3.548-572.2000. PMC 99004Freely accessible. PMID 10974126.

80. Siunov AV, Nikitin DV, Suzina NE, Dmitriev VV, Kuzmin NP, Duda VI (1999). Phylogenetic status of Anaerobacter polyendosporus, an anaerobic, polysporogenic bacterium (PDF). Int J Syst Bacteriol. 49 (3): 1119–24. doi:10.1099/00207713-49-3-1119. PMID 10425769.

81. Nicholson WL, Fajardo-Cavazos P, Rebeil R, Slieman TA, Riesenman PJ, Law JF, Xue Y (2002). Bacterial endospores and their significance in stress resistance. Antonie Van Leeuwenhoek. 81 (1–4): 27–32. doi 10.1023/A:1020561122764. PMID 12448702.

82. Vreeland RH, Rosenzweig WD, Powers DW (2000). Isolation of a 250 million-year-old halotolerant bacterium from a primary salt crystal. Nature. 407 (6806): 897–900. Bibcode:2000Natur.407..897V. doi:10.1038/35038060. PMID 11057666.

83. Cano RJ, Borucki MK (1995). Revival and identification of bacterial spores in 25- to 40-million-year-old Dominican amber. Science. 268 (5213): 1060–4. Bibcode:1995Sci...268.1060C. doi:10.1126/science.7538699. PMID 7538699.

84. Nicholson WL, Schuerger AC, Setlow P (2005). The solar UV environment and bacterial spore UV resistance: considerations for Earth-to-Mars transport by natural processes and human spaceflight. Mutat Res. 571 (1–2): 249–64. doi:10.1016/j.mrfmmm.2004.10.012. PMID 15748651.

85. BBC Staff (23 August 2011). Impacts ‹more likely› to have spread life from Earth. BBC. Retrieved 24 August 2011.

86. Hatheway CL (1990). Toxigenic clostridia. Clinical Microbiology Reviews. 3 (1): 66–98. PMC 358141Freely accessible. PMID 2404569.

87. Nealson KH (1999). Post-Viking microbiology: new approaches, new data, new insights. Origins of Life and Evolution of Biospheres. 29 (1): 73–93. doi:10.1023/A:1006515817767. PMID 11536899.

88. Xu J (2006). Microbial ecology in the age of genomics and metagenomics: concepts, tools, and recent advances. Mol Ecol. 15 (7): 1713–31. doi:10.1111/j.1365-294X.2006.02882.x. PMID 16689892.

89. Zillig W (1991). Comparative biochemistry of Archaea and Bacteria. Current Opinion in Genetics & Development. 1 (4): 544–51. doi:10.1016/S0959-437X(05)80206-0. PMID 1822288.

90. Hellingwerf KJ, Crielaard W, Hoff WD, Matthijs HC, Mur LR, van Rotterdam BJ (1994). Photobiology of bacteria. Antonie Van Leeuwenhoek. 65 (4): 331–47. doi:10.1007/BF00872217. PMID 7832590.
91. Zumft WG (1 December 1997). Cell biology and molecular basis of denitrification. Microbiol Mol Biol Rev. 61 (4): 533–616. PMC 232623Freely accessible. PMID 9409151.
92. Drake HL, Daniel SL, Küsel K, Matthies C, Kuhner C, Braus-Stromeyer S (1997). Acetogenic bacteria: what are the in situ consequences of their diverse metabolic versatilities?. BioFactors. 6 (1): 13–24. doi:10.1002/biof.5520060103. PMID 9233536.
93. Morel FM, Kraepiel AM, Amyot M (1998). The chemical cycle and bioaccumulation of mercury. Annual Review of Ecology and Systematics. 29: 543–566. doi:10.1146/annurev.ecolsys.29.1.543.
94. Dalton H (2005). The Leeuwenhoek Lecture 2000 the natural and unnatural history of methane-oxidizing bacteria. Philosophical Transactions of the Royal Society B. 360 (1458): 1207–22. doi:10.1098/rstb.2005.1657. PMC 1569495Freely accessible. PMID 16147517.
95. Zehr JP, Jenkins BD, Short SM, Steward GF (2003). Nitrogenase gene diversity and microbial community structure: a cross-system comparison. Environ Microbiol. 5 (7): 539–54. doi:10.1046/j.1462-2920.2003.00451.x. PMID 12823187.
96. Lonhienne TG, Sagulenko E, Webb RI, Lee KC, Franke J, Devos DP, Nouwens A, Carroll BJ, Fuerst JA (2010). Endocytosis-like protein uptake in the bacterium Gemmata obscuriglobus. Proceedings of the National Academy of Sciences of the United States of America. 107 (29): 12883–12888. Bibcode:2010PNAS..10712883L. doi:10.1073/pnas.1001085107. PMC 2919973Freely accessible. PMID 20566852.
97. Koch AL (2002). Control of the bacterial cell cycle by cytoplasmic growth. Crit Rev Microbiol. 28 (1): 61–77. doi:10.1080/1040-840291046696. PMID 12003041.
98. Eagon RG (1962). Pseudomonas natriegens, a marine bacterium with a generation time of less than 10 minutes. Journal of Bacteriology. 83 (4): 736–7. PMC 279347Freely accessible. PMID 13888946.
99. Stewart EJ, Madden R, Paul G, Taddei F (2005). Aging and death in an organism that reproduces by morphologically symmetric division. PLoS Biol. 3 (2): e45. doi:10.1371/journal.pbio.0030045. PMC 546039Freely accessible. PMID 15685293.
100. Thomson RB, Bertram H (2001). Laboratory diagnosis of central nervous system infections. Infectious Disease Clinics of North America. 15 (4): 1047–71. doi:10.1016/S0891-5520(05)70186-0. PMID 11780267.
101. Paerl HW, Fulton RS, Moisander PH, Dyble J (2001). Harmful freshwater algal blooms, with an emphasis on cyanobacteria. ScientificWorldJournal. 1: 76–113. doi:10.1100/tsw.2001.16. PMID 12805693.
102. Challis GL, Hopwood DA (2003). Synergy and contingency as driving forces for the evolution of multiple secondary metabolite production by Streptomyces

species. Proceedings of the National Academy of Sciences of the United States of America. 100 Suppl 2 (90002): 14555–61. Bibcode:2003PNAS..10014555C. doi:10.1073/pnas.1934677100. PMC 304118Freely accessible. PMID 12970466.

103. Kooijman SA, Auger P, Poggiale JC, Kooi BW (2003). Quantitative steps in symbiogenesis and the evolution of homeostasis. Biol Rev Camb Philos Soc. 78 (3): 435–63. doi:10.1017/S1464793102006127. PMID 14558592.

104. Prats C, López D, Giró A, Ferrer J, Valls J (2006). Individual-based modelling of bacterial cultures to study the microscopic causes of the lag phase. J Theor Biol. 241 (4): 939–53. doi:10.1016/j.jtbi.2006.01.029. PMID 16524598.

105. Hecker M, Völker U (2001). General stress response of Bacillus subtilis and other bacteria. Adv Microb Physiol. Advances in Microbial Physiology. 44: 35–91. doi:10.1016/S0065-2911(01)44011-2. ISBN 978-0-12-027744-5. PMID 11407115.

106. Genomes Online Database. Genomes Online Database. Joint Genome Institute. Retrieved 14 Sep 2016.

107. Nakabachi A, Yamashita A, Toh H, Ishikawa H, Dunbar HE, Moran NA, Hattori M (2006). The 160-kilobase genome of the bacterial endosymbiont Carsonella. Science. 314 (5797): 267. doi:10.1126/science.1134196. PMID 17038615.

108. Pradella S, Hans A, Spröer C, Reichenbach H, Gerth K, Beyer S (2002). Characterisation, genome size and genetic manipulation of the myxobacterium Sorangium cellulosum So ce56. Arch Microbiol. 178 (6): 484–92. doi:10.1007/s00203-002-0479-2. PMID 12420170.

109. Belfort M, Reaban ME, Coetzee T, Dalgaard JZ (1 July 1995). Prokaryotic introns and inteins: a panoply of form and function. J. Bacteriol. 177 (14): 3897–903. PMC 177115Freely accessible. PMID 7608058.

110. Hinnebusch J, Tilly K (1993). Linear plasmids and chromosomes in bacteria. Mol Microbiol. 10 (5): 917–22. doi:10.1111/j.1365-2958.1993.tb00963.x. PMID 7934868.

111. Fraser, Claire M.; Casjens, Sherwood; Huang, Wai Mun; Sutton, Granger G.; Clayton, Rebecca; Lathigra, Raju; White, Owen; Ketchum, Karen A.; Dodson, Robert (1997-12-11). Genomic sequence of a Lyme disease spirochaete, Borrelia burgdorferi. Nature. 390 (6660): 580–586. doi:10.1038/37551. ISSN 0028-0836. PMID 9403685.

112. The University of Waikato (March 25, 2014). Bacterial DNA – the role of plasmids. Themes — Bacteria in biotech. Biotechnology Learning Hub. Retrieved 2014-09-03.

113. Denamur E, Matic I (2006). Evolution of mutation rates in bacteria. Mol Microbiol. 60 (4): 820–7. doi:10.1111/j.1365-2958.2006.05150.x. PMID 16677295.

114. Wright BE (2004). Stress-directed adaptive mutations and evolution. Mol Microbiol. 52 (3): 643–50. doi:10.1111/j.1365-2958.2004.04012.x. PMID 15101972.

115. Chen I, Dubnau D (2004). DNA uptake during bacterial transformation. Nature

Reviews Microbiology. 2 (3): 241–9. doi:10.1038/nrmicro844. PMID 15083159.

116. Solomon JM, Grossman AD (1996). Who›s competent and when: regulation of natural genetic competence in bacteria. Trends Genet. 12 (4): 150–5. doi:10.1016/0168-9525(96)10014-7. PMID 8901420.

117. Akamatsu T, Taguchi H (2001). Incorporation of the whole chromosomal DNA in protoplast lysates into competent cells of Bacillus subtilis. Biosci. Biotechnol. Biochem. 65 (4): 823–9. doi:10.1271/bbb.65.823. PMID 11388459.

118. Saito Y, Taguchi H, Akamatsu T (2006). Fate of transforming bacterial genome following incorporation into competent cells of Bacillus subtilis: a continuous length of incorporated DNA. J. Biosci. Bioeng. 101 (3): 257–62. doi:10.1263/jbb.101.257. PMID 16716928.

119. Johnsborg O, Eldholm V, Håvarstein LS (2007). Natural genetic transformation: prevalence, mechanisms and function. Res. Microbiol. 158 (10): 767–78. doi:10.1016/j.resmic.2007.09.004. PMID 17997281.

120. Bernstein H, Bernstein C, Michod RE (2012). DNA repair as the primary adaptive function of sex in bacteria and eukaryotes. Chapter 1: pp. 1–49 in: DNA Repair: New Research, Sakura Kimura and Sora Shimizu (eds.). Nova Sci. Publ., Hauppauge, N.Y. ISBN 978-1-62100-808-8.

121. Michod RE, Bernstein H, Nedelcu AM (2008). Adaptive value of sex in microbial pathogens (PDF). Infect. Genet. Evol. 8 (3): 267–85. doi:10.1016/j.meegid.2008.01.002. PMID 18295550.

122. Davison J (1999). Genetic exchange between bacteria in the environment. Plasmid. 42 (2): 73–91. doi:10.1006/plas.1999.1421. PMID 10489325.

123. Hastings PJ, Rosenberg SM, Slack A (2004). Antibiotic-induced lateral transfer of antibiotic resistance. Trends Microbiol. 12 (9): 401–4. doi:10.1016/j.tim.2004.07.003. PMID 15337159.

124. Brüssow H, Canchaya C, Hardt WD (2004). Phages and the evolution of bacterial pathogens: from genomic rearrangements to lysogenic conversion. Microbiology and Molecular Biology Reviews. 68 (3): 560–602. doi:10.1128/MMBR.68.3.560-602.2004. PMC 515249Freely accessible. PMID 15353570.

125. Bickle TA, Krüger DH (1993). Biology of DNA restriction. Microbiol. Rev. 57 (2): 434–50. PMC 372918Freely accessible. PMID 8336674.

126. Barrangou R, Fremaux C, Deveau H, Richards M, Boyaval P, Moineau S, Romero DA, Horvath P (2007). CRISPR provides acquired resistance against viruses in prokaryotes. Science. 315 (5819): 1709–12. Bibcode:2007Sci...315.1709B. doi:10.1126/science.1138140. PMID 17379808.

127. Brouns SJ, Jore MM, Lundgren M, Westra ER, Slijkhuis RJ, Snijders AP, Dickman MJ, Makarova KS, Koonin EV, van der Oost J (2008). Small CRISPR RNAs guide antiviral defense in prokaryotes. Science. 321 (5891): 960–4. Bibcode:2008Sci...321..960B. doi:10.1126/science.1159689. PMID 18703739.

128. Dusenbery, David B. (1996). Life at Small Scale. Scientific American Library. ISBN 0-7167-5060-0.

129. Shapiro JA (1998). Thinking about bacterial populations as multicellular organisms (PDF). Annu. Rev. Microbiol. 52: 81–104. doi:10.1146/annurev.micro.52.1.81. PMID 9891794. Archived from the original (PDF) on 17 July 2011.

130. Costerton JW, Lewandowski Z, Caldwell DE, Korber DR, Lappin-Scott HM (1995). Microbial biofilms. Annu. Rev. Microbiol. 49: 711–45. doi:10.1146/annurev.mi.49.100195.003431. PMID 8561477.

131. Miller MB, Bassler BL (2001). Quorum sensing in bacteria. Annu. Rev. Microbiol. 55: 165–99. doi:10.1146/annurev.micro.55.1.165. PMID 11544353.

132. Bardy S, Ng S, Jarrell K (2003). Prokaryotic motility structures. Microbiology. 149 (Pt 2): 295–304. doi:10.1099/mic.0.25948-0. PMID 12624192.

133. Dusenbery, David B. (2009). Living at Micro Scale p. 136. Harvard University Press, Cambridge, Mass. ISBN 978-0-674-03116-6

134. Merz A, So M, Sheetz M (2000). Pilus retraction powers bacterial twitching motility. Nature. 407 (6800): 98–102. Bibcode:2000Natur.407...98M. doi:10.1038/35024105. PMID 10993081.

135. A re-examination of twitching motility in Pseudomonas aeruginosa – Semmler, Whitchurch & Mattick (1999)

136. Dusenbery, David B. (2009). Living at Micro Scale, Chapter 13. Harvard University Press, Cambridge, Mass. ISBN 978-0-674-03116-6.

137. Macnab RM (1 December 1999). The bacterial flagellum: reversible rotary propellor and type III export apparatus. J. Bacteriol. 181 (23): 7149–53. PMC 103673Freely accessible. PMID 10572114.

138. Wu M, Roberts J, Kim S, Koch D, DeLisa M (2006). Collective bacterial dynamics revealed using a three-dimensional population-scale defocused particle tracking technique. Appl Environ Microbiol. 72 (7): 4987–94. doi:10.1128/AEM.00158-06. PMC 1489374Freely accessible. PMID 16820497.

139. Lux R, Shi W (2004). Chemotaxis-guided movements in bacteria. Crit Rev Oral Biol Med. 15 (4): 207–20. doi:10.1177/154411130401500404. PMID 15284186.

140. Schweinitzer T, Josenhans C (2010). Bacterial energy taxis: a global strategy?. Arch Microbiol. 192 (7): 507–20. doi:10.1007/s00203-010-0575-7. PMC 2886117Freely accessible. PMID 20411245.

141. Frankel R, Bazylinski D, Johnson M, Taylor B (1997). Magneto-aerotaxis in marine coccoid bacteria. Biophys J. 73 (2): 994–1000. Bibcode:1997BpJ....73..994F. doi:10.1016/S0006-3495(97)78132-3. PMC 1180996Freely accessible. PMID 9251816.

142. Goldberg MB (2001). Actin-based motility of intracellular microbial pathogens. Microbiol Mol Biol Rev. 65 (4): 595–626, table of contents. doi:10.1128/MMBR.65.4.595-626.2001. PMC 99042Freely accessible. PMID 11729265.

143. Ciccarelli FD, Doerks T, von Mering C, Creevey CJ, Snel B, Bork P (March 2006). Toward automatic reconstruction of a highly resolved tree of life. Science. 311 (5765): 1283–7. Bibcode:2006Sci...311.1283C. doi:10.1126/science.1123061. PMID 16513982.

144. Boucher Y, Douady CJ, Papke RT, Walsh DA, Boudreau ME, Nesbo CL, Case RJ, Doolittle WF (2003). Lateral gene transfer and the origins of prokaryotic groups. Annu Rev Genet. 37: 283–328. doi:10.1146/annurev.genet.37.050503.084247. PMID 14616063.

145. Olsen GJ, Woese CR, Overbeek R (1994). The winds of (evolutionary) change: breathing new life into microbiology. Journal of Bacteriology. 176 (1): 1–6. doi:10.2172/205047. PMC 205007Freely accessible. PMID 8282683.

146. IJSEM Home. Ijs.sgmjournals.org. 28 October 2011. Retrieved 4 November 2011.

147. Bergey›s Manual Trust. Bergeys.org. Retrieved 4 November 2011.

148. Gupta R (2000). The natural evolutionary relationships among prokaryotes. Crit Rev Microbiol. 26 (2): 111–31. doi:10.1080/10408410091154219. PMID 10890353.

149. Doolittle RF (2005). Evolutionary aspects of whole-genome biology. Current Opinion in Structural Biology. 15 (3): 248–53. doi:10.1016/j.sbi.2005.04.001. PMID 15963888.

150. Cavalier-Smith T (2002). The neomuran origin of archaebacteria, the negibacterial root of the universal tree and bacterial megaclassification. Int J Syst Evol Microbiol. 52 (Pt 1): 7–76. doi:10.1099/00207713-52-1-7. PMID 11837318.

151. Woods GL, Walker DH (1996). Detection of infection or infectious agents by use of cytologic and histologic stains. Clinical Microbiology Reviews. 9 (3): 382–404. PMC 172900Freely accessible. PMID 8809467.

152. Weinstein M (1994). Clinical importance of blood cultures. Clin Lab Med. 14 (1): 9–16. PMID 8181237.

153. Louie M, Louie L, Simor AE (8 August 2000). The role of DNA amplification technology in the diagnosis of infectious diseases. CMAJ. 163 (3): 301–9. PMC 80298Freely accessible. PMID 10951731.

154. Oliver J (2005). The viable but nonculturable state in bacteria. J Microbiol. 43 Spec No: 93–100. PMID 15765062. Archived from the original on 28 September 2007.

155. Euzéby JP (8 December 2011). Number of published names. List of Prokaryotic names with Standing in Nomenclature. Archived from the original on 19 January 2012. Retrieved 10 December 2011.

156. Curtis TP, Sloan WT, Scannell JW (2002). Estimating prokaryotic diversity and its limits. Proceedings of the National Academy of Sciences of the United States of America. 99 (16): 10494–9. Bibcode:2002PNAS...9910494C. doi:10.1073/pnas.142680199. PMC 124953Freely accessible. PMID 12097644.

157. Schloss PD, Handelsman J (2004). Status of the microbial census. Microbiology and Molecular Biology Reviews. 68 (4): 686–91. doi:10.1128/MMBR.68.4.686-691.2004. PMC 539005Freely accessible. PMID 15590780.

158. Fisher B, Harvey RP, Champe PC (2007). Lippincott›s Illustrated Reviews: Microbiology (Lippincott›s Illustrated Reviews Series). Hagerstwon, MD: Lippincott Williams & Wilkins. pp. Chapter 33, pages 367–392. ISBN 0-7817-

8215-5.

159. LEF.org > Bacterial Infections Updated: 19 January 2006. Retrieved on 11 April 2009

160. Martin MO (2002). Predatory prokaryotes: an emerging research opportunity. Journal of Microbiology and Biotechnology. 4 (5): 467–77. PMID 12432957.

161. Velicer GJ, Stredwick KL (2002). Experimental social evolution with Myxococcus xanthus. Antonie Van Leeuwenhoek. 81 (1–4): 155–64. doi:10.1023/A:1020546130033. PMID 12448714.

162. Gromov, BV. Electron Microscope Study of Parasitism by Bdellovibrio Chorellavorus Bacteria on Cells of the Green Alga Chorella Vulgaris. Tsitologiya 14.2 (1972): 256-60. Print.

163. Guerrero R, Pedros-Alio C, Esteve I, Mas J, Chase D, Margulis L (April 1986). Predatory prokaryotes: predation and primary consumption evolved in bacteria. Proceedings of the National Academy of Sciences of the United States of America. 83 (7): 2138–42. Bibcode:1986PNAS...83.2138G. doi:10.1073/pnas.83.7.2138. PMC 323246Freely accessible. PMID 11542073.

164. Velicer GJ, Mendes-Soares H (2009). Bacterial predators. Current Biology. 19 (2): R55–6. doi:10.1016/j.cub.2008.10.043. PMID 19174136.

165. Stams AJ, de Bok FA, Plugge CM, van Eekert MH, Dolfing J, Schraa G (2006). Exocellular electron transfer in anaerobic microbial communities. Environ Microbiol. 8 (3): 371–82. doi:10.1111/j.1462-2920.2006.00989.x. PMID 16478444.

166. Barea JM, Pozo MJ, Azcón R, Azcón-Aguilar C (2005). Microbial co-operation in the rhizosphere. J Exp Bot. 56 (417): 1761–78. doi:10.1093/jxb/eri197. PMID 15911555.

167. O›Hara AM, Shanahan F (2006). The gut flora as a forgotten organ. EMBO Reports. 7 (7): 688–93. doi:10.1038/sj.embor.7400731. PMC 1500832Freely accessible. PMID 16819463.

168. Zoetendal EG, Vaughan EE, de Vos WM (2006). A microbial world within us. Mol Microbiol. 59 (6): 1639–50. doi:10.1111/j.1365-2958.2006.05056.x. PMID 16553872.

169. Gorbach SL (1990). Lactic acid bacteria and human health. Annals of Medicine. 22 (1): 37–41. doi:10.3109/07853899009147239. PMID 2109988.

170. Salminen SJ, Gueimonde M, Isolauri E (1 May 2005). Probiotics that modify disease risk. J Nutr. 135 (5): 1294–8. PMID 15867327.

171. Fish DN (2002). Optimal antimicrobial therapy for sepsis. Am J Health Syst Pharm. 59 Suppl 1: S13–9. PMID 11885408.

172. Belland RJ, Ouellette SP, Gieffers J, Byrne GI (2004). Chlamydia pneumoniae and atherosclerosis. Cell Microbiol. 6 (2): 117–27. doi:10.1046/j.1462-5822.2003.00352.x. PMID 14706098.

173. Heise ER (1982). Diseases associated with immunosuppression. Environmental Health Perspectives. 43: 9–19. doi:10.2307/3429162. JSTOR 3429162. PMC 1568899Freely accessible. PMID 7037390.

174. Saiman L (2004). Microbiology of early CF lung disease. Paediatric Respiratory Reviews. 5 Suppl A: S367–9. doi:10.1016/S1526-0542(04)90065-6. PMID 14980298.

175. Yonath A, Bashan A (2004). Ribosomal crystallography: initiation, peptide bond formation, and amino acid polymerization are hampered by antibiotics. Annu Rev Microbiol. 58: 233–51. doi:10.1146/annurev.micro.58.030603.123822. PMID 15487937.

176. Khachatourians GG (1998). Agricultural use of antibiotics and the evolution and transfer of antibiotic-resistant bacteria. CMAJ. 159 (9): 1129–36. PMC 1229782Freely accessible. PMID 9835883.

177. Johnson ME, Lucey JA (2006). Major technological advances and trends in cheese. J Dairy Sci. 89 (4): 1174–8. doi:10.3168/jds.S0022-0302(06)72186-5. PMID 16537950.

178. Hagedorn S, Kaphammer B (1994). Microbial biocatalysis in the generation of flavor and fragrance chemicals. Annu. Rev. Microbiol. 48: 773–800. doi:10.1146/annurev.mi.48.100194.004013. PMID 7826026.

179. Cohen Y (2002). Bioremediation of oil by marine microbial mats. Int Microbiol. 5 (4): 189–93. doi:10.1007/s10123-002-0089-5. PMID 12497184.

180. Neves LC, Miyamura TT, Moraes DA, Penna TC, Converti A (2006). Biofiltration methods for the removal of phenolic residues. Appl. Biochem. Biotechnol. 129–132: 130–52. doi:10.1385/ABAB:129:1:130. PMID 16915636.

181. Liese A, Filho MV (1999). Production of fine chemicals using biocatalysis. Current Opinion in Biotechnology. 10 (6): 595–603. doi:10.1016/S0958-1669(99)00040-3. PMID 10600695.

182. Aronson AI, Shai Y (2001). Why Bacillus thuringiensis insecticidal toxins are so effective: unique features of their mode of action. FEMS Microbiol. Lett. 195 (1): 1–8. doi:10.1111/j.1574-6968.2001.tb10489.x. PMID 11166987.

183. Bozsik A (2006). Susceptibility of adult Coccinella septempunctata (Coleoptera: Coccinellidae) to insecticides with different modes of action. Pest Manag Sci. 62 (7): 651–4. doi:10.1002/ps.1221. PMID 16649191.

184. Chattopadhyay A, Bhatnagar NB, Bhatnagar R (2004). Bacterial insecticidal toxins. Crit Rev Microbiol. 30 (1): 33–54. doi:10.1080/10408410490270712. PMID 15116762.

185. Serres MH, Gopal S, Nahum LA, Liang P, Gaasterland T, Riley M (2001). A functional update of the Escherichia coli K-12 genome. Genome Biology. 2 (9): research0035.1–research0035.7. doi:10.1186/gb-2001-2-9-research0035. PMC 56896Freely accessible. PMID 11574054.

186. Almaas E, Kovács B, Vicsek T, Oltvai ZN, Barabási AL (2004). Global organization of metabolic fluxes in the bacterium Escherichia coli. Nature. 427 (6977): 839–43. arXiv:q-bio/0403001Freely accessible. Bibcode:2004Natur.427..839A. doi:10.1038/nature02289. PMID 14985762.

187. Reed JL, Vo TD, Schilling CH, Palsson BO (2003). An expanded genome-scale model of Escherichia coli K-12 (iJR904 GSM/GPR). Genome Biol. 4 (9): R54. doi:10.1186/gb-2003-4-9-r54. PMC 193654Freely accessible. PMID 12952533.

188. Walsh G (2005). Therapeutic insulins and their large-scale manufacture. Appl Microbiol Biotechnol. 67 (2): 151–9. doi:10.1007/s00253-004-1809-x. PMID 15580495.

189. Graumann K, Premstaller A (2006). Manufacturing of recombinant therapeutic proteins in microbial systems. Biotechnol J. 1 (2): 164–86. doi:10.1002/biot.200500051. PMID 16892246.

190. Porter JR (1976). Antony van Leeuwenhoek: tercentenary of his discovery of bacteria. Bacteriological Reviews. 40 (2): 260–9. PMC 413956Freely accessible. PMID 786250.

191. van Leeuwenhoek A (1684). An abstract of a letter from Mr. Anthony Leevvenhoek at Delft, dated Sep. 17, 1683, Containing Some Microscopical Observations, about Animals in the Scurf of the Teeth, the Substance Call›d Worms in the Nose, the Cuticula Consisting of Scales. Philosophical Transactions (1683–1775). 14 (155–166): 568–574. doi:10.1098/rstl.1684.0030.

192. van Leeuwenhoek A (1700). Part of a Letter from Mr Antony van Leeuwenhoek, concerning the Worms in Sheeps Livers, Gnats, and Animalcula in the Excrements of Frogs. Philosophical Transactions (1683–1775). 22 (260–276): 509–518. doi:10.1098/rstl.1700.0013.

193. van Leeuwenhoek A (1702). Part of a Letter from Mr Antony van Leeuwenhoek, F. R. S. concerning Green Weeds Growing in Water, and Some Animalcula Found about Them. Philosophical Transactions (1683–1775). 23 (277–288): 1304–11. doi:10.1098/rstl.1702.0042.

194. Asimov, Isaac (1982), Asimov›s Biographical Encyclopedia of Science and Technology, 2nd edition, Garden City, New York: Doubleday and Company, pg 143.

195. Ehrenberg›s Symbolae Physioe. Animalia evertebrata. Decas prima. Berlin, 1828.

196. Breed RS, Conn HJ (1936). The Status of the Generic Term Bacterium Ehrenberg 1828. Journal of Bacteriology. 31 (5): 517–518. PMC 543738Freely accessible. PMID 16559906.

197. EHRENBERG (C.G.): Dritter Beitrag zur Erkenntniss grosser Organisation in der Richtung des kleinsten Raumes. Physikalische Abhandlungen der Koeniglichen Akademie der Wissenschaften zu Berlin aus den Jahren 1833–1835, 1835, pp. 143–336.

198. Pasteur›s Papers on the Germ Theory. LSU Law Center›s Medical and Public Health Law Site, Historic Public Health Articles. Archived from the original on 18 December 2006. Retrieved 23 November 2006.

199. The Nobel Prize in Physiology or Medicine 1905. Nobelprize.org. Archived from the original on 10 December 2006. Retrieved 22 November 2006.

200. O›Brien SJ, Goedert JJ (1996). HIV causes AIDS: Koch›s postulates fulfilled. Current Opinion in Immunology. 8 (5): 613–8. doi:10.1016/S0952-7915(96)80075-6. PMID 8902385.

201. Thurston AJ (2000). Of blood, inflammation and gunshot wounds: the history of the control of sepsis. Aust N Z J Surg. 70 (12): 855–61. doi:10.1046/j.1440-1622.2000.01983.x. PMID 11167573.

202. Schwartz RS (2004). Paul Ehrlich›s magic bullets. N Engl J Med. 350 (11): 1079–80. doi:10.1056/NEJMp048021. PMID 15014180.

203. Biography of Paul Ehrlich. Nobelprize.org. Archived from the original on 28 November 2006. Retrieved 26 November 2006.

CHAPTER 3

Mycology: The Study of Fungi

Chapter Contents

Mycology is the branch of biology that deals with the study of fungi. It includes the research of their genetic and biochemical properties, and their use in medicine and food along with their hazards. The term mycology is a concoction of the Greek words mukēs, meaning fungus, and logia, meaning study.

Fungi are found in almost all types of environments and can be highly beneficial. They help to decompose organisms, they are great sources for antibiotics, and they serve as food. However, some fungi can be harmful and poisonous. Therefore, mycology is necessary to fully understand the properties and suitable uses of mushrooms.

INTRODUCTION

Mycology is the branch of biology concerned with the study of fungi, including their genetic and biochemical properties, their taxonomy and their use to humans as a source for tinder, medicine, food, and entheogens, as well as their dangers, such as poisoning or infection. A biologist specializing in mycology is called a mycologist.

From mycology arose the field of phytopathology, the study of plant diseases, and the two disciplines remain closely related because the vast majority of "plant" pathogens are fungi.

Historically, mycology was a branch of botany because, although fungi are evolutionarily more closely related to animals than to plants, this was not recognized until a few decades ago. Pioneer *mycologists* included Elias Magnus Fries, Christian Hendrik Persoon, Anton de Bary, and Lewis David von Schweinitz.

Many fungi produce toxins, antibiotics, and other secondary metabolites. For example, the cosmopolitan (worldwide) genus *Fusarium* and their toxins associated with fatal outbreaks of alimentary toxic aleukia in humans were extensively studied by Abraham Joffe.

Fungi are fundamental for life on earth in their roles as symbionts, e.g. in the form of mycorrhizae, insect symbionts, and lichens. Many fungi are able to break down complex organic biomolecules such as lignin, the more durable component of wood, and pollutants such as xenobiotics, petroleum, and polycyclic aromatic hydrocarbons. By decomposing these molecules, fungi play a critical role in the global carbon cycle.

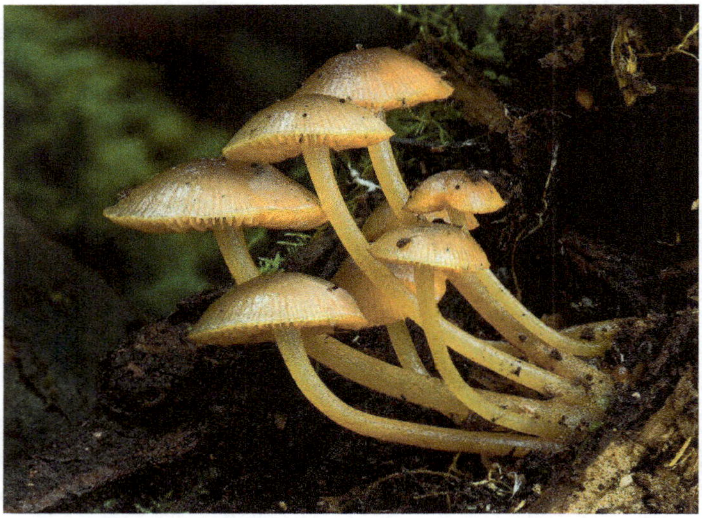

Mushrooms are a kind of fungal reproductive structure.

Fungi and other organisms traditionally recognized as fungi, such as oomycetes and myxomycetes (slime molds), often are economically and socially important, as some cause diseases of animals (such as histoplasmosis) as well as plants (such as Dutch elm disease and Rice blast).

Apart from pathogenic fungi, many fungal species are very important in controlling the plant diseases caused by different pathogens. For example, species of the filamentous fungal genus *Trichoderma* considered as one of the most important biological control agents as an alternative to chemical based products for effective crop diseases management.

Field meetings to find interesting species of fungi are known as 'forays', after the first such meeting organized by the Woolhope Naturalists' Field Club in 1868 and entitled "A foray among the funguses"[*sic*].

Some fungi can cause disease in humans or other organisms. The study of pathogenic fungi is referred to as medical mycology.

HISTORY

It is presumed that humans started collecting mushrooms as food in prehistoric times. Mushrooms were first written about in the works of Euripides (480-406 B.C.). The Greek philosopher Theophrastos of Eressos (371-288 B.C) was perhaps the first to try to systematically classify plants; mushrooms were considered to be plants missing certain organs. It was later Pliny the Elder (23–79 A.D.), who wrote about truffles in his encyclopedia *Naturalis historia*. The word *mycology* comes from the Greek: μύκης (*mukēs*), meaning "fungus" and the suffix -λογία (*-logia*), meaning "study".

The Middle Ages saw little advancement in the body of knowledge about fungi. Rather, the invention of the printing press allowed some authors to disseminate superstitions and misconceptions about the fungi that had been perpetuated by the classical authors.

> "*Fungi and truffles are neither herbs, nor roots, nor flowers, nor seeds, but merely the superfluous moisture or earth, of trees, or rotten wood, and of other rotting things. This is plain from the fact that all fungi and truffles, especially those that are used for eating, grow most commonly in thundery and wet weather*"
>
> — *Jerome Bock (Hieronymus Tragus), 1552*

The start of the modern age of mycology begins with Pier Antonio Micheli's 1737 publication of *Nova plantarum genera*. Published in Florence, this seminal work laid the foundations for the systematic classification of grasses, mosses and fungi. The term *mycology* and the complementary *mycologist* were first used in 1836 by M.J. Berkeley.

MEDICAL MYCOLOGY

For centuries, certain mushrooms have been documented as a folk medicine in China, Japan, and Russia. Although the use of mushrooms in folk medicine is centered largely on the Asian continent, people in other parts of the world like the Middle East, Poland, and Belarus have been documented using mushrooms for medicinal purposes. Certain mushrooms, especially polypores like reishi were thought to be able to benefit a wide variety of health ailments. Medicinal mushroom research in the United States is currently active, with studies taking place at City of Hope National Medical Center, as well as the Memorial Sloan–Kettering Cancer Center.

Current research focuses on mushrooms that may have hypoglycemic activity, anti-cancer activity, anti-pathogenic activity, and immune system-enhancing activity. Recent research has found that the oyster mushroom naturally contains the cholesterol-lowering drug lovastatin, mushrooms produce large amounts of vitamin D when exposed to ultraviolet (UV) light, and that certain fungi may be a future source of taxol. To date, penicillin, lovastatin, ciclosporin, griseofulvin, cephalosporin, ergometrine, and statins are the most famous pharmaceuticals that have been isolated from the fungi kingdom.

FUNGUS

A fungus is any member of the group of eukaryotic organisms that includes unicellular microorganisms such as yeasts and molds, as well as multicellular fungi that produce familiar fruiting forms known as mushrooms. These organisms are classified as a kingdom, Fungi, which is separate from the other eukaryotic life kingdoms of plants and animals.

A characteristic that places fungi in a different kingdom from plants, bacteria and some protists, is chitin in their cell walls. Similar to animals, fungi are heterotrophs; they acquire their food by absorbing dissolved molecules, typically by secreting digestive enzymes into their environment. Fungi do not photosynthesize. Growth is their means of mobility, except for spores (a few of which are flagellated), which may travel through the air or water. Fungi are the principal decomposers in ecological systems. These and other differences place fungi in a single group of related organisms, named the *Eumycota* (*true fungi* or *Eumycetes*), which share a common ancestor (form a *monophyletic group*), an interpretation that is also strongly supported by molecular phylogenetics. This fungal group is distinct from the structurally similar myxomycetes (slime molds) and oomycetes (water molds). The discipline of biology devoted to the study of fungi is known as mycology. In the past, mycology was regarded as a branch of botany, although it is now known fungi are genetically more closely related to animals than to plants.

Abundant worldwide, most fungi are inconspicuous because of the small size of their structures, and their cryptic lifestyles in soil or on dead matter. Fungi include symbionts of plants, animals, or other fungi and also parasites. They may become noticeable when fruiting, either as mushrooms or as molds. Fungi perform an essential role in the decomposition of organic matter and have fundamental roles in nutrient cycling and exchange in the environment. They have long been used as a direct source of human food, in the form of mushrooms and truffles; as a leavening agent for bread; and in the fermentation of various food products, such as wine, beer, and soy sauce. Since the 1940s, fungi have been used for the production of antibiotics, and, more recently, various enzymes produced by fungi are used industrially and in detergents. Fungi are also used as biological pesticides to control weeds, plant diseases and insect pests. Many species produce bioactive compounds called mycotoxins, such as alkaloids and polyketides, that are toxic to animals including humans. The fruiting structures of a few species contain psychotropic compounds and are consumed recreationally or in traditional spiritual ceremonies. Fungi can break down manufactured materials and buildings, and become significant pathogens of humans and other animals. Losses of crops due to fungal diseases (e.g., rice blast disease) or food spoilage can have a large impact on human food supplies and local economies.

The fungus kingdom encompasses an enormous diversity of taxa with varied ecologies, life cycle strategies, and morphologies ranging from unicellular aquatic chytrids to large mushrooms. However, little is known of the true biodiversity of Kingdom Fungi, which has been estimated at 1.5 million to 5 million species, with about 5% of these having been formally classified. Ever since the pioneering 18th and 19th century taxonomical works of Carl Linnaeus, Christian Hendrik Persoon, and Elias Magnus Fries, fungi have been classified according to their morphology (e.g., characteristics such as spore color or microscopic features) or physiology. Advances in molecular genetics have opened the way for DNA analysis to be incorporated into taxonomy, which has sometimes challenged the historical groupings based on morphology and other traits. Phylogenetic studies published in the last decade have helped reshape the classification within Kingdom Fungi, which is divided into one subkingdom, seven phyla, and ten subphyla.

ETYMOLOGY

The English word *fungus* is directly adopted from the Latin *fungus* (mushroom), used in the writings of Horace and Pliny. This in turn is derived from the Greek word *sphongos* ("sponge"), which refers to the macroscopic structures and morphology of mushrooms and molds; the root is also used in other languages, such as the German *Schwamm* ("sponge") and *Schimmel* ("mold"). The use of the word *mycology*, which is derived from the Greek *mykes* ("mushroom") and *logos* ("discourse"), to denote the scientific study of fungi is thought to have originated in 1836 with English naturalist Miles Joseph Berkeley's publication *The English Flora of Sir James Edward Smith, Vol. 5.* A group of all the fungi present in a particular area or geographic region is known as mycobiota (plural noun, no singular), e.g., "the mycobiota of Ireland".

Characteristics

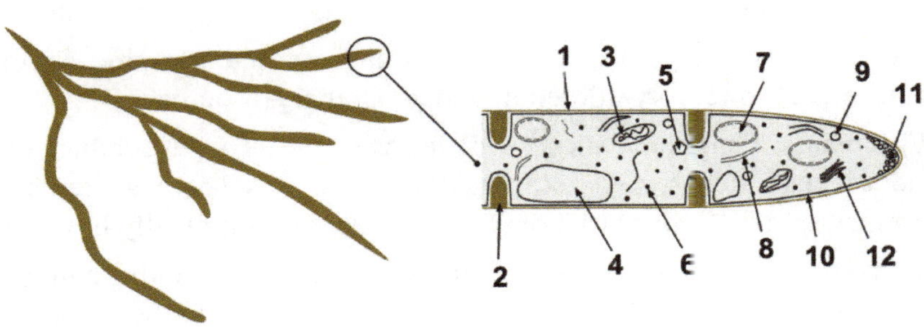

Fungal hyphae cells

- Hyphal wall
- Septum
- Mitochondrion

- Vacuole
- Ergosterol crystal
- Ribosome
- Nucleus
- Endoplasmic reticulum
- Lipid body
- Plasma membrane
- Spitzenkörper
- Golgi apparatus

Before the introduction of molecular methods for phylogenetic analysis, taxonomists considered fungi to be members of the plant kingdom because of similarities in lifestyle: both fungi and plants are mainly immobile, and have similarities in general morphology and growth habitat. Like plants, fungi often grow in soil and, in the case of mushrooms, form conspicuous fruit bodies, which sometimes resemble plants such as mosses. The fungi are now considered a separate kingdom, distinct from both plants and animals, from which they appear to have diverged around one billion years ago. Some morphological, biochemical, and genetic features are shared with other organisms, while others are unique to the fungi, clearly separating them from the other kingdoms:

Shared features:

- With other eukaryotes: Fungal cells contain membrane-bound nuclei with chromosomes that contain DNA with noncoding regions called introns and coding regions called exons. Fungi have membrane-bound cytoplasmic organelles such as mitochondria, sterol-containing membranes, and ribosomes of the 80S type. They have a characteristic range of soluble carbohydrates and storage compounds, including sugar alcohols (e.g., mannitol), disaccharides, (e.g., trehalose), and polysaccharides (e.g., glycogen, which is also found in animals).
- With animals: Fungi lack chloroplasts and are heterotrophic organisms and so require preformed organic compounds as energy sources.
- With plants: Fungi have a cell wall and vacuoles. They reproduce by both sexual and asexual means, and like basal plant groups (such as ferns and mosses) produce spores. Similar to mosses and algae, fungi typically have haploid nuclei.
- With euglenoids and bacteria: Higher fungi, euglenoids, and some bacteria produce the amino acid L-lysine in specific biosynthesis steps, called the α-aminoadipate pathway.
- The cells of most fungi grow as tubular, elongated, and thread-like (filamentous) structures called hyphae, which may contain multiple nuclei and extend by growing at their tips. Each tip contains a set of aggregated vesicles—cellular structures consisting of proteins, lipids, and other organic molecules—called the Spitzenkörper. Both fungi and oomycetes grow as filamentous hyphal cells. In contrast, similar-looking organisms, such as filamentous green algae, grow by repeated cell division within a chain of cells. There are also single-celled

fungi (yeasts) that do not form hyphae, and some fungi have both hyphal and yeast forms.

- In common with some plant and animal species, more than 70 fungal species display bioluminescence.

Unique features:

- Some species grow as unicellular yeasts that reproduce by budding or binary fission. Dimorphic fungi can switch between a yeast phase and a hyphal phase in response to environmental conditions.
- The fungal cell wall is composed of glucans and chitin; while glucans are also found in plants and chitin in the exoskeleton of arthropods, fungi are the only organisms that combine these two structural molecules in their cell wall. Unlike those of plants and oomycetes, fungal cell walls do not contain cellulose.

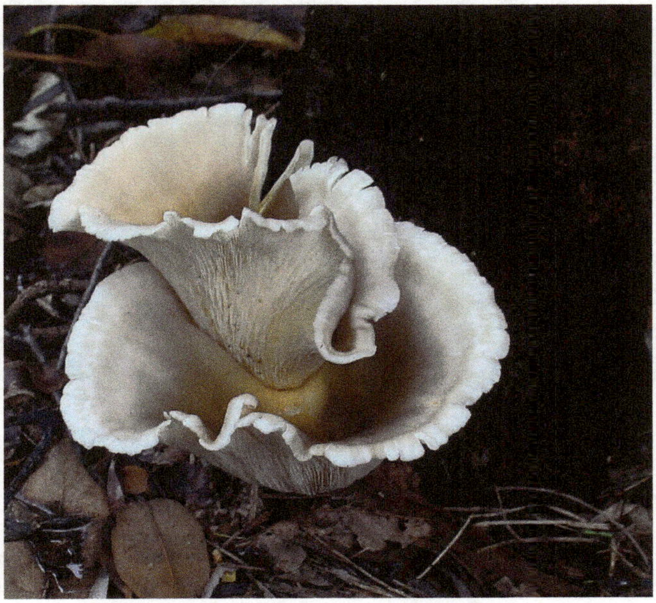

Omphalotus nidiformis, a bioluminescent mushroom.

Most fungi lack an efficient system for the long-distance transport of water and nutrients, such as the xylem and phloem in many plants. To overcome this limitation, some fungi, such as *Armillaria*, form rhizomorphs, which resemble and perform functions similar to the roots of plants. As eukaryotes, fungi possess a biosynthetic pathway for producing terpenes that uses mevalonic acid and pyrophosphate as chemical building blocks. Plants and some other organisms have an additional terpene biosynthesis pathway in their chloroplasts, a structure fungi and animals do not have. Fungi produce several secondary metabolites that are similar or identical in structure to those made by plants. Many of the plant and fungal enzymes that make these compounds differ from each other in sequence and other characteristics, which indicates separate origins and convergent evolution of these enzymes in the fungi and plants.

DIVERSITY

Fungi have a worldwide distribution, and grow in a wide range of habitats, including extreme environments such as deserts or areas with high salt concentrations or ionizing radiation, as well as in deep sea sediments. Some can survive the intense UV and cosmic radiation encountered during space travel. Most grow in terrestrial environments, though several species live partly or solely in aquatic habitats, such as the chytrid fungus *Batrachochytrium dendrobatidis*, a parasite that has been responsible for a worldwide decline in amphibian populations. This organism spends part of its life cycle as a motile zoospore, enabling it to propel itself through water and enter its amphibian host. Other examples of aquatic fungi include those living in hydrothermal areas of the ocean.

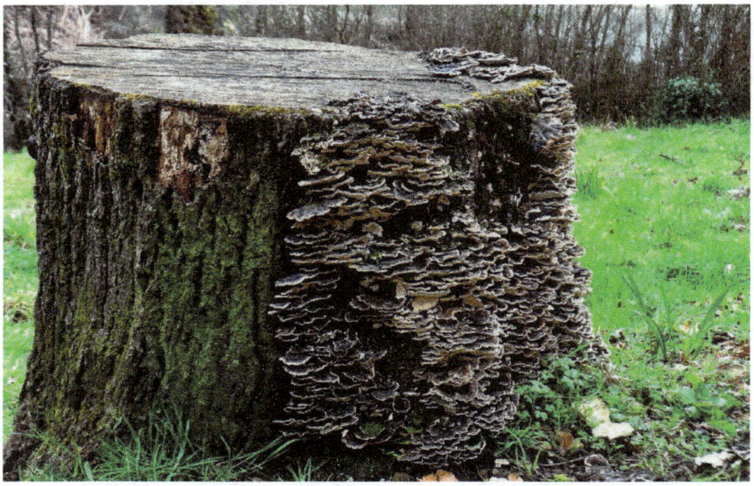

Bracket fungi on a tree stump.

Around 100,000 species of fungi have been formally described by taxonomists, but the global biodiversity of the fungus kingdom is not fully understood. On the basis of observations of the ratio of the number of fungal species to the number of plant species in selected environments, the fungal kingdom has been estimated to contain about 1.5 million species. A recent (2011) estimate suggests there may be over 5 million species. In mycology, species have historically been distinguished by a variety of methods and concepts. Classification based on morphological characteristics, such as the size and shape of spores or fruiting structures, has traditionally dominated fungal taxonomy. Species may also be distinguished by their biochemical and physiological characteristics, such as their ability to metabolize certain biochemicals, or their reaction to chemical tests. The biological species concept discriminates species based on their ability to mate. The application of molecular tools, such as DNA sequencing and phylogenetic analysis, to study diversity has greatly enhanced the resolution and added robustness to estimates of genetic diversity within various taxonomic groups.

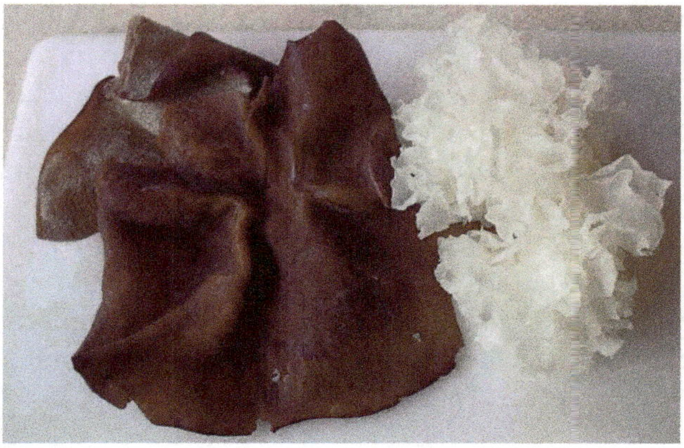

Two types of edible fungi.

HISTORY

Mycology is a relatively new science that became systematic after the development of the microscope in the 17th century. Although fungal spores were first observed by Giambattista della Porta in 1588, the seminal work in the development of mycology is considered to be the publication of Pier Antonio Micheli's 1729 work *Nova plantarum genera*. Micheli not only observed spores but also showed that, under the proper conditions, they could be induced into growing into the same species of fungi from which they originated. Extending the use of the binomial system of nomenclature introduced by Carl Linnaeus in his *Species plantarum* (1753), the Dutch Christian Hendrik Persoon (1761–1836) established the first classification of mushrooms with such skill so as to be considered a founder of modern mycology. Later, Elias Magnus Fries (1794–1878) further elaborated the classification of fungi, using spore color and various microscopic characteristics, methods still used by taxonomists today. Other notable early contributors to mycology in the 17th–19th and early 20th centuries include Miles Joseph Berkeley, August Carl Joseph Corda, Anton de Bary, the brothers Louis René and Charles Tulasne, Arthur H. R. Buller, Curtis G. Lloyd, and Pier Andrea Saccardo. The 20th century has seen a modernization of mycology that has come from advances in biochemistry, genetics, molecular biology, and biotechnology. The use of DNA sequencing technologies and phylogenetic analysis has provided new insights into fungal relationships and biodiversity, and has challenged traditional morphology-based groupings in fungal taxonomy.

MORPHOLOGY

Microscopic Structures

Most fungi grow as hyphae, which are cylindrical, thread-like structures 2–10 µm in diameter and up to several centimeters in length. Hyphae grow at their tips (apices); new hyphae are typically formed by emergence of new tips along existing hyphae by a process called *branching*, or occasionally growing hyphal tips fork, giving rise to two parallel-growing hyphae. Hyphae also sometimes fuse when they come into contact, a process called hyphal fusion (or anastamosis). These growth processes lead to the development of a mycelium, an interconnected network of hyphae. Hyphae can be either septate or coenocytic. Septate hyphae are divided into compartments separated by cross walls (internal cell walls, called septa, that are formed at right angles to the cell wall giving the hypha its shape), with each compartment containing one or more nuclei; coenocytic hyphae are not compartmentalized. Septa have pores that allow cytoplasm, organelles, and sometimes nuclei to pass through; an example is the dolipore septum in fungi of the phylum Basidiomycota. Coenocytic hyphae are in essence multinucleate supercells.

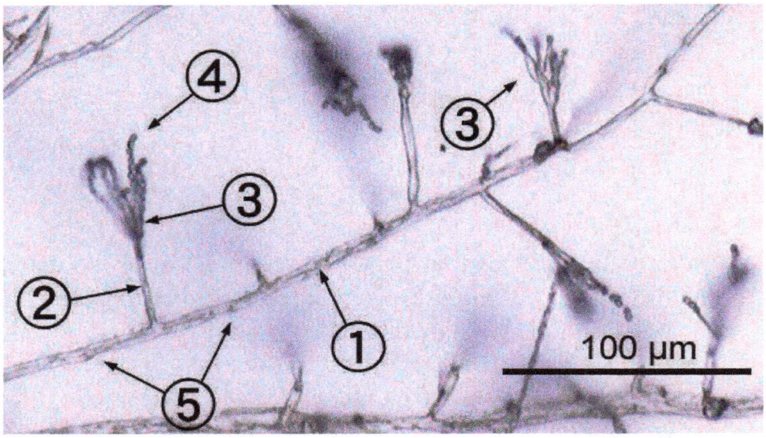

An environmental isolate of *Penicillium*

1. hypha
2. conidiophore
3. phialide
4. conidia
5. septa

Many species have developed specialized hyphal structures for nutrient uptake from living hosts; examples include haustoria in plant-parasitic species of most fungal phyla, and arbuscules of several mycorrhizal fungi, which penetrate into the host cells to consume nutrients.

Although fungi are opisthokonts—a grouping of evolutionarily related organisms broadly characterized by a single posterior flagellum—all phyla except for the chytrids have lost their posterior flagella. Fungi are unusual among the eukaryotes in having a cell wall that, in addition to glucans (e.g., β-1,3-glucan) and other typical components, also contains the biopolymer chitin.

Macroscopic Structures

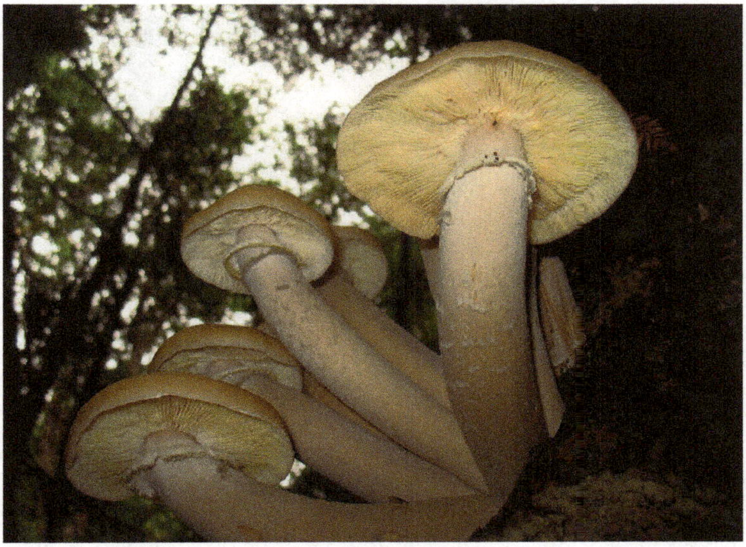

Armillaria solidipes

Fungal mycelia can become visible to the naked eye, for example, on various surfaces and substrates, such as damp walls and spoiled food, where they are commonly called molds. Mycelia grown on solid agar media in laboratory petri dishes are usually referred to as colonies. These colonies can exhibit growth shapes and colors (due to spores or pigmentation) that can be used as diagnostic features in the identification of species or groups. Some individual fungal colonies can reach extraordinary dimensions and ages as in the case of a clonal colony of *Armillaria solidipes*, which extends over an area of more than 900 ha (3.5 square miles), with an estimated age of nearly 9,000 years.

The apothecium—a specialized structure important in sexual reproduction in the ascomycetes—is a cup-shaped fruit body that is often macroscopic and holds the hymenium, a layer of tissue containing the spore-bearing cells. The fruit bodies of the basidiomycetes (basidiocarps) and some ascomycetes can sometimes grow very large, and many are well known as mushrooms.

GROWTH AND PHYSIOLOGY

The growth of fungi as hyphae on or in solid substrates or as single cells in aquatic environments is adapted for the efficient extraction of nutrients, because these growth forms have high surface area to volume ratios. Hyphae are specifically adapted for growth on solid surfaces, and to invade substrates and tissues. They can exert large penetrative mechanical forces; for example, many plant pathogens, including *Magnaporthe grisea*, form a structure called an appressorium that evolved to puncture plant tissues. The pressure generated by the appressorium, directed against the plant epidermis, can exceed

8 megapascals (1,200 psi). The filamentous fungus *Paecilomyces lilacinus* uses a similar structure to penetrate the eggs of nematodes.

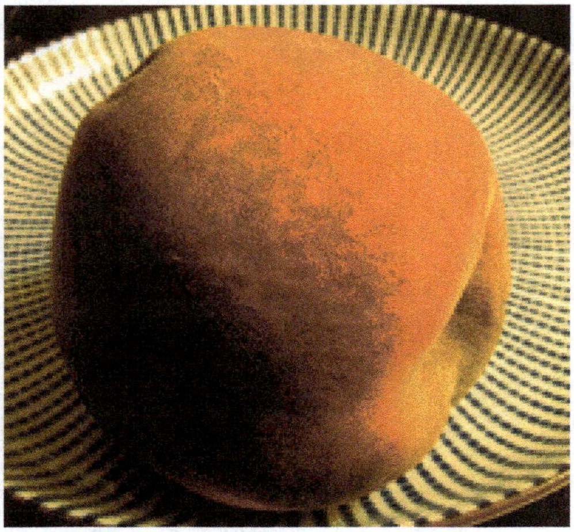

Mold growth covering a decaying peach. The frames were taken approximately 12 hours apart over a period of six days.

The mechanical pressure exerted by the appressorium is generated from physiological processes that increase intracellular turgor by producing osmolytes such as glycerol. Adaptations such as these are complemented by hydrolytic enzymes secreted into the environment to digest large organic molecules—such as polysaccharides, proteins, and lipids—into smaller molecules that may then be absorbed as nutrients. The vast majority of filamentous fungi grow in a polar fashion (extending in one direction) by elongation at the tip (apex) of the hypha. Other forms of fungal growth include intercalary extension (longitudinal expansion of hyphal compartments that are below the apex) as in the case of some endophytic fungi,or growth by volume expansion during the development of mushroom stipes and other large organs. Growth of fungi as multicellular structures consisting of somatic and reproductive cells—a feature independently evolved in animals and plants—has several functions, including the development of fruit bodies for dissemination of sexual spores (see above) and biofilms for substrate colonization and intercellular communication.

The fungi are traditionally considered heterotrophs, organisms that rely solely on carbon fixed by other organisms for metabolism. Fungi have evolved a high degree of metabolic versatility that allows them to use a diverse range of organic substrates for growth, including simple compounds such as nitrate, ammonia, acetate, or ethanol. In some species the pigment melanin may play a role in extracting energy from ionizing radiation, such as gamma radiation. This form of "radiotrophic" growth has been described for only a few species, the effects on growth rates are small, and the underlying biophysical and biochemical processes are not well known. This process might bear similarity to CO_2 fixation via visible light, but instead uses ionizing radiation as a source of energy.

REPRODUCTION

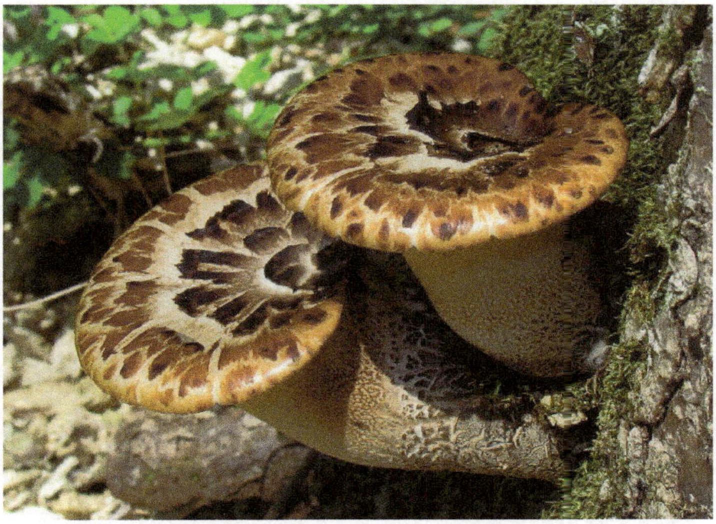

Polyporus squamosus

Fungal reproduction is complex, reflecting the differences in lifestyles and genetic makeup within this diverse kingdom of organisms. It is estimated that a third of all fungi reproduce using more than one method of propagation; for example, reproduction may occur in two well-differentiated stages within the life cycle of a species, the teleomorph and the anamorph. Environmental conditions trigger genetically determined developmental states that lead to the creation of specialized structures for sexual or asexual reproduction. These structures aid reproduction by efficiently dispersing spores or spore-containing propagules.

Asexual Reproduction

Asexual reproduction occurs via vegetative spores (conidia) or through mycelial fragmentation. Mycelial fragmentation occurs when a fungal mycelium separates into pieces, and each component grows into a separate mycelium. Mycelial fragmentation and vegetative spores maintain clonal populations adapted to a specific niche, and allow more rapid dispersal than sexual reproduction. The "Fungi imperfecti" (fungi lacking the perfect or sexual stage) or Deuteromycota comprise all the species that lack an observable sexual cycle. Deuteromycota is not an accepted taxonomic clade, and is now taken to mean simply fungi that lack a known sexual stage.

Sexual Reproduction

Sexual reproduction with meiosis has been directly observed in all fungal phyla except Glomeromycota (genetic analysis suggests meiosis in Glomeromycota as well). It differs in many aspects from sexual reproduction in animals or plants. Differences also exist between fungal groups and can be used to discriminate species by morphological differences in sexual structures and reproductive strategies. Mating experiments between fungal isolates may identify species on the basis of biological species concepts. The major fungal groupings have initially been delineated based on the morphology of their sexual structures and spores; for example, the spore-containing structures, asci and basidia, can be used in the identification of ascomycetes and basidiomycetes, respectively. Some species may allow mating only between individuals of opposite mating type, whereas others can mate and sexually reproduce with any other individual or itself. Species of the former mating system are called heterothallic, and of the latter homothallic.

Most fungi have both a haploid and a diploid stage in their life cycles. In sexually reproducing fungi, compatible individuals may combine by fusing their hyphae together into an interconnected network; this process, anastomosis, is required for the initiation of the sexual cycle. Many ascomycetes and basidiomycetes go through a dikaryotic stage, in which the nuclei inherited from the two parents do not combine immediately after cell fusion, but remain separate in the hyphal cells.

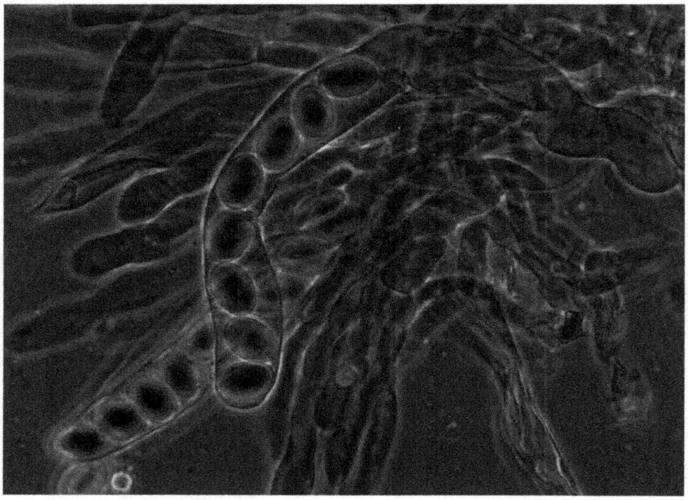

The 8-spore asci of *Morchella elata*, viewed with phase contrast microscopy.

In ascomycetes, dikaryotic hyphae of the hymenium (the spore-bearing tissue layer) form a characteristic *hook* at the hyphal septum. During cell division, formation of the hook ensures proper distribution of the newly divided nuclei into the apical and basal hyphal compartments. An ascus (plural *asci*) is then formed, in which karyogamy (nuclear fusion) occurs. Asci are embedded in an ascocarp, or fruiting body. Karyogamy in the asci is followed immediately by meiosis and the production of ascospores. After dispersal, the ascospores may germinate and form a new haploid mycelium.

Sexual reproduction in basidiomycetes is similar to that of the ascomycetes. Compatible haploid hyphae fuse to produce a dikaryotic mycelium. However, the dikaryotic phase is more extensive in the basidiomycetes, often also present in the vegetatively growing mycelium. A specialized anatomical structure, called a clamp connection, is formed at each hyphal septum. As with the structurally similar hook in the ascomycetes, the clamp connection in the basidiomycetes is required for controlled transfer of nuclei during cell division, to maintain the dikaryotic stage with two genetically different nuclei in each hyphal compartment. A basidiocarp is formed in which club-like structures known as basidia generate haploid basidiospores after karyogamy and meiosis. The most commonly known basidiocarps are mushrooms, but they may also take other forms.

In glomeromycetes (formerly zygomycetes), haploid hyphae of two individuals fuse, forming a gametangium, a specialized cell structure that becomes a fertile gamete-producing cell. The gametangium develops into a zygospore, a thick-walled spore formed by the union of gametes. When the zygospore germinates, it undergoes meiosis, generating new haploid hyphae, which may then form asexual sporangiospores. These sporangiospores allow the fungus to rapidly disperse and germinate into new genetically identical haploid fungal mycelia.

Spore Dispersal

Both asexual and sexual spores or sporangiospores are often actively dispersed by forcible ejection from their reproductive structures. This ejection ensures exit of the spores from the reproductive structures as well as traveling through the air over long distances.

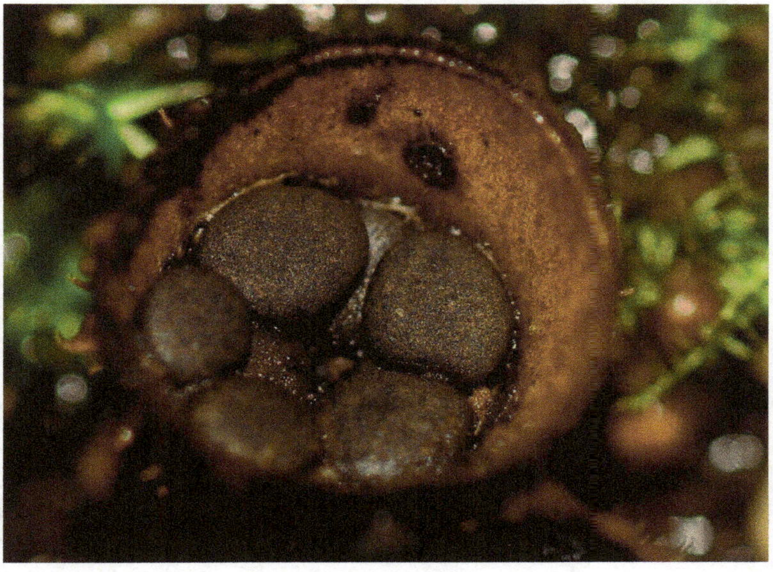

The bird's nest fungus *Cyathus stercoreus.*

Specialized mechanical and physiological mechanisms, as well as spore surface structures (such as hydrophobins), enable efficient spore ejection. For example, the structure of the spore-bearing cells in some ascomycete species is such that the buildup of substances affecting cell volume and fluid balance enables the explosive discharge of spores into the air. The forcible discharge of single spores termed *ballistospores* involves formation of a small drop of water (Buller's drop), which upon contact with the spore leads to its projectile release with an initial acceleration of more than 10,000 g; the net result is that the spore is ejected 0.01–0.02 cm, sufficient distance for it to fall through the gills or pores into the air below. Other fungi, like the puffballs, rely on alternative mechanisms for spore release, such as external mechanical forces. The bird's nest fungi use the force of falling water drops to liberate the spores from cup-shaped fruiting bodies. Another strategy is seen in the stinkhorns, a group of fungi with lively colors and putrid odor that attract insects to disperse their spores.

Other Sexual Processes

Besides regular sexual reproduction with meiosis, certain fungi, such as those in the genera *Penicillium* and *Aspergillus*, may exchange genetic material via parasexual processes, initiated by anastomosis between hyphae and plasmogamy of fungal cells. The frequency and relative importance of parasexual events is unclear and may be lower than other sexual processes. It is known to play a role in intraspecific hybridization and is likely required for hybridization between species, which has been associated with major events in fungal evolution.

EVOLUTION

In contrast to plants and animals, the early fossil record of the fungi is meager. Factors that likely contribute to the under-representation of fungal species among fossils include the nature of fungal fruiting bodies, which are soft, fleshy, and easily degradable tissues and the microscopic dimensions of most fungal structures, which therefore are not readily evident. Fungal fossils are difficult to distinguish from those of other microbes, and are most easily identified when they resemble extant fungi. Often recovered from a permineralized plant or animal host, these samples are typically studied by making thin-section preparations that can be examined with light microscopy or transmission electron microscopy. Researchers study compression fossils by dissolving the surrounding matrix with acid and then using light or scanning electron microscopy to examine surface details.

The earliest fossils possessing features typical of fungi date to the Proterozoic eon, some 1,430 million years ago (Ma); these multicellular benthic organisms had filamentous structures with septa, and were capable of anastomosis. More recent studies (2009) estimate the arrival of fungal organisms at about 760–1060 Ma on the basis of comparisons of the rate of evolution in closely related groups. For much of the Paleozoic Era (542–251 Ma), the fungi appear to have been aquatic and consisted of organisms similar to the extant chytrids in having flagellum-bearing spores. The evolutionary adaptation from an aquatic to a terrestrial lifestyle necessitated a diversification of ecological strategies for obtaining nutrients, including parasitism, saprobism, and the development of mutualistic relationships such as mycorrhiza and lichenization. Recent (2009) studies suggest that the ancestral ecological state of the Ascomycota was saprobism, and that independent lichenization events have occurred multiple times.

It is presumed that the fungi colonized the land during the Cambrian (542–488.3 Ma), long before land plants. Fossilized hyphae and spores recovered from the Ordovician of Wisconsin (460 Ma) resemble modern-day Glomerales, and existed at a time when the land flora likely consisted of only non-vascular bryophyte-like plants. Prototaxites, which was probably a fungus or lichen, would have been the tallest organism of the late Silurian. Fungal fossils do not become common and uncontroversial until the early Devonian (416–359.2 Ma), when they occur abundantly in the Rhynie chert, mostly as Zygomycota and Chytridiomycota.At about this same time, approximately 400 Ma, the Ascomycota and Basidiomycota diverged, and all modern classes of fungi were present by the Late Carboniferous (Pennsylvanian, 318.1–299 Ma).

Lichen-like fossils have been found in the Doushantuo Formation in southern China dating back to 635–551 Ma. Lichens formed a component of the early terrestrial ecosystems, and the estimated age of the oldest terrestrial lichen fossil is 400 Ma; this date corresponds to the age of the oldest known sporocarp fossil, a *Paleopyrenomycites* species found in the Rhynie Chert. The oldest fossil with microscopic features resembling modern-day basidiomycetes is *Palaeoancistrus*, found permineralized with a fern from the Pennsylvanian. Rare in the fossil record are the Homobasidiomycetes (a taxon roughly equivalent to the mushroom-producing species of the Agaricomycetes). Two amber-preserved specimens provide evidence that the earliest known mushroom-forming fungi (the extinct species *Archaeomarasmius leggetti*) appeared during the late Cretaceous, 90 Ma.

Some time after the Permian–Triassic extinction event (251.4 Ma), a fungal spike (originally thought to be an extraordinary abundance of fungal spores in sediments) formed, suggesting that fungi were the dominant life form at this time, representing nearly 100% of the available fossil record for this period.However, the relative proportion of fungal spores relative to spores formed by algal species is difficult to assess, the spike did not appear worldwide, and in many places it did not fall on the Permian–Triassic boundary.

TAXONOMY

Although commonly included in botany curricula and textbooks, fungi are more closely related to animals than to plants and are placed with the animals in the monophyletic group of opisthokonts. Analyses using molecular phylogenetics support a monophyletic origin of the Fungi. The taxonomy of the Fungi is in a state of constant flux, especially due to recent research based on DNA comparisons. These current phylogenetic analyses often overturn classifications based on older and sometimes less discriminative methods based on morphological features and biological species concepts obtained from experimental matings.

There is no unique generally accepted system at the higher taxonomic levels and there are frequent name changes at every level, from species upwards. Efforts among researchers are now underway to establish and encourage usage of a unified and more consistent nomenclature. Fungal species can also have multiple scientific names depending on their life cycle and mode (sexual or asexual) of reproduction. Web sites such as Index Fungorum and ITIS list current names of fungal species (with cross-references to older synonyms).

The 2007 classification of Kingdom Fungi is the result of a large-scale collaborative research effort involving dozens of mycologists and other scientists working on fungal taxonomy. It recognizes seven phyla, two of which—the Ascomycota and the Basidiomycota—are contained within a branch representing subkingdom Dikarya, the most species rich and familiar group, including all the mushrooms, most food-spoilage molds, most plant pathogenic fungi, and the beer, wine, and bread yeasts. The accompanying cladogram depicts the major fungal taxa and their relationship to opisthokont and unikont organisms, based on the work of Philippe Silar and "The Mycota: A Comprehensive Treatise on Fungi as Experimental Systems for Basic and Applied Research". The lengths of the branches are not proportional to evolutionary distances.

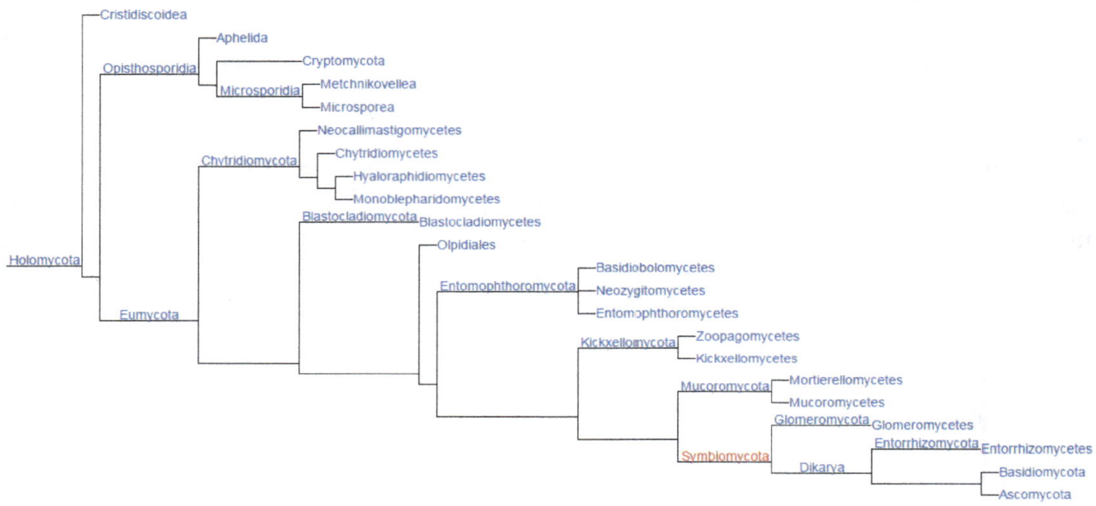

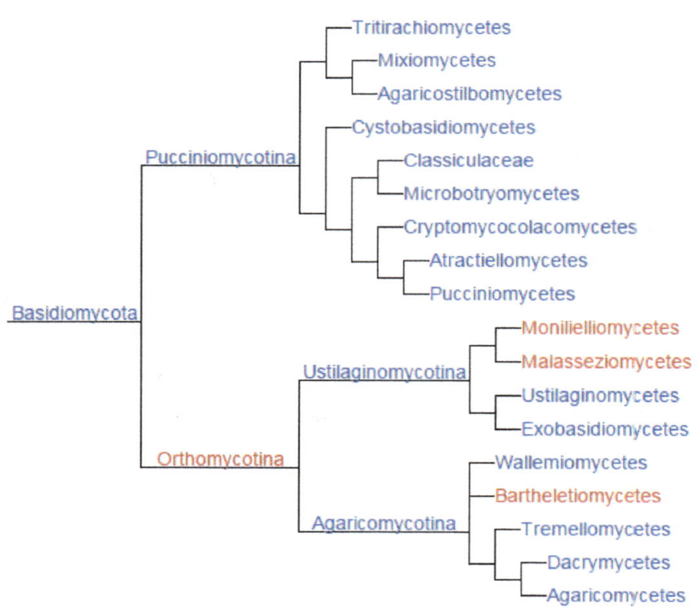

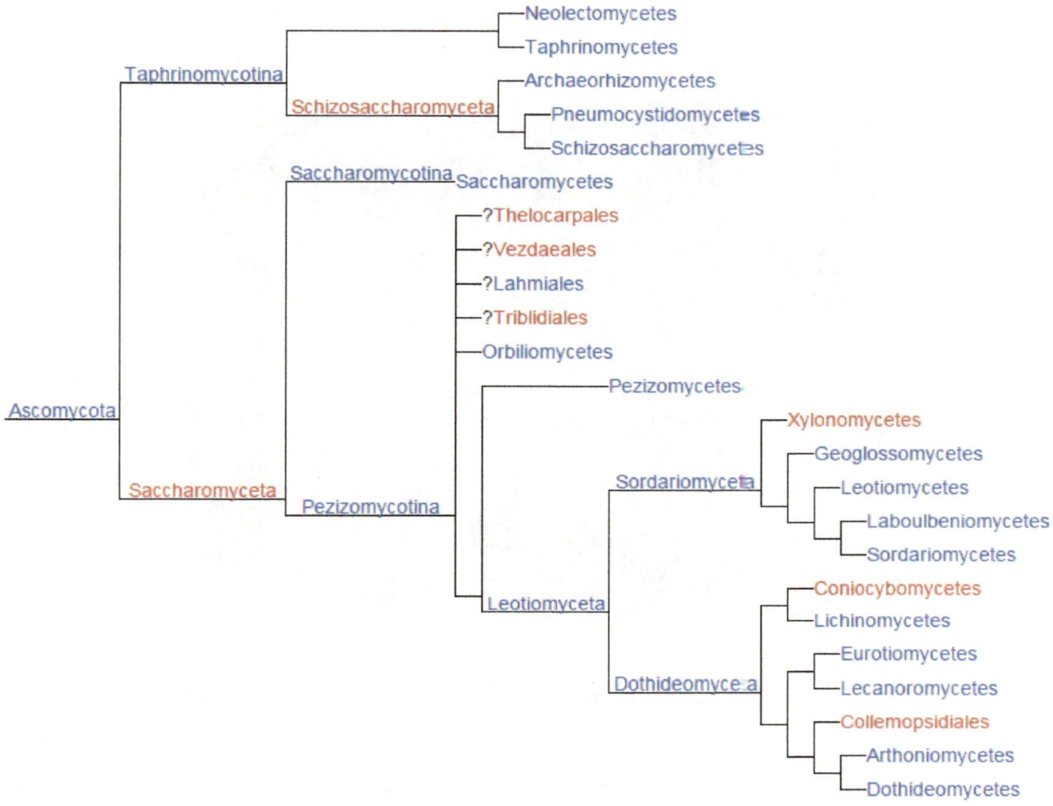

Taxonomic Groups

The major phyla (sometimes called divisions) of fungi have been classified mainly on the basis of characteristics of their sexual reproductive structures. Currently, seven phyla are proposed: Microsporidia, Chytridiomycota, Blastocladiomycota, Neocallimastigomycota, Glomeromycota, Ascomycota, and Basidiomycota.

Phylogenetic analysis has demonstrated that the Microsporidia, unicellular parasites of animals and protists, are fairly recent and highly derived endobiotic fungi (living within the tissue of another species). One 2006 study concludes that the Microsporidia are a sister group to the true fungi; that is, they are each other's closest evolutionary relative. Hibbett and colleagues suggest that this analysis does not clash with their classification of the Fungi, and although the Microsporidia are elevated to phylum status, it is acknowledged that further analysis is required to clarify evolutionary relationships within this group.

The Chytridiomycota are commonly known as chytrids. These fungi are distributed worldwide. Chytrids and their close relatives Neocallimastigomycota and Blastocladiomycota (below) are the only fungi with active motility, producing zoospores that are capable of active movement through aqueous phases with a single flagellum, leading early taxonomists to classify them as protists. Molecular phylogenies, inferred from rRNA sequences in ribosomes, suggest that the Chytrids are a basal group divergent from the other fungal phyla, consisting of four major clades with suggestive evidence for paraphyly or possibly polyphyly.

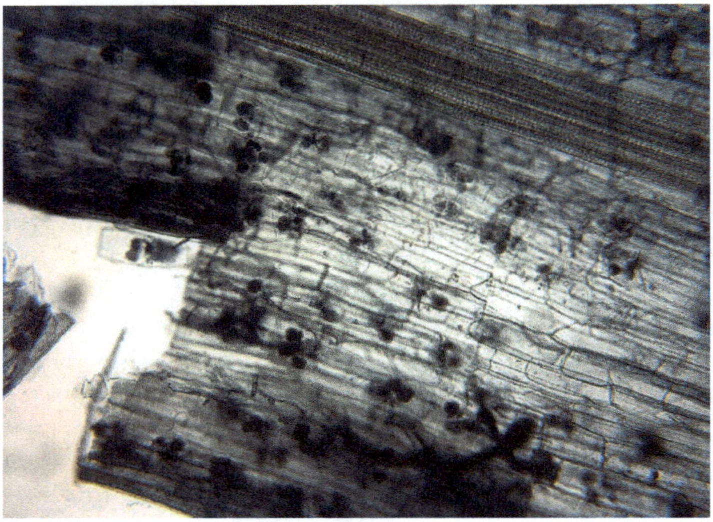

Arbuscular mycorrhiza seen under microscope. Flax root cortical cells containing paired arbuscules.

The Blastocladiomycota were previously considered a taxonomic clade within the Chytridiomycota. Recent molecular data and ultrastructural characteristics, however, place the Blastocladiomycota as a sister clade to the Zygomycota, Glomeromycota, and Dikarya (Ascomycota and Basidiomycota). The blastocladiomycetes are saprotrophs, feeding on decomposing organic matter, and they are parasites of all eukaryotic groups. Unlike their close relatives, the chytrids, most of which exhibit zygotic meiosis, the blastocladiomycetes undergo sporic meiosis.

The Neocallimastigomycota were earlier placed in the phylum Chytridomycota. Members of this small phylum are anaerobic organisms, living in the digestive system of larger herbivorous mammals and in other terrestrial and aquatic environments enriched in cellulose (e.g., domestic waste landfill sites). They lack mitochondria but contain hydrogenosomes of mitochondrial origin. As in the related chrytrids, neocallimastigomycetes form zoospores that are posteriorly uniflagellate or polyflagellate.

Members of the Glomeromycota form arbuscular mycorrhizae, a form of mutualist symbiosis wherein fungal hyphae invade plant root cells and both species benefit from the resulting increased supply of nutrients. All known Glomeromycota species reproduce asexually. The symbiotic association between the Glomeromycota and plants is ancient, with evidence dating to 400 million years ago. Formerly part of the Zygomycota (commonly known as 'sugar' and 'pin' molds), the Glomeromycota were elevated to phylum status in 2001 and now replace the older phylum Zygomycota. Fungi that were placed in the Zygomycota are now being reassigned to the Glomeromycota, or the subphyla incertae sedis Mucoromycotina, Kickxellomycotina, the Zoopagomycotina and the Entomophthoromycotina. Some well-known examples of fungi formerly in the

Zygomycota include black bread mold (*Rhizopus stolonifer*), and *Pilobolus* species, capable of ejecting spores several meters through the air. Medically relevant genera include *Mucor*, *Rhizomucor*, and *Rhizopus*.

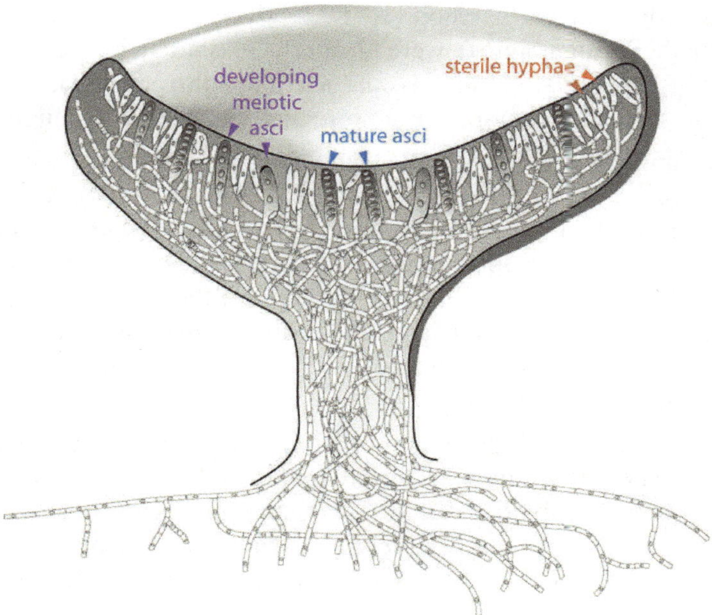

Diagram of an apothecium (the typical cup-like reproductive structure of Ascomycetes) showing sterile tissues as well as developing and mature asci.

The Ascomycota, commonly known as sac fungi or ascomycetes, constitute the largest taxonomic group within the Eumycota. These fungi form meiotic spores called ascospores, which are enclosed in a special sac-like structure called an ascus. This phylum includes morels, a few mushrooms and truffles, unicellular yeasts (e.g., of the genera *Saccharomyces*, *Kluyveromyces*, *Pichia*, and *Candida*), and many filamentous fungi living as saprotrophs, parasites, and mutualistic symbionts (e.g. lichens). Prominent and important genera of filamentous ascomycetes include *Aspergillus*, *Penicillium*, *Fusarium*, and *Claviceps*. Many ascomycete species have only been observed undergoing asexual reproduction (called anamorphic species), but analysis of molecular data has often been able to identify their closest teleomorphs in the Ascomycota. Because the products of meiosis are retained within the sac-like ascus, ascomycetes have been used for elucidating principles of genetics and heredity (e.g., *Neurospora crassa*).

Members of the Basidiomycota, commonly known as the club fungi or basidiomycetes, produce meiospores called basidiospores on club-like stalks called basidia. Most common mushrooms belong to this group, as well as rust and smut fungi, which are major pathogens of grains. Other important basidiomycetes include the maize pathogen *Ustilago maydis*, human commensal species of the genus *Malassezia*, and the opportunistic human pathogen, *Cryptococcus neoformans*.

Fungus-like Organisms

Because of similarities in morphology and lifestyle, the slime molds (mycetozoans, plasmodiophorids, acrasids, *Fonticula* and labyrinthulids, now in Amoebozoa, Rhizaria, Excavata, Opisthokonta and Stramenopiles, respectively), water molds (oomycetes) and hyphochytrids (both Stramenopiles) were formerly classified in the kingdom Fungi, in groups like Mastigomycotina, Gymnomycota and Phycomycetes. The slime molds were studied also as protozoans, leading to a ambiregnal, duplicated taxonomy.

Unlike true fungi, the cell walls of oomycetes contain cellulose and lack chitin. Hyphochytrids have both chitin and cellulose. Slime molds lack a cell wall during the assimilative phase (except labyrinthulids, which have a wall of scales), and ingest nutrients by ingestion (phagocytosis, except labyrinthulids) rather than absorption (osmotrophy, as fungi, labyrinthulids, oomycetes and hyphochytrids). Neither water molds nor slime molds are closely related to the true fungi, and, therefore, taxonomists no longer group them in the kingdom Fungi. Nonetheless, studies of the oomycetes and myxomycetes are still often included in mycology textbooks and primary research literature.

The Eccrinales and Amoebidiales are opisthokont protists, previously thought to be zygomycete fungi. Other groups now in Opisthokonta (e.g., *Corallochytrium*, Ichthyosporea) were also at given time classified as fungi. The genus *Blastocystis*, now in Stramenopiles, was originally classified as a yeast. *Ellobiopsis*, now in Alveolata, was considered a chytrid. The bacteria were also included in fungi in some classifications, as the group Schizomycetes.

The Rozellida clade, including the "ex-chytrid" *Rozella*, is a genetically disparate group known mostly from environmental DNA sequences that is a sister group to fungi. Members of the group that have been isolated lack the chitinous cell wall that is characteristic of fungi.

The nucleariids, protists currently grouped in the Choanozoa (Opisthokonta), may be the next sister group to the eumycete clade, and as such could be included in an expanded fungal kingdom.

Many Actinomycetales (Actinobacteria), a group with many filamentous bacteria, were also long believed to be fungi.

ECOLOGY

Although often inconspicuous, fungi occur in every environment on Earth and play very important roles in most ecosystems. Along with bacteria, fungi are the major decomposers in most terrestrial (and some aquatic) ecosystems, and therefore play a critical role in biogeochemical cycles and in many food webs. As decomposers, they play an essential role in nutrient cycling, especially as saprotrophs and symbionts, degrading organic matter to inorganic molecules, which can then re-enter anabolic metabolic pathways in plants or other organisms.

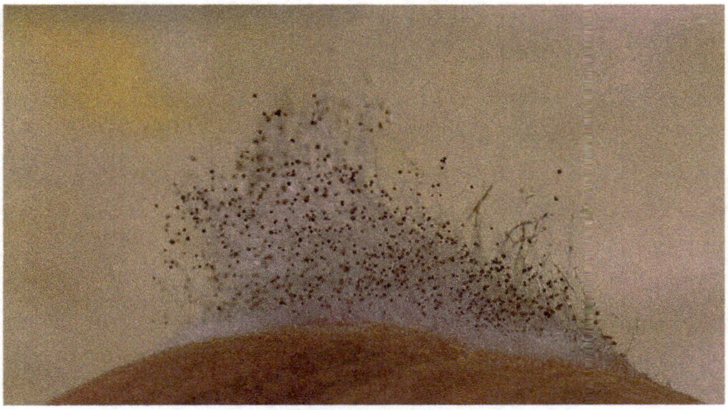

A pin mold decomposing a peach.

Symbiosis

Many fungi have important symbiotic relationships with organisms from most if not all Kingdoms. These interactions can be mutualistic or antagonistic in nature, or in the case of commensal fungi are of no apparent benefit or detriment to the host.

With Plants

Mycorrhizal symbiosis between plants and fungi is one of the most well-known plant–fungus associations and is of significant importance for plant growth and persistence in many ecosystems; over 90% of all plant species engage in mycorrhizal relationships with fungi and are dependent upon this relationship for survival.

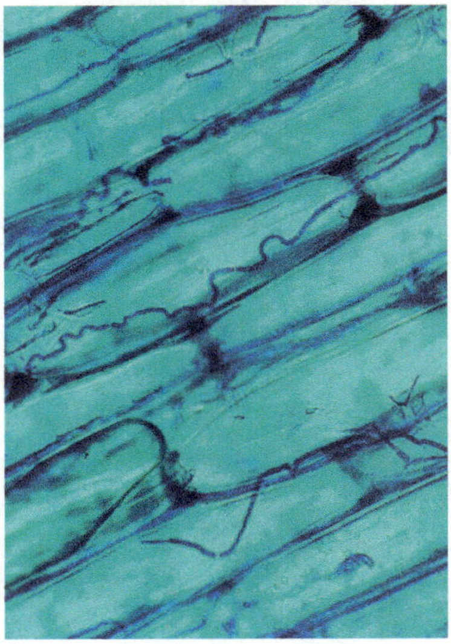

The dark filaments are hyphae of the endophytic fungus *Neotyphodium coenophialum* in the intercellular spaces of tall fescue leaf sheath tissue.

The mycorrhizal symbiosis is ancient, dating to at least 400 million years ago. It often increases the plant's uptake of inorganic compounds, such as nitrate and phosphate from soils having low concentrations of these key plant nutrients. The fungal partners may also mediate plant-to-plant transfer of carbohydrates and other nutrients. Such mycorrhizal communities are called "common mycorrhizal networks". A special case of mycorrhiza is myco-heterotrophy, whereby the plant parasitizes the fungus, obtaining all of its nutrients from its fungal symbiont. Some fungal species inhabit the tissues inside roots, stems, and leaves, in which case they are called endophytes. Similar to mycorrhiza, endophytic colonization by fungi may benefit both symbionts; for example, endophytes of grasses impart to their host increased resistance to herbivores and other environmental stresses and receive food and shelter from the plant in return.

With Algae and Cyanobacteria

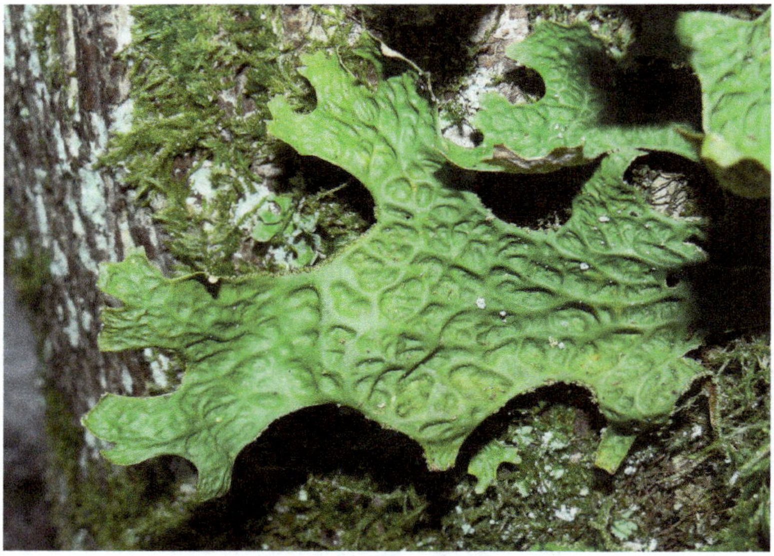

The lichen *Lobaria pulmonaria*, a symbiosis of fungal, algal, and cyanobacterial species.

Lichens are a symbiotic relationship between fungi and photosynthetic algae or cyanobacteria. The photosynthetic partner in the relationship is referred to in lichen terminology as a "photobiont". The fungal part of the relationship is composed mostly of various species of ascomycetes and a few basidiomycetes. Lichens occur in every ecosystem on all continents, play a key role in soil formation and the initiation of biological succession, and are prominent in some extreme environments, including polar, alpine, and semiarid desert regions. They are able to grow on inhospitable surfaces, including bare soil, rocks, tree bark, wood, shells, barnacles and leaves. As in mycorrhizas, the photobiont provides sugars and other carbohydrates via photosynthesis to the fungus, while the fungus provides minerals and water to the photobiont. The functions of both symbiotic organisms are so closely intertwined that they function almost as a single organism; in most cases the resulting organism differs greatly from the individual components. Lichenization is a common mode of nutrition for fungi; around 20% of fungi—between 17,500 and 20,000 described species—are lichenized. Characteristics common to most lichens include obtaining organic carbon by photosynthesis, slow growth, small size, long life, long-lasting (seasonal) vegetative reproductive structures, mineral nutrition obtained largely from airborne sources, and greater tolerance of desiccation than most other photosynthetic organisms in the same habitat.

With Insects

Many insects also engage in mutualistic relationships with fungi. Several groups of ants cultivate fungi in the order Agaricales as their primary food source, while ambrosia beetles cultivate various species of fungi in the bark of trees that they infest. Likewise, females of several wood wasp species (genus *Sirex*) inject their eggs together with spores of the wood-rotting fungus *Amylostereum areolatum* into the sapwood of pine trees; the growth of the fungus provides ideal nutritional conditions for the development of the wasp larvae. At least one species of stingless bee has a relationship with a fungus in the genus *Monascus*, where the larvae consume and depend on fungus transferred from old to new nests. Termites on the African savannah are also known to cultivate fungi, and yeasts of the genera *Candida* and *Lachancea* inhabit the gut of a wide range of insects, including neuropterans, beetles, and cockroaches; it is not known whether these fungi benefit their hosts. Fungi ingrowing dead wood are essential for xylophagous insects (e.g. woodboring beetles). They deliver nutrients needed by xylophages to nutritionally scarce dead wood. Thanks to this nutritional enrichment the larvae of woodboring insect is able to grow and develop to adulthood. The larvae of many families of fungicolous flies, particularly those within the superfamily Sciaroidea such as the Mycetophilidae and some Keroplatidae feed on fungal fruiting bodies and sterile mycorrhizae.

As Pathogens and Parasites

Many fungi are parasites on plants, animals (including humans), and other fungi. Serious pathogens of many cultivated plants causing extensive damage and losses to agriculture and forestry include the rice blast fungus *Magnaporthe oryzae*, tree pathogens such as *Ophiostoma ulmi* and *Ophiostoma novo-ulmi* causing Dutch elm disease and *Cryphonectria parasitica* responsible for chestnut blight, and plant pathogens in the genera *Fusarium*, *Ustilago*, *Alternaria*, and *Cochliobolus*. Some carnivorous fungi, like *Paecilomyces lilacinus*, are predators of nematodes, which they capture using an array of specialized structures such as constricting rings or adhesive nets.

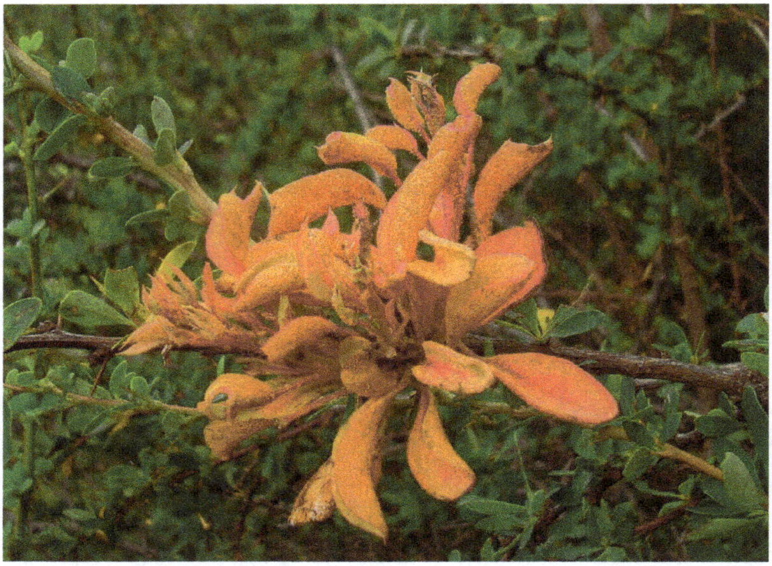

The plant pathogen *Aecidium magellanicum* causes calafate rust, seen here on a *Berberis* shrub in Chile.

Some fungi can cause serious diseases in humans, several of which may be fatal if untreated. These include aspergillosis, candidiasis, coccidioidomycosis, cryptococcosis, histoplasmosis, mycetomas, and paracoccidioidomycosis. Furthermore, persons with immuno-deficiencies are particularly susceptible to disease by genera such as *Aspergillus*, *Candida*, *Cryptoccocus*, *Histoplasma*, and *Pneumocystis*. Other fungi can attack eyes, nails, hair, and especially skin, the so-called dermatophytic and keratinophilic fungi, and cause local infections such as ringworm and athlete's foot.Fungal spores are also a cause of allergies, and fungi from different taxonomic groups can evoke allergic reactions.

As Targets of Mycoparasites

The organisms which parasitize fungi are known as mycoparasitic organisms. Certain species of the *Pythium* genus, which are oomycetes, have potential as biocontrol agents against certain fungi. Fungi can also act as mycoparasites or antagonists of other fungi, such as *Hypomyces chrysospermus*, which grows on bolete mushrooms.

Fungi can become the target of infection by mycoviruses.

MYCOTOXINS

Many fungi produce biologically active compounds, several of which are toxic to animals or plants and are therefore called mycotoxins. Of particular relevance to humans are mycotoxins produced by molds causing food spoilage, and poisonous mushrooms (see above). Particularly infamous are the lethal amatoxins in some *Amanita* mushrooms, and ergot alkaloids, which have a long history of causing serious epidemics of ergotism (St

Anthony's Fire) in people consuming rye or related cereals contaminated with sclerotia of the ergot fungus, *Claviceps purpurea*. Other notable mycotoxins include the aflatoxins, which are insidious liver toxins and highly carcinogenic metabolites produced by certain *Aspergillus* species often growing in or on grains and nuts consumed by humans, ochratoxins, patulin, and trichothecenes (e.g., T-2 mycotoxin) and fumonisins, which have significant impact on human food supplies or animal livestock.

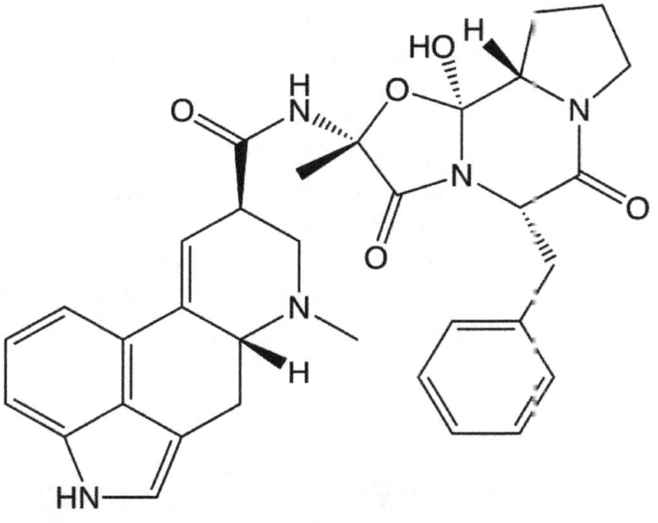

Ergotamine, a major mycotoxin produced by *Claviceps* species, which if ingested can cause gangrene, convulsions, and hallucinations.

Mycotoxins are secondary metabolites (or natural products) and research has established the existence of biochemical pathways solely for the purpose of producing mycotoxins and other natural products in fungi. Mycotoxins may provide fitness benefits in terms of physiological adaptation, competition with other microbes and fungi, and protection from consumption (fungivory). Many fungal secondary metabolites (or derivatives) are used medically, as described under Human Use below.

PATHOGENIC MECHANISMS

Ustilago maydis is a pathogenic plant fungus that causes smut disease in maize and teosinte. Plants have evolved efficient defense systems against pathogenic microbes such as *U. maydis*. A rapid defense reaction after pathogen attack is the oxidative burst where the plant produces reactive oxygen species at the site of the attempted invasion. *U. maydis* can respond to the oxidative burst with an oxidative stress response, regulated by the gene *YAP1*. The response protects *U. maydis* from the host defense, and is necessary for the pathogen's virulence. Furthermore, *U. maydis* has a well-established recombinational DNA repair system which acts during mitosis and meiosis. The system may assist the pathogen in surviving DNA damage arising from the host plant's oxidative defensive response to infection.

Cryptococcus neoformans is an encapsulated yeast that can live in both plants and animals. *C. neoformans* usually infects the lungs, where it is phagocytosed by alveolar macrophages. Some *C. neoformans* can survive inside macrophages, which appears to be the basis for latency, disseminated disease, and resistance to antifungal agents. One mechanism by which *C. neoformans* survives the hostile macrophage environment is by up-regulating the expression of genes involved in the oxidative stress response. Another mechanism involves meiosis. The majority of *C. neoformans* are mating "type a". Filaments of mating "type a" ordinarily have haploid nuclei, but they can become diploid (perhaps by endoduplication or by stimulated nuclear fusion) to form blastospores. The diploid nuclei of blastospores can undergo meiosis, including recombination, to form haploid basidiospores that can be dispersed. This process is referred to as monokaryotic fruiting. this process requires a gene called *DMC1*, which is a conserved homologue of genes *recA* in bacteria and *RAD51* in eukaryotes, that mediates homologous chromosome pairing during meiosis and repair of DNA double-strand breaks. Thus, *C. neoformans* can undergo a meiosis, monokaryotic fruiting, that promotes recombinational repair in the oxidative, DNA damaging environment of the host macrophage, and the repair capability may contribute to its virulence.

Human Use

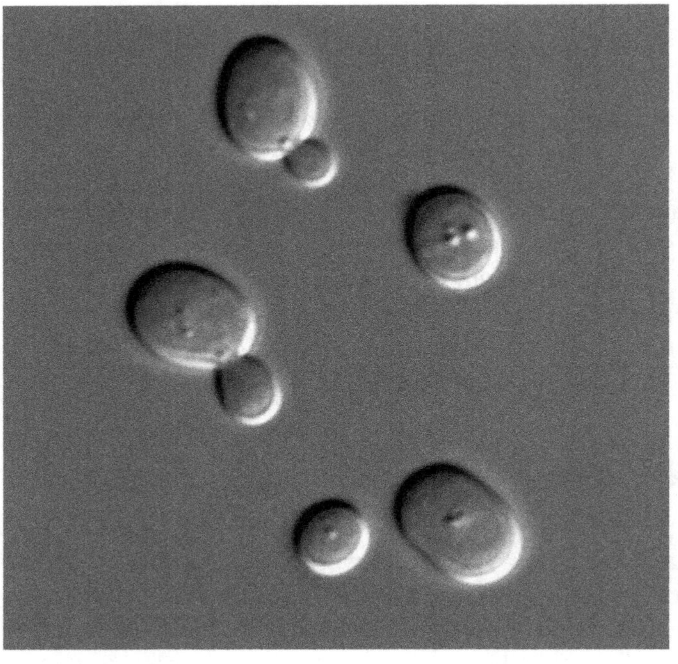

Saccharomyces cerevisiae cells shown with DIC microscopy.

The human use of fungi for food preparation or preservation and other purposes is extensive and has a long history. Mushroom farming and mushroom gathering are large industries in many countries. The study of the historical uses and sociological impact of fungi is known as ethnomycology. Because of the capacity of this group to produce an enormous range of natural products with antimicrobial or other biological activities, many species have long been used or are being developed for industrial production of antibiotics, vitamins, and anti-cancer and cholesterol-lowering drugs. More recently, methods have been developed for genetic engineering of fungi, enabling metabolic engineering of fungal species. For example, genetic modification of yeast species—which are easy to grow at fast rates in large fermentation vessels—has opened up ways of pharmaceutical production that are potentially more efficient than production by the original source organisms.

Therapeutic Uses

Modern Chemotherapeutics

Many species produce metabolites that are major sources of pharmacologically active drugs. Particularly important are the antibiotics, including the penicillins, a structurally related group of β-lactam antibiotics that are synthesized from small peptides. Although naturally occurring penicillins such as penicillin G (produced by *Penicillium chrysogenum*) have a relatively narrow spectrum of biological activity, a wide range of other penicillins can be produced by chemical modification of the natural penicillins. Modern penicillins are semisynthetic compounds, obtained initially from fermentation cultures, but then structurally altered for specific desirable properties. Other antibiotics produced by fungi include: ciclosporin, commonly used as an immunosuppressant during transplant surgery; and fusidic acid, used to help control infection from methicillin-resistant *Staphylococcus aureus* bacteria. Widespread use of antibiotics for the treatment of bacterial diseases, such as tuberculosis, syphilis, leprosy, and others began in the early 20th century and continues to date. In nature, antibiotics of fungal or bacterial origin appear to play a dual role: at high concentrations they act as chemical defense against competition with other microorganisms in species-rich environments, such as the rhizosphere, and at low concentrations as quorum-sensing molecules for intra- or interspecies signaling. Other drugs produced by fungi include griseofulvin isolated from *Penicillium griseofulvum*, used to treat fungal infections, and statins (HMG-CoA reductase inhibitors), used to inhibit cholesterol synthesis. Examples of statins found in fungi include mevastatin from *Penicillium citrinum* and lovastatin from *Aspergillus terreus* and the oyster mushroom.

Traditional and Folk Medicine

Certain mushrooms enjoy usage as therapeutics in folk medicines, such as Traditional Chinese medicine. Notable medicinal mushrooms with a well-documented history of use include *Agaricus subrufescens*, *Ganoderma lucidum*, and *Ophiocordyceps sinensis*. Research has identified compounds produced by these and other fungi that have inhibitory biological effects against viruses and cancer cells. Specific metabolites such as polysaccharide-K, ergotamine, and β-lactam antibiotics, are routinely used in clinical medicine. The shiitake mushroom is a source of lentinan, a clinical drug approved for use in cancer treatments in several countries, including Japan. In Europe and Japan, polysaccharide-K (brand name Krestin), a chemical derived from *Trametes versicolor*, is an approved adjuvant for cancer therapy.

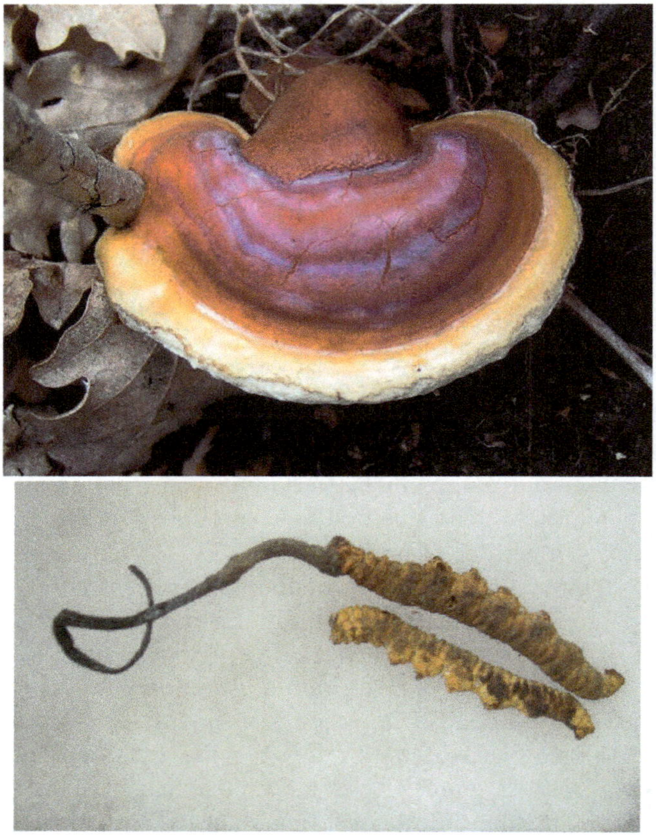

The medicinal fungi *Ganoderma lucidum* (left) and *Ophiocordyceps sinensis* (right).

Cultured Foods

Baker's yeast or *Saccharomyces cerevisiae*, a unicellular fungus, is used to make bread and other wheat-based products, such as pizza dough and dumplings.Yeast species of the genus *Saccharomyces* are also used to produce alcoholic beverages through fermentation. Shoyu koji mold (*Aspergillus oryzae*) is an essential ingredient in brewing Shoyu (soy sauce) and sake, and the preparation of miso, while *Rhizopus* species are used for making tempeh. Several of these fungi are domesticated species that were bred or selected according to their capacity to ferment food without producing harmful mycotoxins (see below), which are produced by very closely related *Aspergilli*. Quorn, a meat substitute, is made from *Fusarium venenatum*.

Edible and Poisonous Species

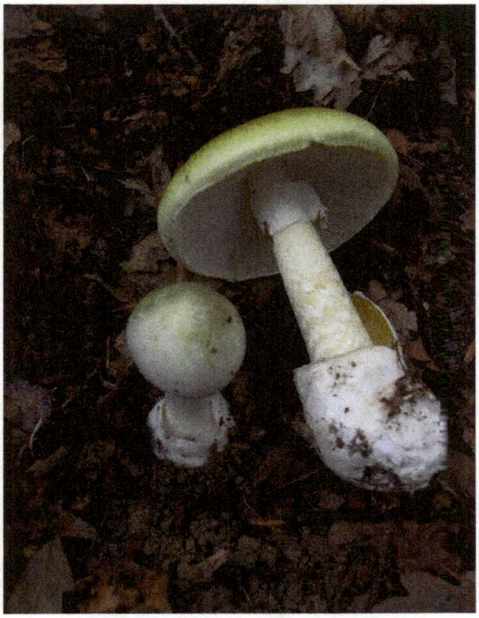

Amanita phalloides accounts for the majority of fatal mushroom poisonings worldwide.

Edible mushrooms are well-known examples of fungi. Many are commercially raised, but others must be harvested from the wild. *Agaricus bisporus*, sold as button mushrooms when small or Portobello mushrooms when larger, is a commonly eaten species, used in salads, soups, and many other dishes. Many Asian fungi are commercially grown and have increased in popularity in the West. They are often available fresh in grocery stores and markets, including straw mushrooms (*Volvariella volvacea*), oyster mushrooms (*Pleurotus ostreatus*), shiitakes (*Lentinula edodes*), and enokitake (*Flammulina* spp.).

There are many more mushroom species that are harvested from the wild for personal consumption or commercial sale. Milk mushrooms, morels, chanterelles, truffles, black trumpets, and *porcini* mushrooms (*Boletus edulis*) (also known as king boletes) demand a high price on the market. They are often used in gourmet dishes.

Certain types of cheeses require inoculation of milk curds with fungal species that impart a unique flavor and texture to the cheese. Examples include the blue color in cheeses such as Stilton or Roquefort, which are made by inoculation with *Penicillium roqueforti*. Molds used in cheese production are non-toxic and are thus safe for human consumption; however, mycotoxins (e.g., aflatoxins, roquefortine C, patulin, or others) may accumulate because of growth of other fungi during cheese ripening or storage.

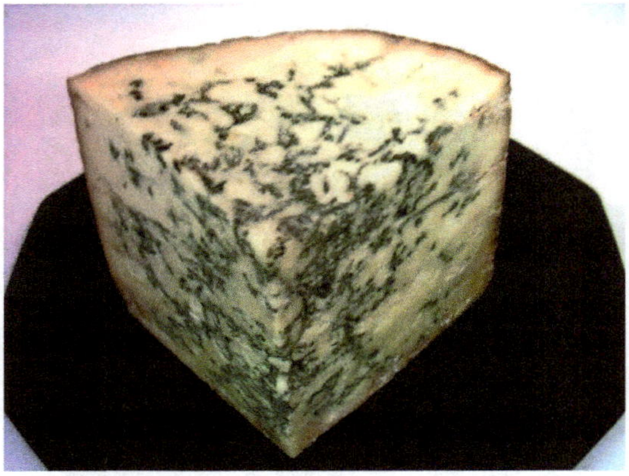

Stilton cheese veined with *Penicillium roqueforti.*

Many mushroom species are poisonous to humans, with toxicities ranging from slight digestive problems or allergic reactions as well as hallucinations to severe organ failures and death. Genera with mushrooms containing deadly toxins include *Conocybe*, *Galerina*, *Lepiota*, and, the most infamous, *Amanita*. The latter genus includes the destroying angel *(A. virosa)* and the death cap *(A. phalloides)*, the most common cause of deadly mushroom poisoning. The false morel (*Gyromitra esculenta*) is occasionally considered a delicacy when cooked, yet can be highly toxic when eaten raw. *Tricholoma equestre* was considered edible until it was implicated in serious poisonings causing rhabdomyolysis. Fly agaric mushrooms (*Amanita muscaria*) also cause occasional non-fatal poisonings, mostly as a result of ingestion for its hallucinogenic properties. Historically, fly agaric was used by different peoples in Europe and Asia and its present usage for religious or shamanic purposes is reported from some ethnic groups such as the Koryak people of north-eastern Siberia.

As it is difficult to accurately identify a safe mushroom without proper training and knowledge, it is often advised to assume that a wild mushroom is poisonous and not to consume it.

Pest Control

In agriculture, fungi may be useful if they actively compete for nutrients and space with pathogenic microorganisms such as bacteria or other fungi via the competitive exclusion principle, or if they are parasites of these pathogens. For example, certain species may be used to eliminate or suppress the growth of harmful plant pathogens, such as insects, mites, weeds, nematodes, and other fungi that cause diseases of important crop plants. This has generated strong interest in practical applications that use these fungi in the biological control of these agricultural pests. Entomopathogenic fungi can be used as biopesticides, as they actively kill insects. Examples that have been used as biological insecticides are *Beauveria bassiana*, *Metarhizium* spp, *Hirsutella* spp, *Paecilomyces* (*Isaria*) spp, and *Lecanicillium lecanii*. Endophytic fungi of grasses of the genus *Neotyphodium*, such as *N. coenophialum*, produce alkaloids that are toxic to a range of invertebrate and vertebrate herbivores. These alkaloids protect grass plants from herbivory, but several endophyte alkaloids can poison grazing animals, such as cattle and sheep. Infecting cultivars of pasture or forage grasses with *Neotyphodium* endophytes is one approach being used in grass breeding programs; the fungal strains are selected for producing only alkaloids that increase resistance to herbivores such as insects, while being non-toxic to livestock.

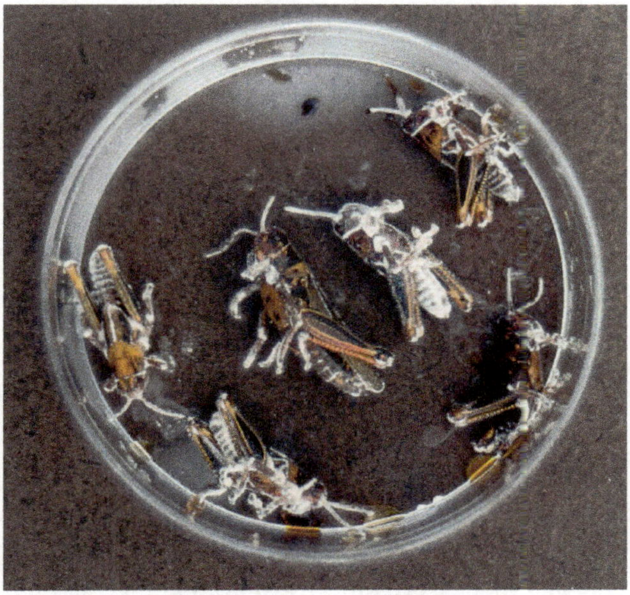

Grasshoppers killed by *Beauveria bassiana.*

Bioremediation

Certain fungi, in particular "white rot" fungi, can degrade insecticides, herbicides, pentachlorophenol, creosote, coal tars, and heavy fuels and turn them into carbon dioxide, water, and basic elements. Fungi have been shown to biomineralize uranium oxides, suggesting they may have application in the bioremediation of radioactively polluted sites.

Model Organisms

Several pivotal discoveries in biology were made by researchers using fungi as model organisms, that is, fungi that grow and sexually reproduce rapidly in the laboratory. For example, the one gene-one enzyme hypothesis was formulated by scientists using the bread mold *Neurospora crassa* to test their biochemical theories. Other important model fungi are *Aspergillus nidulans* and the yeasts *Saccaromyces cerevisiae* and *Schizosaccharomyces pombe*, each of which with a long history of use to investigate issues in eukaryotic cell biology and genetics, such as cell cycle regulation, chromatin structure, and gene regulation. Other fungal models have more recently emerged that address specific biological questions relevant to medicine, plant pathology, and industrial uses; examples include

Candida albicans, a dimorphic, opportunistic human pathogen, *Magnaporthe grisea*, a plant pathogen, and *Pichia pastoris*, a yeast widely used for eukaryotic protein production.

Others

Fungi are used extensively to produce industrial chemicals like citric, gluconic, lactic, and malic acids, and industrial enzymes, such as lipases used in biological detergents, cellulases used in making cellulosic ethanol and stonewashed jeans, and amylases, invertases, proteases and xylanases. Several species, most notably *Psilocybin mushrooms* (colloquially known as *magic mushrooms*), are ingested for their psychedelic properties, both recreationally and religiously.

REFERENCES

1. Ruano-Rosa, David; Prieto, Pilar; Rincón, Ana María; Gómez-Rodríguez, María Victoria; Valderrama, Raquel; Barroso, Juan Bautista; Mercado-Blanco, Jesús (2015-11-07). "Fate of Trichoderma harzianum in the olive rhizosphere: time course of the root colonization process and interaction with the fungal pathogen Verticillium dahliae". BioControl. 61 (3): 269–282. doi:10.1007/s10526-015-9706-z. ISSN 1386-6141.
2. Anon (1868). "A foray among the funguses". Transactions of the Woolhope Naturalists' Field Club: 184–192.
3. San-Blas G; Calderone RA (editors). (2008). Pathogenic Fungi. Caister Academic Press. ISBN 978-1-904455-32-5.
4. Ainsworth, p. 13.
5. De stirpium maxime earum quae in Germania nostra nascuntur, usitatis nomenclaturis. Strasbourg. In Ainsworth, p. 13, quoting Buller, AHR. (1915). Micheli and the discovery of reproduction in fungi. Transactions of the royal Society of Canada, series 3 9: 1–25.
6. Ainsworth, p. 4.
7. Ainsworth, p. 2.
8. Smith JE, Rowan NJ, Sullivan R (May 2002). "Medicinal Mushrooms: Their therapeutic properties and current medical usage with special emphasis on cancer treatments". Cancer Research UK. p. 5.
9. Sarfaraz Khan Marwat; Mir Ajab Khan; Muhammad Aslam Khan; Mushtaq Ahmad; Muhammad Zafar; Fazal-ur-Rehman and Shazia Sultana (2009). "Aromatic Plant Species Mentioned in the Holy Qura'n and Ahadith and Their Ethnomedicinal Importance" (PDF). Pakistan Journal of Nutrition. 8 (9): 1472–1479. doi:10.3923/pjn.2009.1472.1479. Sahih Muslim, Book 23, Chapter 27, Hadiths
10. Shashkina MIa; Shashkin PN; Sergeev AV (October 2006). "[Chemical and medicobiological properties of Chaga (review)]". Farmatsevtychnyĭ zhurnal. 40 (10): 560–568. doi:10.1007/s11094-006-0194-4.

11. Di Rado, Alicia (July 2008). "A salad fixin' with medical benefits?". EHope. City of Hope National Medical Center. 7 (7).
12. Di Rado, Alicia (November 2008). "Can a mushroom help fight lung cancer?". EHope. City of Hope National Medical Center. 7 (11).
13. Deng G, Lin H, Seidman A (September 2009). "A phase I/II trial of a polysaccharide extract from Grifola frondosa (Maitake mushroom) in breast cancer patients: immunological effects". Journal of Cancer Research and Clinical Oncology. 135 (9): 1215–21. doi:10.1007/s00432-009-0562-z. PMID 19253021.
14. Bowerman, Susan (March 31, 2008), "If mushrooms see the light", The Los Angeles Times
15. Ji, Y; Bi; Yan; Zhu (Jan 2006), "Taxol-producing fungi: a new approach to industrial production of taxol" (Free full text), Sheng wu gong cheng xue bao = Chinese journal of biotechnology, 22 (1): 1–6, doi:10 1016/s1872-2075(06)60001-0, ISSN 1000-3061, PMID 16572833
16. Moore RT (1980). "Taxonomic proposals for the classification of marine yeasts and other yeast-like fungi including the smuts". Botanica Marina. 23: 361–373.
17. The classification system presented here is based on the 2007 phylogenetic study by Hibbett et al.
18. "Fungus". Oxford Dictionaries. Retrieved 26 February 2011.
19. Simpson DP (1979). Cassell's Latin Dictionary (5 ed.). London, UK: Cassell Ltd. p. 883. ISBN 0-304-52257-0.
20. Mitzka W, ed. (1960). Etymologisches Wörterbuch der deutschen Sprache. Berlin: Walter de Gruyter.
21. Alexopoulos et al., p. 1.
22. "LIAS Glossary". Retrieved 14 August 2013.
23. Bruns T (October 2006). "Evolutionary biology: a kingdom revised". Nature. 443 (7113): 758–61. Bibcode:2006Natur.443..758B. doi:10.1038/443758a. PMID 17051197.
24. Baldauf SL, Palmer JD (December 1993). "Animals and fungi are each other's closest relatives: congruent evidence from multiple proteins". Proceedings of the National Academy of Sciences of the United States of America. 90 (24): 11558–62. Bibcode:1993PNAS...9011558B. doi:10.1073/pnas.90.24.11558. PMC 48023Freely accessible. PMID 8265589.
25. Shoji JY, Arioka M, Kitamoto K (2006). "Possible involvement of pleiomorphic vacuolar networks in nutrient recycling in filamentous fungi". Autophagy. 2 (3): 226–7. doi:10.4161/auto.2695. PMID 16874107.
26. Deacon, p. 58.
27. Zabriskie TM, Jackson MD (February 2000). "Lysine biosynthesis and metabolism in fungi". Natural Product Reports. 17 (1): 85–97. doi:10.1039/a801345d. PMID 10714900.

28. Xu H, Andi B, Qian J, West AH, Cook PF (2006). "The alpha-aminoadipate pathway for lysine biosynthesis in fungi". Cell Biochemistry and Biophysics. 46 (1): 43–64. doi:10.1385/CBB:46:1:43. PMID 16943623.
29. Desjardin DE, Perry BA, Lodge DJ, Stevani CV, Nagasawa E (2010). "Luminescent Mycena: new and noteworthy species". Mycologia. 102 (2): 459–77. doi:10.3852/09-197. PMID 20361513.
30. Alexopoulos et al., pp. 32–33.
31. Bowman SM, Free SJ (August 2006). "The structure and synthesis of the fungal cell wall". BioEssays. 28 (8): 799–808. doi:10.1002/bies.20441. PMID 16927300.
32. Alexopoulos et al., p. 33.
33. Mihail JD, Bruhn JN (November 2005). "Foraging behaviour of Armillaria rhizomorph systems". Mycological Research. 109 (Pt 11): 1195–207. doi:10.1017/S0953756205003606. PMID 16279413.
34. Keller NP, Turner G, Bennett JW (December 2005). "Fungal secondary metabolism - from biochemistry to genomics". Nature Reviews. Microbiology. 3 (12): 937–47. doi:10.1038/nrmicro1286. PMID 16322742.
35. Wu S, Schalk M, Clark A, Miles RB, Coates R, Chappell J (November 2006). "Redirection of cytosolic or plastidic isoprenoid precursors elevates terpene production in plants". Nature Biotechnology. 24 (11): 1441–7. doi:10.1038/nbt1251. PMID 17057703.
36. Tudzynski B (March 2005). "Gibberellin biosynthesis in fungi: genes, enzymes, evolution, and impact on biotechnology". Applied Microbiology and Biotechnology. 66 (6): 597–611. doi:10.1007/s00253-004-1805-1. PMID 15578178.
37. Vaupotic T, Veranic P, Jenoe P, Plemenitas A (June 2008). "Mitochondrial mediation of environmental osmolytes discrimination during osmoadaptation in the extremely halotolerant black yeast Hortaea werneckii". Fungal Genetics and Biology. 45 (6): 994–1007. doi:10.1016/j.fgb.2008.01.006. PMID 18343697.
38. Dadachova E, Bryan RA, Huang X, Moadel T, Schweitzer AD, Aisen P, Nosanchuk JD, Casadevall A (2007). "Ionizing radiation changes the electronic properties of melanin and enhances the growth of melanized fungi". PloS One. 2 (5): e457. Bibcode:2007PLoSO...2..457D. doi:10.1371/journal.pone.0000457. PMC 1866175Freely accessible. PMID 17520016. open access publication - free to read
39. Raghukumar C, Raghukumar S (1998). "Barotolerance of fungi isolated from deep-sea sediments of the Indian Ocean". Aquatic Microbial Ecology. 15 (2): 153–163. doi:10.3354/ame015153.
40. Sancho LG, de la Torre R, Horneck G, Ascaso C, de Los Rios A, Pintado A, Wierzchos J, Schuster M (June 2007). "Lichens survive in space: results from the 2005 LICHENS experiment". Astrobiology. 7 (3): 443–54. Bibcode:2007AsBio...7..443S. doi:10.1089/ast.2006.0046. PMID 17630840.
41. Brem FM, Lips KR (September 2008). "Batrachochytrium dendrobatidis infection patterns among Panamanian amphibian species, habitats and elevations during epizootic and enzootic stages". Diseases of Aquatic Organisms. 81 (3): 189–202.

doi:10.3354/dao01960. PMID 18998584.

42. Le Calvez T, Burgaud G, Mahé S, Barbier G, Vandenkoornhuyse P (October 2009). "Fungal diversity in deep-sea hydrothermal ecosystems". Applied and Environmental Microbiology. 75 (20): 6415–21. doi:10.1128/AEM.00653-09. PMC 2765129Freely accessible. PMID 19633124.
43. This estimation is determined by combining the species count for each phyla, based on values obtained from the 10th edition of the Dictionary of the Fungi (Kirk et al., 2008): Ascomycota, 64163 species (p. 55); Basidiomycota, 31515 (p. 78); Blastocladiomycota, 179 (p. 94); Chytridiomycota, 706 (p. 142); Glomeromycota, 169 (p. 287); Microsporidia, >1300 (p. 427); Neocallimastigomycota, 20 (p. 463).
44. Mueller GM, Schmit JP (2006). "Fungal biodiversity: what do we know? What can we predict?". Biodiversity and Conservation. 16: 1–5. doi:10.1007/s10531-006-9117-7.
45. Hawksworth DL (2006). "The fungal dimension of biodiversity: magnitude, significance, and conservation". Mycological Research. 95 (6): 641–655. doi:10.1016/S0953-7562(09)80810-1.
46. Blackwell M (March 2011). "The fungi: 1, 2, 3 ... 5.1 million species?". American Journal of Botany. 98 (3): 426–38. doi:10.3732/ajb.1000298. PMID 21613136.
47. Hibbett DS, Binder M, Bischoff JF, Blackwell M, Cannon PF, Eriksson OE, et al. (May 2007). "A higher-level phylogenetic classification of the Fungi" (PDF). Mycological Research. 111 (Pt 5): 509–47. doi:10.1016/j.mycres.2007.03.004. PMID 17572334. Archived from the original (PDF) on 26 March 2009.
48. According to one 2001 estimate, some 10,000 fungal diseases are known. Struck C (2006). "Infection strategies of plant parasitic fungi". In Cooke BM, Jones DG, Kaye B. The Epidemiology of Plant Diseases. Berlin, Germany: Springer. p. 117. ISBN 1-4020-4580-8.
49. Peintner U, Pöder R, Pümpel T (1998). "The Iceman's fungi". Mycological Research. 102 (10): 1153–1162. doi:10.1017/S0953756298006546.
50. Ainsworth, p. 1.
51. Alexopoulos et al., pp. 1–2.
52. Ainsworth, p. 18.
53. Hawksworth DL (September 2006). "Pandora's mycological box: molecular sequences vs. morphology in understanding fungal relationships and biodiversity". Revista Iberoamericana de MicologíA. 23 (3): 127–33. doi:10.1016/S1130-1406(06)70031-6. PMID 17196017.
54. Harris SD (2008). "Branching of fungal hyphae: regulation, mechanisms and comparison with other branching systems". Mycologia. 100 (6): 823–32. doi:10.3852/08-177. PMID 19202837.
55. Deacon, p. 51.
56. Deacon, p. 57.
57. Chang S-T, Miles PG (2004). Mushrooms: Cultivation, Nutritional Value, Medicinal Effect and Environmental Impact. Boca Raton, Florida: CRC Press.

ISBN 0-8493-1043-1.

58. Parniske M (October 2008). "Arbuscular mycorrhiza: the mother of plant root endosymbioses". Nature Reviews. Microbiology. 6 (10): 763–75. doi:10.1038/nrmicro1987. PMID 18794914.
59. Steenkamp ET, Wright J, Baldauf SL (January 2006). "The protistan origins of animals and fungi". Molecular Biology and Evolution. 23 (1): 93–106. doi:10.1093/molbev/msj011. PMID 16151185.
60. Stevens DA, Ichinomiya M, Koshi Y, Horiuchi H (September 2006). "Escape of Candida from caspofungin inhibition at concentrations above the MIC (paradoxical effect) accomplished by increased cell wall chitin; evidence for beta-1,6-glucan synthesis inhibition by caspofungin". Antimicrobial Agents and Chemotherapy. 50 (9): 3160–1. doi:10.1128/AAC.00563-06. PMC 1563524Freely accessible. PMID 16940118.
61. Hanson, pp. 127–141.
62. Ferguson BA, Dreisbach TA, Parks CG, Filip GM, Schmitt CL (2003). "Coarse-scale population structure of pathogenic Armillaria species in a mixed-conifer forest in the Blue Mountains of northeast Oregon". Canadian Journal of Forest Research. 33 (4): 612–623. doi:10.1139/x03-065.
63. Alexopoulos et al., pp. 204–205.
64. Moss ST (1986). The Biology of Marine Fungi. Cambridge, UK: Cambridge University Press. p. 76. ISBN 0-521-30899-2.
65. Peñalva MA, Arst HN (September 2002). "Regulation of gene expression by ambient pH in filamentous fungi and yeasts". Microbiology and Molecular Biology Reviews. 66 (3): 426–46, table of contents. doi:10.1128/MMBR.66.3.426-446.2002. PMC 120796Freely accessible. PMID 12208998.
66. Howard RJ, Ferrari MA, Roach DH, Money NP (December 1991). "Penetration of hard substrates by a fungus employing enormous turgor pressures". Proceedings of the National Academy of Sciences of the United States of America. 88 (24): 11281–4. Bibcode:1991PNAS...8811281H. doi:10.1073/pnas.88.24.11281. PMC 53118Freely accessible. PMID 1837147.
67. Money NP (1998). "Mechanics of invasive fungal growth and the significance of turgor in plant infection". Molecular Genetics of Host-Specific Toxins in Plant Disease: Proceedings of the 3rd Tottori International Symposium on Host-Specific Toxins, Daisen, Tottori, Japan, August 24–29, 1997. Netherlands: Kluwer Academic Publishers. pp. 261–271. ISBN 0-7923-4981-4.
68. Wang ZY, Jenkinson JM, Holcombe LJ, Soanes DM, Veneault-Fourrey C, Bhambra GK, Talbot NJ (April 2005). "The molecular biology of appressorium turgor generation by the rice blast fungus Magnaporthe grisea". Biochemical Society Transactions. 33 (Pt 2): 384–8. doi:10.1042/BST0330384. PMID 15787612.
69. Pereira JL, Noronha EF, Miller RN, Franco OL (June 2007). "Novel insights in the use of hydrolytic enzymes secreted by fungi with biotechnological potential". Letters in Applied Microbiology. 44 (6): 573–81. doi:10.1111/j.1472-765X.2007.02151.x. PMID 17576216.

70. Schaller M, Borelli C, Korting HC, Hube B (November 2005). "Hydrolytic enzymes as virulence factors of Candida albicans'. Mycoses. 48 (6): 365–77. doi:10.1111/j.1439-0507.2005.01165.x. PMID 16262871.

71. Farrar JF (October 1985). "Carbohydrate metabolism in biotrophic plant pathogens". Microbiological Sciences. 2 (10): 314–7. PMID 3939987.

72. Fischer R, Zekert N, Takeshita N (May 2008). "Polarized growth in fungi--interplay between the cytoskeleton, positional markers and membrane domains". Molecular Microbiology. 68 (4): 813–26. doi:10.1111/j.1365-2958.2008.06193.x. PMID 18399939.

73. Christensen MJ, Bennett RJ, Ansari HA, Koga H, Johnson RD, Bryan GT, Simpson WR, Koolaard JP, Nickless EM, Voisey CR (February 2008). "Epichloë endophytes grow by intercalary hyphal extension in elongating grass leaves". Fungal Genetics and Biology. 45 (2): 84–93. doi:10.1016/j.fgb.2007.07.013. PMID 17919950.

74. Money NP (October 2002). "Mushroom stem cells". BioEssays. 24 (10): 949–52. doi:10.1002/bies.10160. PMID 12325127.

75. Willensdorfer M (February 2009). "On the evolution of differentiated multicellularity". Evolution; International Journal of Organic Evolution. 63 (2): 306–23. doi:10.1111/j.1558-5646.2008.00541.x. PMID 19154376.

76. Daniels KJ, Srikantha T, Lockhart SR, Pujol C, Soll DR (May 2006). "Opaque cells signal white cells to form biofilms in Candida albicans". The EMBO Journal. 25 (10): 2240–52. doi:10.1038/sj.emboj.7601099. PMC 1462973Freely accessible. PMID 16628217.

77. Marzluf GA (September 1981). "Regulation of nitrogen metabolism and gene expression in fungi". Microbiological Reviews. 45 (3) 437–61. PMC 281519Freely accessible. PMID 6117784.

78. Hynes MJ (1994). "Regulatory circuits of the amdS gene of Aspergillus nidulans". Antonie Van Leeuwenhoek. 65 (3): 179–82. doi:10.1007/BF00871944. PMID 7847883.

79. Dadachova E, Casadevall A (December 2008). "Ionizing radiation: how fungi cope, adapt, and exploit with the help of melanin". Current Opinion in Microbiology. 11 (6): 525–31. doi:10.1016/j.mib.2008.09.013. PMC 2677413Freely accessible. PMID 18848901.

80. Alexopoulos et al., pp. 48–56.

81. Kirk et al., p. 633.

82. Heitman J (September 2006). "Sexual reproduction and the evolution of microbial pathogens". Current Biology. 16 (17): R711–25. doi:10.1016/j.cub.2006.07.064. PMID 16950098.

83. Alcamo IE, Pommerville J (2004). Alcamo's Fundamentals of Microbiology. Boston, Massachusetts: Jones and Bartlett. p. 590. ISBN 0-7637-0067-3.

84. Redecker D, Raab P (2006). "Phylogeny of the glomeromycota (arbuscular mycorrhizal fungi): recent developments and new gene markers". Mycologia.

98 (6): 885–95. doi:10.3852/mycologia.98.6.885. PMID 17486965.

85. Guarro J, Stchigel AM (July 1999). "Developments in fungal taxonomy". Clinical Microbiology Reviews. 12 (3): 454–500. PMC 100249Freely accessible. PMID 10398676.
86. Taylor JW, Jacobson DJ, Kroken S, Kasuga T, Geiser DM, Hibbett DS, Fisher MC (October 2000). "Phylogenetic species recognition and species concepts in fungi". Fungal Genetics and Biology. 31 (1): 21–32. doi:10.1006/fgbi.2000.1228. PMID 11118132.
87. Metzenberg RL, Glass NL (February 1990). "Mating type and mating strategies in Neurospora". BioEssays. 12 (2): 53–9. doi:10.1002/bies.950120202. PMID 2140508.
88. Jennings and Lysek, pp. 107–114.
89. Deacon, p. 31.
90. Alexopoulos et al., pp. 492–493.
91. Jennings and Lysek, p. 142.
92. Deacon, pp. 21–24.
93. Linder MB, Szilvay GR, Nakari-Setälä T, Penttilä ME (November 2005). "Hydrophobins: the protein-amphiphiles of filamentous fungi". FEMS Microbiology Reviews. 29 (5): 877–96. doi:10.1016/j.femsre.2005.01.004. PMID 16219510.
94. Trail F (November 2007). "Fungal cannons: explosive spore discharge in the Ascomycota". FEMS Microbiology Letters. 276 (1): 12–8. doi:10.1111/j.1574-6968.2007.00900.x. PMID 17784861.
95. Pringle A, Patek SN, Fischer M, Stolze J, Money NP (2005). "The captured launch of a ballistospore". Mycologia. 97 (4): 866–71. doi:10.3852/mycologia.97.4.866. PMID 16457355.
96. Kirk et al., p. 495.
97. Brodie HJ (1975). The Bird's Nest Fungi. Toronto, Ontario: University of Toronto Press. p. 80. ISBN 0-8020-5307-6.
98. Alexopoulos et al., p. 545.
99. Jennings and Lysek, pp. 114–115.
100. Furlaneto MC, Pizzirani-Kleiner AA (January 1992). "Intraspecific hybridisation of Trichoderma pseudokoningii by anastomosis and by protoplast fusion". FEMS Microbiology Letters. 69 (2): 191–5. doi:10.1111/j.1574-6968.1992.tb05150.x. PMID 1537549.
101. Schardl CL, Craven KD (November 2003). "Interspecific hybridization in plant-associated fungi and oomycetes: a review". Molecular Ecology. 12 (11): 2861–73. doi:10.1046/j.1365-294X.2003.01965.x. PMID 14629368.
102. Donoghue MJ, Cracraft J (2004). Assembling the Tree of Life. Oxford (Oxfordshire), UK: Oxford University Press. p. 187. ISBN 0-19-517234-5.

103. Taylor and Taylor, p. 19.

104. Taylor and Taylor, pp. 7–12.

105. Butterfield NJ (2005). "Probable Proterozoic fungi". Paleobiology. 31 (1): 165–182. doi:10.1666/0094-8373(2005)031<0165:PPF>2.0.CO;2.

106. Lücking R, Huhndorf S, Pfister DH, Plata ER, Lumbsch HT (2009). "Fungi evolved right on track". Mycologia. 101 (6): 810–22. doi:10.3852/09-016. PMID 19927746.

107. James TY, Kauff F, Schoch CL, Matheny PB, Hofstetter V, Cox CJ, et al. (October 2006). "Reconstructing the early evolution of Fungi using a six-gene phylogeny". Nature. 443 (7113): 818–22. Bibcode:2006Natur.443..818J. doi:10.1038/nature05110. PMID 17051209.

108. Taylor and Taylor, pp. 84–94 and 106–107.

109. Schoch CL, Sung GH, López-Giráldez F, Townsend JP, Miadlikowska J, Hofstetter V, et al. (April 2009). "The Ascomycota tree of life: a phylum-wide phylogeny clarifies the origin and evolution of fundamental reproductive and ecological traits". Systematic Biology. 58 (2): 224–39. doi:10.1093/sysbio/syp020. PMID 20525580.

110. Brundrett MC (2002). "Coevolution of roots and mycorrhizas of land plants". New Phytologist. 154 (2): 275–304. doi:10.1046/j.1469-8137.2002.00397.x.

111. Redecker D, Kodner R, Graham LE (September 2000). "Glomalean fungi from the Ordovician". Science. 289 (5486): 1920–1. Bibcode:2000Sci...289.1920R. doi:10.1126/science.289.5486.1920. PMID 10988069.

112. Taylor TN, Taylor EL (1996). "The distribution and interactions of some Paleozoic fungi". Review of Palaeobotany and Palynology. 95 (1–4): 83–94. doi:10.1016/S0034-6667(96)00029-2.

113. Dotzler N, Walker C, Krings M, Hass H, Kerp H, Taylor TN, Agerer R (2009). "Acaulosporoid glomeromycotan spores with a germination shield from the 400-million-year-old Rhynie chert". Mycological Progress. 8 (1): 9–18. doi:10.1007/s11557-008-0573-1.

114. Taylor JW, Berbee ML (2006). "Dating divergences in the Fungal Tree of Life: review and new analyses". Mycologia. 98 (6): 838–49. doi:10.3852/mycologia.98.6.838. PMID 17486961.

115. Blackwell M, Vilgalys R, James TY, Taylor JW (2009). "Fungi. Eumycota: mushrooms, sac fungi, yeast, molds, rusts, smuts, etc.". Tree of Life Web Project. Retrieved 25 April 2009.

116. Yuan X, Xiao S, Taylor TN (May 2005). "Lichen-like symbiosis 600 million years ago". Science. 308 (5724): 1017–20. Bibcode:2005Sci...308.1017Y. doi:10.1126/science.1111347. PMID 15890881.

117. Karatygin IV, Snigirevskaya NS, Vikulin SV (2009). "The most ancient terrestrial lichen Winfrenatia reticulata: A new find and new interpretation". Paleontological Journal. 43 (1): 107–114. doi:10.1134/S0031030109010110.

118. Taylor TN, Hass H, Kerp H, Krings M, Hanlin RT (2005). "Perithecial

ascomycetes from the 400 million year old Rhynie chert: an example of ancestral polymorphism". Mycologia. 97 (1): 269–85. doi:10.3852/mycologia.97.1.269. PMID 16389979.

119. Dennis RL (1970). "A Middle Pennsylvanian basidiomycete mycelium with clamp connections". Mycologia. 62 (3): 578–584. doi:10.2307/3757529. JSTOR 3757529.
120. Hibbett DS, Grimaldi D, Donoghue MJ (1995). "Cretaceous mushrooms in amber". Nature. 377 (6549): 487. Bibcode:1995Natur.377..487H. doi:10.1038/377487a0.
121. Hibbett DS, Grimaldi D, Donoghue MJ (1997). "Fossil mushrooms from Miocene and Cretaceous ambers and the evolution of homobasidiomycetes". American Journal of Botany. 84 (7): 981–991. doi:10.2307/2446289. JSTOR 2446289.
122. Eshet Y, Rampino MR, Visscher H (1995). "Fungal event and palynological record of ecological crisis and recovery across the Permian-Triassic boundary". Geology. 23 (1): 967–970. Bibcode:1995Geo....23..967E. doi:10.1130/0091-7613(1995)023<0967:FEAPRO>2.3.CO;2.
123. Foster CB, Stephenson MH, Marshall C, Logan GA, Greenwood PF (2002). "A revision of Reduviasporonites Wilson 1962: description, illustration, comparison and biological affinities". Palynology. 26 (1): 35–58. doi:10.2113/0260035.
124. López-Gómez J, Taylor EL (2005). "Permian-Triassic transition in Spain: a multidisciplinary approach". Palaeogeography, Palaeoclimatology, Palaeoecology. 229 (1–2): 1–2. doi:10.1016/j.palaeo.2005.06.028.
125. Looy CV, Twitchett RJ, Dilcher DL, Van Konijnenburg-Van Cittert JH, Visscher H (July 2001). "Life in the end-Permian dead zone". Proceedings of the National Academy of Sciences of the United States of America. 98 (14): 7879–83. Bibcode:2001PNAS...98.7879L. doi:10.1073/pnas.131218098. PMC 35436Freely accessible. PMID 11427710. See image 2
126. Ward PD, Botha J, Buick R, De Kock MO, Erwin DH, Garrison GH, Kirschvink JL, Smith R (February 2005). "Abrupt and gradual extinction among Late Permian land vertebrates in the Karoo basin, South Africa". Science. 307 (5710): 709–14. Bibcode:2005Sci...307..709W. doi:10.1126/science.1107068. PMID 15661973.
127. Shalchian-Tabrizi K, Minge MA, Espelund M, Orr R, Ruden T, Jakobsen KS, Cavalier-Smith T (2008). "Multigene phylogeny of choanozoa and the origin of animals". PloS One. 3 (5): e2098. Bibcode:2008PLoSO...3.2098S. doi:10.1371/journal.pone.0002098. PMC 2346548Freely accessible. PMID 18461162. open access publication - free to read
128. See Palaeos Fungi: Fungi for an introduction to fungal taxonomy, including recent controversies. archive
129. Celio GJ, Padamsee M, Dentinger BT, Bauer R, McLaughlin DJ (2006). "Assembling the Fungal Tree of Life: constructing the structural and biochemical database". Mycologia. 98 (6): 850–9. doi:10.3852/mycologia.98.6.850. PMID 17486962.
130. Silar P (2016). "Protistes Eucaryotes: Origine, Evolution et Biologie des Microbes Eucaryotes". HAL: 462. ISBN 978-2-9555841-0-1.

131. Esser K (2014). The Mycota VII A: Systematics and Evolution (2nd ed.). Springer. p. 461. ISBN 978-3-642-55317-2.

132. Gill EE, Fast NM (June 2006). "Assessing the microsporidia-fungi relationship: Combined phylogenetic analysis of eight genes". Gene. 375: 103–9. doi:10.1016/j.gene.2006.02.023. PMID 16626896.

133. Liu YJ, Hodson MC, Hall BD (2006). "Loss of the flagellum happened only once in the fungal lineage: phylogenetic structure of kingdom Fungi inferred from RNA polymerase II subunit genes". BMC Evolutionary Biology. 6: 74. doi:10.1186/1471-2148-6-74. PMC 1599754Freely accessible. PMID 17010206.

134. James TY, Letcher PM, Longcore JE, Mozley-Standridge SE, Porter D, Powell MJ, Griffith GW, Vilgalys R (2006). "A molecular phylogeny of the flagellated fungi (Chytridiomycota) and description of a new phylum (Blastocladiomycota)". Mycologia. 98 (6): 860–71. doi:10.3852/mycologia.98.6.860. PMID 17486963.

135. Lockhart RJ, Van Dyke MI, Beadle IR, Humphreys P, McCarthy AJ (August 2006). "Molecular biological detection of anaerobic gut fungi (Neocallimastigales) from landfill sites". Applied and Environmental Microbiology. 72 (8): 5659–61. doi:10.1128/AEM.01057-06. PMC 1538735Freely accessible. PMID 16885325.

136. Remy W, Taylor TN, Hass H, Kerp H (December 1994). "Four hundred-million-year-old vesicular arbuscular mycorrhizae". Proceedings of the National Academy of Sciences of the United States of America. 91 (25): 11841–3. Bibcode:1994PNAS...9111841R. doi:10.1073/pnas.91 25.11841. PMC 45331Freely accessible. PMID 11607500.

137. Schüssler A, Schwarzott D, Walker C (2001). "A new fungal phylum, the Glomeromycota: phylogeny and evolution". Mycological Research. 105 (12): 1413–1421. doi:10.1017/S0953756201005196.

138. Alexopoulos et al., p. 145.

139. For an example, see Samuels GJ (February 2006). "Trichoderma: systematics, the sexual state, and ecology". Phytopathology. 96 (2): 195–206. doi:10.1094/PHYTO-96-0195. PMID 18943925.

140. Radford A, Parish JH (June 1997). "The genome and genes of Neurospora crassa". Fungal Genetics and Biology. 21 (3): 258–66. doi:10.1006/fgbi.1997.0979. PMID 9290240.

141. Valverde ME, Paredes-López O, Pataky JK, Guevara-Lara F (January 1995). "Huitlacoche (Ustilago maydis) as a food source--biology, composition, and production". Critical Reviews in Food Science and Nutrition. 35 (3): 191–229. doi:10.1080/10408399509527699. PMID 7632354.

142. Zisova LG (2009). "Malassezia species and seborrheic dermatitis". Folia Medica. 51 (1): 23–33. PMID 19437895.

143. Perfect JR (June 2006). "Cryptococcus neoformans: the yeast that likes it hot". FEMS Yeast Research. 6 (4): 463–8. doi:10.1111/j.1567-1364.2006.00051.x. PMID 16696642.

144. Blackwell M, Spatafora JW (2004). "Fungi and their allies". In Bills GF, Mueller

GM, Foster MS. Biodiversity of Fungi: Inventory and Monitoring Methods. Amsterdam: Elsevier Academic Press. pp. 18–20. ISBN 0-12-509551-1.

145. Gadd GM (January 2007). "Geomycology: biogeochemical transformations of rocks, minerals, metals and radionuclides by fungi, bioweathering and bioremediation". Mycological Research. 111 (Pt 1): 3–49. doi:10.1016/j.mycres.2006.12.001. PMID 17307120.
146. Lindahl BD, Ihrmark K, Boberg J, Trumbore SE, Högberg P, Stenlid J, Finlay RD (2007). "Spatial separation of litter decomposition and mycorrhizal nitrogen uptake in a boreal forest". The New Phytologist. 173 (3): 611–20. doi:10.1111/j.1469-8137.2006.01936.x. PMID 17244056.
147. Barea JM, Pozo MJ, Azcón R, Azcón-Aguilar C (July 2005). "Microbial co-operation in the rhizosphere". Journal of Experimental Botany. 56 (417): 1761–78. doi:10.1093/jxb/eri197. PMID 15911555.
148. Aanen DK (June 2006). "As you reap, so shall you sow: coupling of harvesting and inoculating stabilizes the mutualism between termites and fungi". Biology Letters. 2 (2): 209–12. doi:10.1098/rsbl.2005.0424. PMC 1618886Freely accessible. PMID 17148364.
149. Nikoh N, Fukatsu T (April 2000). "Interkingdom host jumping underground: phylogenetic analysis of entomoparasitic fungi of the genus cordyceps". Molecular Biology and Evolution. 17 (4): 629–38. doi:10.1093/oxfordjournals.molbev.a026341. PMID 10742053.
150. Perotto S, Bonfante P (December 1997). "Bacterial associations with mycorrhizal fungi: close and distant friends in the rhizosphere". Trends in Microbiology. 5 (12): 496–501. doi:10.1016/S0966-842X(97)01154-2. PMID 9447662.
151. Arnold AE, Mejía LC, Kyllo D, Rojas EI, Maynard Z, Robbins N, Herre EA (December 2003). "Fungal endophytes limit pathogen damage in a tropical tree". Proceedings of the National Academy of Sciences of the United States of America. 100 (26): 15649–54. Bibcode:2003PNAS..10015649A. doi:10.1073/pnas.2533483100. PMC 307622Freely accessible. PMID 14671327.
152. Paszkowski U (August 2006). "Mutualism and parasitism: the yin and yang of plant symbioses". Current Opinion in Plant Biology. 9 (4): 364–70. doi:10.1016/j.pbi.2006.05.008. PMID 16713732.
153. Hube B (August 2004). "From commensal to pathogen: stage- and tissue-specific gene expression of Candida albicans". Current Opinion in Microbiology. 7 (4): 336–41. doi:10.1016/j.mib.2004.06.003. PMID 15288621.
154. Bonfante P (April 2003). "Plants, mycorrhizal fungi and endobacteria: a dialog among cells and genomes". The Biological Bulletin. 204 (2): 215–20. doi:10.2307/1543562. JSTOR 1543562. PMID 12700157.
155. van der Heijden MG, Streitwolf-Engel R, Riedl R, Siegrist S, Neudecker A, Ineichen K, Boller T, Wiemken A, Sanders IR (2006). "The mycorrhizal contribution to plant productivity, plant nutrition and soil structure in experimental grassland". The New Phytologist. 172 (4): 739–52. doi:10.1111/j.1469-8137.2006.01862.x. PMID 17096799.

156. Selosse MA, Richard F, He X, Simard SW (November 2006). "Mycorrhizal networks: des liaisons dangereuses?". Trends in Ecology & Evolution. 21 (11): 621–8. doi:10.1016/j.tree.2006.07.003. PMID 16843567.

157. Merckx V, Bidartondo MI, Hynson NA (December 2009). "Myco-heterotrophy: when fungi host plants". Annals of Botany. 104 (7) 1255–61. doi:10.1093/aob/mcp235. PMC 2778383Freely accessible. PMID 19767309.

158. Schulz B, Boyle C (June 2005). "The endophytic continuum". Mycological Research. 109 (Pt 6): 661–86. doi:10.1017/S095375620500273X. PMID 16080390.

159. Clay K, Schardl C (October 2002). "Evolutionary origins and ecological consequences of endophyte symbiosis with grasses". The American Naturalist. 160 Suppl 4 (suppl. 4): S99–S127. doi:10.1086/342161. PMID 18707456.

160. Brodo IM, Sharnoff SD (2001). Lichens of North America. New Haven, Connecticut: Yale University Press. ISBN 0-300-08249-5.

161. Raven PH, Evert RF, Eichhorn, SE (2005). "14—Fungi". Biology of Plants (7 ed.). W. H. Freeman. p. 290. ISBN 978-0-7167-1007-3.

162. Deacon, p. 267.

163. Purvis W (2000). Lichens. Washington, D.C.: Smithsonian Institution Press in association with the Natural History Museum, London. pp. 49–75. ISBN 1-56098-879-7.

164. Kirk et al., p. 378.

165. Deacon, pp. 267–276.

166. Douglas AE (November 1989). "Mycetocyte symbiosis in insects". Biological Reviews of the Cambridge Philosophical Society. 64 (4): 409–34. doi:10.1111/j.1469-185X.1989.tb00682.x. PMID 2696562.

167. Deacon, p. 277.

168. "Entomologists: Brazilian Stingless Bee Must Cultivate Special Type of Fungus to Survive". Sci-News.com. 23 October 2015. Retrieved 25 October 2015.

169. Nguyen NH, Suh SO, Blackwell M (2007). "Five novel Candida species in insect-associated yeast clades isolated from Neuroptera and other insects". Mycologia. 99 (6): 842–58. doi:10.3852/mycologia.99.6.842. PMID 18333508.

170. Filipiak, Michał; Weiner, January (2016-09-01). "Nutritional dynamics during the development of xylophagous beetles related to changes in the stoichiometry of 11 elements". Physiological Entomology: n/a–n/a. doi:10.1111/phen.12168. ISSN 1365-3032.

171. Filipiak, Michał; Sobczyk, Łukasz; Weiner, January (2016-04-09). Fungal Transformation of Tree Stumps into a Suitable Resource for Xylophagous Beetles via Changes in Elemental Ratios. Insects. 7 (2): 13. doi:10.3390/insects7020013.

172. Chandler PJ (2010). A Dipterist›s Handbook (2nd Edition). U.K.: The Amateur Entomologists› Society. pp. 1–525.

173. Talbot NJ (2003). On the trail of a cereal killer Exploring the biology of Magnaporthe grisea. Annual Review of Microbiology. 57: 177–202. doi:10.1146/

annurev.micro.57.030502.090957. PMID 14527276.

174. Paoletti M, Buck KW, Brasier CM (January 2006). Selective acquisition of novel mating type and vegetative incompatibility genes via interspecies gene transfer in the globally invading eukaryote Ophiostoma novo-ulmi. Molecular Ecology. 15 (1): 249–62. doi:10.1111/j.1365-294X.2005.02728.x. PMID 16367844.
175. Gryzenhout M, Wingfield BD, Wingfield MJ (May 2006). New taxonomic concepts for the important forest pathogen Cryphonectria parasitica and related fungi. FEMS Microbiology Letters. 258 (2): 161–72. doi:10.1111/j.1574-6968.2006.00170.x. PMID 16640568.
176. Yang Y, Yang E, An Z, Liu X (May 2007). Evolution of nematode-trapping cells of predatory fungi of the Orbiliaceae based on evidence from rRNA-encoding DNA and multiprotein sequences. Proceedings of the National Academy of Sciences of the United States of America. 104 (20): 8379–84. Bibcode:2007PNAS..104.8379Y. doi:10.1073/pnas.0702770104. PMC 1895958Freely accessible. PMID 17494736.
177. Nielsen K, Heitman J (2007). Sex and virulence of human pathogenic fungi. Advances in Genetics. Advances in Genetics. 57: 143–73. doi:10.1016/S0065-2660(06)57004-X. ISBN 978-0-12-017657-1. PMID 17352904.
178. Brakhage AA (December 2005). Systemic fungal infections caused by Aspergillus species: epidemiology, infection process and virulence determinants. Current Drug Targets. 6 (8): 875–86. doi:10.2174/138945005774912717. PMID 16375671.
179. Kauffman CA (January 2007). Histoplasmosis: a clinical and laboratory update. Clinical Microbiology Reviews. 20 (1): 115–32. doi:10.1128/CMR.00027-06. PMC 1797635Freely accessible. PMID 17223625.
180. Cushion MT, Smulian AG, Slaven BE, Sesterhenn T, Arnold J, Staben C, Porollo A, Adamczak R, Meller J (2007). Transcriptome of Pneumocystis carinii during fulminate infection: carbohydrate metabolism and the concept of a compatible parasite. PloS One. 2 (5): e423. Bibcode:2007PLoSO...2..423C. doi:10.1371/journal.pone.0000423. PMC 1855432Freely accessible. PMID 17487271. open access publication - free to read
181. Cook GC, Zumla AI (2008). Manson›s Tropical Diseases: Expert Consult. Edinburgh, Scotland: Saunders Ltd. p. 347. ISBN 1-4160-4470-1.
182. Simon-Nobbe B, Denk U, Pöll V, Rid R, Breitenbach M (2008). The spectrum of fungal allergy. International Archives of Allergy and Immunology. 145 (1): 58–86. doi:10.1159/000107578. PMID 17709917.
183. Le Floch G, Rey P, Benizri E, Benhamou N, Tirilly Y (2003). Impact of auxin-compounds produced by the antagonistic fungus Pythium oligandrum or the minor pathogen Pythium group F on plant growth.. Plant Soil. 257 (2): 459–470. doi:10.1023/a:1027330024834.
184. Schardl CL, Panaccione DG, Tudzynski P (2006). Ergot alkaloids--biology and molecular biology. The Alkaloids. Chemistry and Biology. The Alkaloids: Chemistry and Biology. 63: 45–86. doi:10.1016/S1099-4831(06)63002-2. ISBN 978-0-12-469563-4. PMID 17133714.

185. van Egmond HP, Schothorst RC, Jonker MA (September 2007). Regulations relating to mycotoxins in food: perspectives in a global and European context. Analytical and Bioanalytical Chemistry. 389 (1): 147–57. doi:10.1007/s00216-007-1317-9. PMID 17508207.

186. Demain AL, Fang A (2000). The natural functions of secondary metabolites. Advances in Biochemical Engineering/Biotechnology. Advances in Biochemical Engineering/Biotechnology. 69: 1–39. doi:10.1007/3-540-44964-7_1. ISBN 978-3-540-67793-2. PMID 11036689.

187. Rohlfs M, Albert M, Keller NP, Kempken F (October 2007). Secondary chemicals protect mould from fungivory. Biology Letters. 3 (5): 523–5. doi:10.1098/rsbl.2007.0338. PMC 2391202Freely accessible. PMID 17686752.

188. Molina L, Kahmann R (July 2007). An Ustilago maydis gene involved in H2O2 detoxification is required for virulence. The Plant Cell. 19 (7): 2293–309. doi:10.1105/tpc.107.052332. PMC 1955693Freely accessible. PMID 17616735.

189. Kojic M, Zhou Q, Lisby M, Holloman WK (January 2006). Rec2 interplay with both Brh2 and Rad51 balances recombinational repair in Ustilago maydis. Molecular and Cellular Biology. 26 (2): 678–88. doi:10.1128/MCB.26.2.678-688.2006. PMC 1346908Freely accessible. PMID 16382157.

190. Michod RE, Bernstein H, Nedelcu AM (May 2008). Adaptive value of sex in microbial pathogens (PDF). Infection, Genetics and Evolution. 8 (3): 267–85. doi:10.1016/j.meegid.2008.01.002. PMID 18295550.

191. Fan W, Kraus PR, Boily MJ, Heitman J (August 2005). Cryptococcus neoformans gene expression during murine macrophage infection. Eukaryotic Cell. 4 (8): 1420–33. doi:10.1128/EC.4.8.1420-1433.2005. PMC 1214536Freely accessible. PMID 16087747.

192. Lin X, Hull CM, Heitman J (April 2005). Sexual reproduction between partners of the same mating type in Cryptococcus neoformans. Nature. 434 (7036): 1017–21. Bibcode:2005Natur.434.1017L. doi:10.1038/nature03448. PMID 15846346.

193. Fincham JR (March 1989). Transformation in fungi. Microbiological Reviews. 53 (1): 148–70. PMC 372721Freely accessible. PMID 2651864.

194. Hawkins KM, Smolke CD (September 2008). Production of benzylisoquinoline alkaloids in Saccharomyces cerevisiae. Nature Chemical Biology. 4 (9): 564–73. doi:10.1038/nchembio.105. PMC 2830865Freely accessible. PMID 18690217.

195. Huang B, Guo J, Yi B, Yu X, Sun L, Chen W (July 2008). Heterologous production of secondary metabolites as pharmaceuticals in Saccharomyces cerevisiae. Biotechnology Letters. 30 (7): 1121–37. doi:10.1007/s10529-008-9663-z. PMID 18512022.

196. Brakhage AA, Spröte P, Al-Abdallah Q, Gehrke A, Plattner H, Tüncher A (2004). Regulation of penicillin biosynthesis in filamentous fungi. Advances in Biochemical Engineering/Biotechnology. 88: 45–90. doi:10.1007/b99257. PMID 15719552.

197. Pan A, Lorenzotti S, Zoncada A (January 2008). Registered and investigational drugs for the treatment of methicillin-resistant Staphylococcus aureus

infection. Recent Patents on Anti-Infective Drug Discovery. 3 (1): 10–33. doi:10.2174/157489108783413173. PMID 18221183.

198. Fajardo A, Martínez JL (April 2008). Antibiotics as signals that trigger specific bacterial responses. Current Opinion in Microbiology. 11 (2): 161–7. doi:10.1016/j.mib.2008.02.006. PMID 18373943.

199. Loo DS (2006). Systemic antifungal agents: an update of established and new therapies. Advances in Dermatology. 22: 101–24. doi:10.1016/j.yadr.2006.07.001. PMID 17249298.

200. Manzoni M, Rollini M (April 2002). Biosynthesis and biotechnological production of statins by filamentous fungi and application of these cholesterol-lowering drugs. Applied Microbiology and Biotechnology. 58 (5): 555–64. doi:10.1007/s00253-002-0932-9. PMID 11956737.

201. Hetland G, Johnson E, Lyberg T, Bernardshaw S, Tryggestad AM, Grinde B (October 2008). Effects of the medicinal mushroom Agaricus blazei Murill on immunity, infection and cancer. Scandinavian Journal of Immunology. 68 (4): 363–70. doi:10.1111/j.1365-3083.2008.02156.x. PMID 18782264.

202. Firenzuoli F, Gori L, Lombardo G (March 2008). The Medicinal Mushroom Agaricus blazei Murrill: Review of Literature and Pharmaco-Toxicological Problems. Evidence-Based Complementary and Alternative Medicine. 5 (1): 3–15. doi:10.1093/ecam/nem007. PMC 2249742Freely accessible. PMID 18317543.

203. Paterson RR (September 2006). Ganoderma - a therapeutic fungal biofactory. Phytochemistry. 67 (18): 1985–2001. doi:10.1016/j.phytochem.2006.07.004. PMID 16905165.

204. Paterson RR (May 2008). Cordyceps: a traditional Chinese medicine and another fungal therapeutic biofactory?. Phytochemistry. 69 (7): 1469–95. doi:10.1016/j.phytochem.2008.01.027. PMID 18343466.

205. el-Mekkawy S, Meselhy MR, Nakamura N, Tezuka Y, Hattori M, Kakiuchi N, Shimotohno K, Kawahata T, Otake T (November 1998). Anti-HIV-1 and anti-HIV-1-protease substances from Ganoderma lucidum. Phytochemistry. 49 (6): 1651–7. doi:10.1016/S0031-9422(98)00254-4. PMID 9862140.

206. El Dine RS, El Halawany AM, Ma CM, Hattori M (June 2008). Anti-HIV-1 protease activity of lanostane triterpenes from the vietnamese mushroom Ganoderma colossum. Journal of Natural Products. 71 (6): 1022–6. doi:10.1021/np8001139. PMID 18547117.

207. Yuen JW, Gohel MD (2005). Anticancer effects of Ganoderma lucidum: a review of scientific evidence. Nutrition and Cancer. 53 (1): 11–7. doi:10.1207/s15327914nc5301_2. PMID 16351502.

208. Sullivan R, Smith JE, Rowan NJ (2006). Medicinal mushrooms and cancer therapy: translating a traditional practice into Western medicine. Perspectives in Biology and Medicine. 49 (2): 159–70. doi:10.1353/pbm.2006.0034. PMID 16702701.

209. Halpern GM, Miller A (2002). Medicinal Mushrooms: Ancient Remedies for Modern Ailments. New York, New York: M. Evans and Co. p. 116. ISBN 0-87131-981-0.

210. Fisher M, Yang LX (2002). Anticancer effects and mechanisms of polysaccharide-K (PSK): implications of cancer immunotherapy. Anticancer Research. 22 (3): 1737–54. PMID 12168863.

211. Kulp K (2000). Handbook of Cereal Science and Technology. CRC Press. ISBN 0-8247-8294-1.

212. Piskur J, Rozpedowska E, Polakova S, Merico A, Compagno C (April 2006). How did Saccharomyces evolve to become a good brewer?. Trends in Genetics. 22 (4): 183–6. doi:10.1016/j.tig.2006.02.002. PMID 16499989.

213. Abe K, Gomi K, Hasegawa F, Machida M (September 2006). Impact of Aspergillus oryzae genomics on industrial production of metabolites. Mycopathologia. 162 (3): 143–53. doi:10.1007/s11046-006-0049-2. PMID 16944282.

214. Hachmeister KA, Fung DY (1993). Tempeh: a mold-modified indigenous fermented food made from soybeans and/or cereal grains. Critical Reviews in Microbiology. 19 (3): 137–88. doi:10.3109/10408419309113527. PMID 8267862.

215. Jørgensen TR (December 2007). Identification and toxigenic potential of the industrially important fungi, Aspergillus oryzae and Aspergillus sojae. Journal of Food Protection. 70 (12): 2916–34. PMID 18095455.

216. O›Donnell K, Cigelnik E, Casper HH (February 1998). Molecular phylogenetic, morphological, and mycotoxin data support reidentification of the Quorn mycoprotein fungus as Fusarium venenatum. Fungal Genetics and Biology. 23 (1): 57–67. doi:10.1006/fgbi.1997.1018. PMID 9501477.

217. Stamets P (2000). Growing Gourmet and Medicinal Mushrooms = [Shokuyō oyobi yakuyō kinoko no saibai]. Berkeley, California: Ten Speed Press. pp. 233–248. ISBN 1-58008-175-4.

218. Hall, pp. 13–26.

219. Kinsella JE, Hwang DH (November 1976). Enzymes of Penicillium roqueforti involved in the biosynthesis of cheese flavor. CRC Critical Reviews in Food Science and Nutrition. 8 (2): 191–228. doi:10.1080/10408397609527222. PMID 21770.

220. Erdogan A, Gurses M, Sert S (August 2003). Isolation of moulds capable of producing mycotoxins from blue mouldy Tulum cheeses produced in Turkey. International Journal of Food Microbiology. 85 (1-2): 83–5. doi:10.1016/S0168-1605(02)00485-3. PMID 12810273.

221. Orr DB, Orr RT (1979). Mushrooms of Western North America. Berkeley, California: University of California Press. p. 17. ISBN 0-520-03656-5.

222. Vetter J (January 1998). Toxins of Amanita phalloides. Toxicon. 36 (1): 13–24. doi:10.1016/S0041-0101(97)00074-3. PMID 9604278.

223. Leathem AM, Dorran TJ (March 2007). Poisoning due to raw Gyromitra

esculenta (false morels) west of the Rockies. Cjem. 9 (2): 127–30. doi:10.1017/s1481803500014937. PMID 17391587.

224. Karlson-Stiber C, Persson H (September 2003). Cytotoxic fungi--an overview. Toxicon. 42 (4): 339–49. doi:10.1016/S0041-0101(03)00238-1. PMID 14505933.

225. Michelot D, Melendez-Howell LM (February 2003). Amanita muscaria: chemistry, biology, toxicology, and ethnomycology. Mycological Research. 107 (Pt 2): 131–46. doi:10.1017/S0953756203007305. PMID 12747324.

226. Hall, p. 7.

227. Ammirati JF, McKenny M, Stuntz DE (1987). The New Savory Wild Mushroom. Seattle, Washington: University of Washington Press. pp. xii–xiii. ISBN 0-295-96480-4.

228. López-Gómez J, Molina-Meyer M (February 2006). The competitive exclusion principle versus biodiversity through competitive segregation and further adaptation to spatial heterogeneities. Theoretical Population Biology. 69 (1): 94–109. doi:10.1016/j.tpb.2005.08.004. PMID 16223517.

229. Becker H (1998). Setting the Stage To Screen Biocontrol Fungi. United States Department of Agriculture, Agricultural Research Service. Retrieved 23 February 2009.

230. Keiller TS. Whey-based fungal microfactory technology for enhanced biological pest management using fungi (PDF). UVM Innovations. Retrieved 29 October 2011.

231. Deshpande MV (1999). Mycopesticide production by fermentation: potential and challenges. Critical Reviews in Microbiology. 25 (3): 229–43. doi:10.1080/10408419991299220. PMID 10524330.

232. Thomas MB, Read AF (May 2007). Can fungal biopesticides control malaria?. Nature Reviews. Microbiology. 5 (5): 377–83. doi:10.1038/nrmicro1638. PMID 17426726.

233. Bush LP, Wilkinson HH, Schardl CL (May 1997). Bioprotective Alkaloids of Grass-Fungal Endophyte Symbioses. Plant Physiology. 114 (1): 1–7. doi:10.1104/pp.114.1.1. PMC 158272Freely accessible. PMID 12223685.

234. Bouton JH, Latch GCM, Hill NS, Hoveland CS, McCannc MA, Watson RH, Parish JA, Hawkins LL, Thompson FN (2002). Use of nonergot alkaloid-producing endophytes for alleviating tall fescue toxicosis in sheep. Agronomy Journal. 94: 567–574. Review by Parish JA, McCann MA, Watson RH, Hoveland CS, Hawkins LL, Hill NS, Bouton JH (May 2003). Use of nonergot alkaloid-producing endophytes for alleviating tall fescue toxicosis in sheep. Journal of Animal Science. 81 (5): 1316–22. PMID 12772860.

235. Christian V, Shrivastava R, Shukla D, Modi HA, Vyas BR (April 2005). Degradation of xenobiotic compounds by lignin-degrading white-rot fungi: enzymology and mechanisms involved. Indian Journal of Experimental Biology. 43 (4): 301–12. PMID 15875713.

236. Fungi to fight ‹toxic war zones›. BBC News. 5 May 2008.

237. Fomina M, Charnock JM, Hillier S, Alvarez R, Gadd GM (July 2007). Fungal transformations of uranium oxides. Environmental Microbiology. 9 (7): 1696–710. doi:10.1111/j.1462-2920.2007.01288.x. PMID 17564604.

238. Fomina M, Charnock JM, Hillier S, Alvarez R, Livens F, Gadd GM (May 2008). Role of fungi in the biogeochemical fate of depleted uranium. Current Biology. 18 (9): R375–7. doi:10.1016/j.cub.2008.03.011. PMID 18460315.

239. Beadle GW, Tatum EL (November 1941). Genetic Control of Biochemical Reactions in Neurospora. Proceedings of the National Academy of Sciences of the United States of America. 27 (11): 499–506. Bibcode:1941PNAS...27..499B. doi:10.1073/pnas.27.11.499. PMC 1078370Freely accessible. PMID 16588492.

240. Datta A, Ganesan K, Natarajan K (1989). Current trends in Candida albicans research. Advances in Microbial Physiology. Advances in Microbial Physiology. 30: 53–88. doi:10.1016/S0065-2911(08)60110-1. ISBN 978-0-12-027730-8. PMID 2700541.

241. Dean RA, Talbot NJ, Ebbole DJ, Farman ML, Mitchell TK, Orbach MJ, et al. (April 2005). The genome sequence of the rice blast fungus Magnaporthe grisea. Nature. 434 (7036): 980–6. Bibcode:2005Natur.434..980D. doi:10.1038/nature03449. PMID 15846337.

242. Daly R, Hearn MT (2005). Expression of heterologous proteins in Pichia pastoris: a useful experimental tool in protein engineering and production. Journal of Molecular Recognition. 18 (2): 119–38. doi:10.1002/jmr.687. PMID 15565717.

243. Schlegel HG (1993). General Microbiology. Cambridge, UK: Cambridge University Press. p. 360. ISBN 0-521-43980-9.

244. Joseph B, Ramteke PW, Thomas G (2008). Cold active microbial lipases: some hot issues and recent developments. Biotechnology Advances. 26 (5): 457–70. doi:10.1016/j.biotechadv.2008.05.003. PMID 18571355.

245. Kumar R, Singh S, Singh OV (May 2008). Bioconversion of lignocellulosic biomass: biochemical and molecular perspectives. Journal of Industrial Microbiology & Biotechnology. 35 (5): 377–91. doi:10.1007/s10295-008-0327-8. PMID 18338189.

246. Trichoderma spp., including T. harzianum, T. viride, T. koningii, T. hamatum and other spp. Deuteromycetes, Moniliales (asexual classification system). Biological Control: A Guide to Natural Enemies in North America. Retrieved 10 July 2007.

247. Olempska-Beer ZS, Merker RI, Ditto MD, DiNovi MJ (July 2006). Food-processing enzymes from recombinant microorganisms--a review. Regulatory Toxicology and Pharmacology. 45 (2): 144–158. doi:10.1016/j.yrtph.2006.05.001. PMID 16769167.

248. Polizeli ML, Rizzatti AC, Monti R, Terenzi HF, Jorge JA, Amorim DS (June 2005). Xylanases from fungi: properties and industrial applications. Applied Microbiology and Biotechnology. 67 (5): 577–91. doi:10.1007/s00253-005-1904-7. PMID 15944805.

CHAPTER 4

Virology: Study of Viruses

Chapter Contents

- **Introduction**
- **Virus Structure and Classification**
- **Viral Diseases and Host Defenses**
- **Molecular Biology Research and Viral Therapy**
- **History of Virology**
- **Virus**
- **Origins**
- **Classification**
- **Applications**

Virology is the study of viruses and virus-like agents, including (but not limited to) their taxonomy, disease-producing properties, cultivation and genetics. It is often considered a part of microbiology or pathology. In the early years this discipline was dependent upon advances in the chemical and physical sciences, but viruses soon became tools for probing basic biochemical processes of cells.

Viruses have traditionally been viewed in a rather negative context as agents responsible for disease that must be controlled or eliminated. However, viruses also have certain beneficial properties that can be exploited for useful purposes (for example in gene therapy or vaccinology).

INTRODUCTION

Virology is the study of viruses – submicroscopic, parasitic particles of genetic material contained in a protein coat – and virus-like agents. It focuses on the following aspects of viruses: their structure, classification and evolution, their ways to infect and exploit host cells for reproduction, their interaction with host organism physiology and immunity, the diseases they cause, the techniques to isolate and culture them, and their use in research and therapy. Virology is considered to be a subfield of microbiology or of medicine.

VIRUS STRUCTURE AND CLASSIFICATION

A major branch of virology is virus classification. Viruses can be classified according to the host cell they infect: animal viruses, plant viruses, fungal viruses, and bacteriophages (viruses infecting bacterium, which include the most complex viruses). Another classification uses the geometrical shape of their capsid (often a helix or an icosahedron) or the virus's structure (e.g. presence or absence of a lipid envelope). Viruses range in size from about 30 nm to about 450 nm, which means that most of them cannot be seen with light microscopes. The shape and structure of viruses has been studied by electron microscopy, NMR spectroscopy, and X-ray crystallography.

The most useful and most widely used classification system distinguishes viruses according to the type of nucleic acid they use as genetic material and the viral replication method they employ to coax host cells into producing more viruses:

- DNA viruses (divided into double-stranded DNA viruses and single-stranded DNA viruses),
- RNA viruses (divided into positive-sense single-stranded RNA viruses, negative-sense single-stranded RNA viruses and the much less common double-stranded RNA viruses),
- reverse transcribing viruses (double-stranded reverse-transcribing DNA viruses and single-stranded reverse-transcribing RNA viruses including retroviruses).

The latest report by the International Committee on Taxonomy of Viruses (2005) lists 5450 viruses, organized in over 2,000 species, 287 genera, 73 families and 3 orders.

Virologists also study subviral particles, infectious entities notably smaller and simpler than viruses:

- viroids (naked circular RNA molecules infecting plants),
- satellites (nucleic acid molecules with or without a capsid that require a helper virus for infection and reproduction), and
- prions (proteins that can exist in a pathological conformation that induces other prion molecules to assume that same conformation).

Taxa in virology are not necessarily monophyletic, as the evolutionary relationships of the various virus groups remain unclear. Three hypotheses regarding their origin exist:

- Viruses arose from non-living matter, separately from yet in parallel to cells, perhaps in the form of self-replicating RNA ribozymes similar to viroids.
- Viruses arose by genome reduction from earlier, more competent cellular life forms that became parasites to host cells and subsequently lost most of their functionality; examples of such tiny parasitic prokaryotes are Mycoplasma and Nanoarchaea.

- Viruses arose from mobile genetic elements of cells (such as transposons, retrotransposons or plasmids) that became encapsulated in protein capsids, acquired the ability to "break free" from the host cell and infect other cells.

Of particular interest here is mimivirus, a giant virus that infects amoebae and encodes much of the molecular machinery traditionally associated with bacteria. Is it a simplified version of a parasitic prokaryote, or did it originate as a simpler virus that acquired genes from its host?

The evolution of viruses, which often occurs in concert with the evolution of their hosts, is studied in the field of viral evolution.

While viruses reproduce and evolve, they do not engage in metabolism, do not move, and depend on a host cell for reproduction. The often-debated question of whether they are alive or not is a matter of definition that does not affect the biological reality of viruses.

VIRAL DISEASES AND HOST DEFENSES

One main motivation for the study of viruses is the fact that they cause many important infectious diseases, among them the common cold, influenza, rabies, measles, many forms of diarrhea, hepatitis, Dengue fever, yellow fever, polio, smallpox and AIDS. Herpes simplex causes cold sores and genital herpes and is under investigation as a possible factor in Alzheimer's.

Some viruses, known as oncoviruses, contribute to the development of certain forms of cancer. The best studied example is the association between Human papillomavirus and cervical cancer: almost all cases of cervical cancer are caused by certain strains of this sexually transmitted virus. Another example is the association of infection with hepatitis B and hepatitis C viruses and liver cancer.

Some subviral particles also cause disease: the transmissible spongiform encephalopathies, which include Kuru, Creutzfeldt–Jakob disease and bovine spongiform encephalopathy ("mad cow disease"), are caused by prions, hepatitis D is due to a satellite virus.

The study of the manner in which viruses cause disease is viral pathogenesis. The degree to which a virus causes disease is its virulence.

When the immune system of a vertebrate encounters a virus, it may produce specific antibodies which bind to the virus and neutralize its infectivity or mark it for destruction. Antibody presence in blood serum is often used to determine whether a person has been exposed to a given virus in the past, with tests such as ELISA. Vaccinations protect against viral diseases, in part, by eliciting the production of antibodies. Monoclonal antibodies, specific to the virus, are also used for detection, as in fluorescence microscopy.

A second defense of vertebrates against viruses, cell-mediated immunity, involves immune cells known as T cells: the body's cells constantly display short fragments of their proteins on the cell's surface, and if a T cell recognizes a suspicious viral fragment there, the host cell is destroyed and the virus-specific T-cells proliferate. This mechanism is jump-started by certain vaccinations.

RNA interference, an important cellular mechanism found in plants, animals and many other eukaryotes, most likely evolved as a defense against viruses. An elaborate machinery of interacting enzymes detects double-stranded RNA molecules (which occur as part of the life cycle of many viruses) and then proceeds to destroy all single-stranded versions of those detected RNA molecules.

Every lethal viral disease presents a paradox: killing its host is obviously of no benefit to the virus, so how and why did it evolve to do so? Today it is believed that most viruses are relatively benign in their natural hosts; some viral infection might even be beneficial to the host. The lethal viral diseases are believed to have resulted from an "accidental" jump of the virus from a species in which it is benign to a new one that is not accustomed to it (see zoonosis). For example, viruses that cause serious influenza in humans probably have pigs or birds as their natural host, and HIV is thought to derive from the benign non-human primate virus SIV.

While it has been possible to prevent (certain) viral diseases by vaccination for a long time, the development of antiviral drugs to treat viral diseases is a comparatively recent development. The first such drug was interferon, a substance that is naturally produced when an infection is detected and stimulates other parts of the immune system.

MOLECULAR BIOLOGY RESEARCH AND VIRAL THERAPY

Bacteriophages, the viruses which infect bacteria, can be relatively easily grown as viral plaques on bacterial cultures. Bacteriophages occasionally move genetic material from one bacterial cell to another in a process known as transduction, and this horizontal gene transfer is one reason why they served as a major research tool in the early development of molecular biology. The genetic code, the function of ribozymes, the first recombinant DNA and early genetic libraries were all arrived at using bacteriophages. Certain genetic elements derived from viruses, such as highly effective promoters, are commonly used in molecular biology research today.

Growing animal viruses outside of the living host animal is more difficult. Classically, fertilized chicken eggs have often been used, but cell cultures are increasingly employed for this purpose today.

Since some viruses that infect eukaryotes need to transport their genetic material into the host cell's nucleus, they are attractive tools for introducing new genes into the host (known as transformation or transfection). Modified retroviruses are often used for this purpose, as they integrate their genes into the host's chromosomes.

This approach of using viruses as gene vectors is being pursued in the gene therapy of genetic diseases. An obvious problem to be overcome in viral gene therapy is the rejection of the transforming virus by the immune system.

Phage therapy, the use of bacteriophages to combat bacterial diseases, was a popular research topic before the advent of antibiotics and has recently seen renewed interest.

Oncolytic viruses are viruses that preferably infect cancer cells. While early efforts to employ these viruses in the therapy of cancer failed, there have been reports in 2005 and 2006 of encouraging preliminary results.

Other Uses of Viruses

A new application of genetically engineered viruses in nanotechnology was recently described; see the uses of viruses in material science and nanotechnology. For a use in mapping neurons see the applications of pseudorabies in neuroscience.

HISTORY OF VIROLOGY

The word virus appeared in 1599 and originally meant "venom".

A very early form of vaccination known as variolation was developed several thousand years ago in China. It involved the application of materials from smallpox sufferers in order to immunize others. In 1717 Lady Mary Wortley Montagu observed the practice in Istanbul and attempted to popularize it in Britain, but encountered considerable resistance. In 1796 Edward Jenner developed a much safer method, using cowpox to successfully immunize a young boy against smallpox, and this practice was widely adopted. Vaccinations against other viral diseases followed, including the successful rabies vaccination by Louis Pasteur in 1886. The nature of viruses however was not clear to these researchers.

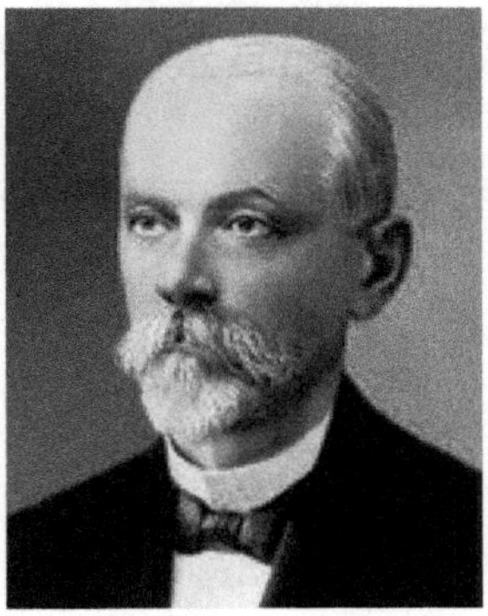

Dmitri Ivanovsky

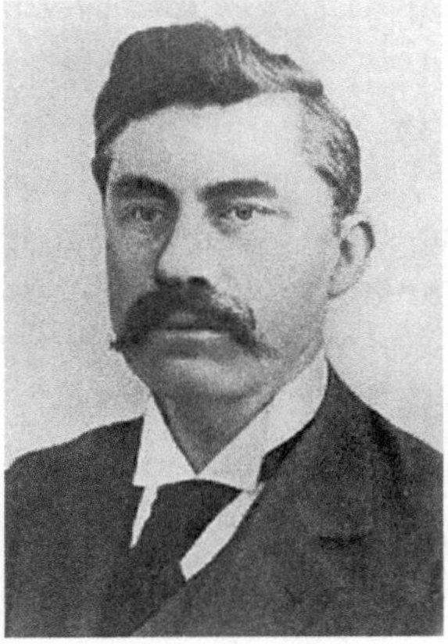

Martinus Beijerinck.

In 1892, the Russian biologist Dmitry Ivanovsky used a Chamberland filter to try to isolate the bacteria that caused tobacco mosaic disease. His experiments showed that crushed leaf extracts from infected tobacco plants remained infectious after filtration. Ivanovsky reported a minuscule infectious agent or toxin, capable of passing the filter, may be being produced by a bacterium.

In 1898 Martinus Beijerinck repeated Ivanovski's work but went further and passed the "filterable agent" from plant to plant, found the action undiminished, and concluded it infectious—replicating in the host—and thus not a mere toxin. He called it contagium vivum fluidum. The question of whether the agent was a "living fluid" or a particle was however still open.

In 1903 it was suggested for the first time that transduction by viruses might cause cancer. In 1908 Bang and Ellerman showed that a filterable virus could transmit chicken leukemia, data largely ignored till the 1930s when leukemia became regarded as cancerous. In 1911 Peyton Rous reported the transmission of chicken sarcoma, a solid tumor, with a virus, and thus Rous became "father of tumor virology". The virus was later called Rous sarcoma virus 1 and understood to be a retrovirus. Several other cancer-causing retroviruses have since been described.

The existence of viruses that infect bacteria (bacteriophages) was first recognized by Frederick Twort in 1911, and, independently, by Félix d'Herelle in 1917. As bacteria could be grown easily in culture, this led to an explosion of virology research.

The cause of the devastating Spanish flu pandemic of 1918 was initially unclear. In late 1918, French scientists showed that a "filter-passing virus" could transmit the disease to people and animals, fulfilling Koch's postulates.

In 1926 it was shown that scarlet fever is caused by a bacterium that is infected by a certain bacteriophage.

While plant viruses and bacteriophages can be grown comparatively easily, animal viruses normally require a living host animal, which complicates their study immensely. In 1931 it was shown that influenza virus could be grown in fertilized chicken eggs, a method that is still used today to produce vaccines. In 1937, Max Theiler managed to grow the yellow fever virus in chicken eggs and produced a vaccine from an attenuated virus strain; this vaccine saved millions of lives and is still being used today.

Max Delbrück, an important investigator in the area of bacteriophages, described the basic "life cycle" of a virus in 1937: rather than "growing", a virus particle is assembled from its constituent pieces in one step; eventually it leaves the host cell to infect other cells. The Hershey–Chase experiment in 1952 showed that only DNA and not protein enters a bacterial cell upon infection with bacteriophage T2. Transduction of bacteria by bacteriophages was first described in the same year.

In 1949 John F. Enders, Thomas Weller and Frederick Robbins reported growth of poliovirus in cultured human embryonal cells, the first significant example of an animal virus grown outside of animals or chicken eggs. This work aided Jonas Salk in deriving a polio vaccine from deactivated polio viruses; this vaccine was shown to be effective in 1955.

The first virus that could be crystalized and whose structure could therefore be elucidated in detail was tobacco mosaic virus (TMV), the virus that had been studied earlier by Ivanovski and Beijerink. In 1935, Wendell Stanley achieved its crystallization for electron microscopy and showed that it remains active even after crystallization. Clear X-ray diffraction pictures of the crystallized virus were obtained by Bernal and Fankuchen in 1941. Based on such pictures, Rosalind Franklin proposed the full structure of the tobacco mosaic virus in 1955. Also in 1955, Heinz Fraenkel-Conrat and Robley Williams showed that purified TMV RNA and its capsid (coat) protein can self-assemble into functional virions, suggesting that this assembly mechanism is also used within the host cell, as Delbrück had proposed earlier.

From the 1950s-60's, Chester M. Southam, a leading virologist and cancer researcher, injected cancer patients, healthy individuals, and prison inmates from the Ohio Penitentiary with HeLa cancer cells in order to observe if cancer could be transmitted. Additionally, in hopes of creating a vaccine for cancer, he observed if the subjects could become immune to cancer by developing an acquired immune response. This experiment was highly controversial, as the cancer patient subjects were unaware that they were being injected with cancer cells.

In 1963, the Hepatitis B virus was discovered by Baruch Blumberg who went on to develop a hepatitis B vaccine.

In 1965, Howard Temin described the first retrovirus: a virus whose RNA genome was reverse transcribed into complementary DNA (cDNA), then integrated into the host's genome and expressed from that template. The viral enzyme reverse transcriptase, which along with integrase is a distinguishing trait of retroviruses, was first described in 1970, independently by Howard Temin and David Baltimore. The first retrovirus infecting humans was identified by Robert Gallo in 1974. Later it was found that reverse transcriptase is not specific to retroviruses; retrotransposons which code for reverse transcriptase are abundant in the genomes of all eukaryotes. About 10-40% of the human genome derives from such retrotransposons.

In 1975 the functioning of oncoviruses was clarified considerably. Until that time, it was thought that these viruses carried certain genes called oncogenes which, when inserted into the host's genome, would cause cancer. Michael Bishop and Harold Varmus showed that the oncogene of Rous sarcoma virus is in fact not specific to the virus but is contained in the genome of healthy animals of many species. The oncovirus can switch this pre-existing benign proto-oncogene on, turning it into a true oncogene that causes cancer.

1976 saw the first recorded outbreak of Ebola virus disease, a highly lethal virally transmitted disease.

In 1977, Frederick Sanger achieved the first complete sequencing of the genome of any organism, the bacteriophage Phi X 174. In the same year, Richard Roberts and Phillip Sharp independently showed that the genes of adenovirus contain introns and therefore require gene splicing. It was later realized that almost all genes of eukaryotes have introns as well.

A worldwide vaccination campaign led by the UN World Health Organization resulted in the eradication of smallpox in 1979.

In 1982, Stanley Prusiner discovered prions and showed that they cause scrapie.

The first cases of AIDS were reported in 1981, and HIV, the retrovirus causing it, was identified in 1983 by Luc Montagnier, Françoise Barré-Sinoussi and Robert Gallo. Tests detecting HIV infection by detecting the presence of HIV antibody were developed. Subsequent tremendous research efforts turned HIV into the best studied virus. Human Herpes Virus 8, the cause of Kaposi's sarcoma which is often seen in AIDS patients, was identified in 1994. Several antiretroviral drugs were developed in the late 1990s, decreasing AIDS mortality dramatically in developed countries.

The Hepatitis C virus was identified using novel molecular cloning techniques in 1987, leading to screening tests that dramatically reduced the incidence of post-transfusion hepatitis.

The first attempts at gene therapy involving viral vectors began in the early 1980s, when retroviruses were developed that could insert a foreign gene into the host's genome. They contained the foreign gene but did not contain the viral genome and therefore could not reproduce. Tests in mice were followed by tests in humans, beginning in 1989. The first human studies attempted to correct the genetic disease severe combined immunodeficiency (SCID), but clinical success was limited. In the period from 1990 to 1995, gene therapy was tried on several other diseases and with different viral vectors, but it became clear that the initially high expectations were overstated. In 1999 a further setback occurred when 18-year-old Jesse Gelsinger died in a gene therapy trial. He suffered a severe immune response after having received an adenovirus vector. Success in the gene therapy of two cases of X-linked SCID was reported in 2000.

In 2002 it was reported that poliovirus had been synthetically assembled in the laboratory, representing the first synthetic organism. Assembling the 7741-base genome from scratch, starting with the virus's published RNA sequence, took about two years. In 2003 a faster method was shown to assemble the 5386-base genome of the bacteriophage Phi X 174 in 2 weeks.

The giant mimivirus, in some sense an intermediate between tiny prokaryotes and ordinary viruses, was described in 2003 and sequenced in 2004.

The strain of Influenza A virus subtype H1N1 that killed up to 50 million people during the Spanish flu pandemic in 1918 was reconstructed in 2005. Sequence information was pieced together from preserved tissue samples of flu victims; viable virus was then synthesized from this sequence. The 2009 flu pandemic involved another strain of Influenza A H1N1, commonly known as "swine flu".

By 1985, Harald zur Hausen had shown that two strains of Human papillomavirus (HPV) cause most cases of cervical cancer. Two vaccines protecting against these strains were released in 2006.

In 2006 and 2007 it was reported that introducing a small number of specific transcription factor genes into normal skin cells of mice or humans can turn these cells into pluripotent stem cells, known as induced pluripotent stem cells. The technique uses modified retroviruses to transform the cells; this is a potential problem for human therapy since these viruses integrate their genes at a random location in the host's genome, which can interrupt other genes and potentially causes cancer.

In 2008, Sputnik virophage was described, the first known virophage: it uses the machinery of a helper virus to reproduce and inhibits reproduction of that helper virus. Sputnik reproduces in amoeba infected by mamavirus, a relative of the mimivirus mentioned above and the largest known virus to date.

An endogenous retrovirus (ERV) is a retrovirus whose genome has been permanently incorporated into the germ-line genome of some organism and that is therefore copied with each reproduction of that organism. It is estimated that about 9 percent of the human genome have their origin in ERVs. In 2015 it was shown that proteins from an ERV are actively expressed in 3-day-old human embryos and appear to play a role in embryonal development and protect embryos from infection by other viruses.

VIRUS

A virus is a small infectious agent that replicates only inside the living cells of other organisms. Viruses can infect all types of life forms, from animals and plants to microorganisms, including bacteria and archaea.

Since Dmitri Ivanovsky's 1892 article describing a non-bacterial pathogen infecting tobacco plants, and the discovery of the tobacco mosaic virus by Martinus Beijerinck in 1898, about 5,000 virus species have been described in detail, although there are millions of types. Viruses are found in almost every ecosystem on Earth and are the most abundant type of biological entity. The study of viruses is known as virology, a sub-speciality of microbiology.

While not inside an infected cell or in the process of infecting a cell, viruses exist in the form of independent particles. These viral particles, also known as virions, consist of two or three parts: (i) the genetic material made from either DNA or RNA, long molecules that carry genetic information; (ii) a protein coat, called the capsid, which surrounds and protects the genetic material; and in some cases (iii) an envelope of lipids that surrounds the protein coat when they are outside a cell. The shapes of these virus particles range from simple helical and icosahedral forms for some virus species to more complex structures for others. Most virus species have virions that are too small to be seen with an optical microscope. The average virion is about one one-hundredth the size of the average bacterium.

The origins of viruses in the evolutionary history of life are unclear: some may have evolved from plasmids—pieces of DNA that can move between cells—while others may have evolved from bacteria. In evolution, viruses are an important means of horizontal gene transfer, which increases genetic diversity. Viruses are considered by some to be a life form, because they carry genetic material, reproduce, and evolve through natural selection. However they lack key characteristics (such as cell structure) that are generally considered necessary to count as life. Because they possess some but not all such qualities, viruses have been described as "organisms at the edge of life", and as replicators.

Viruses spread in many ways; viruses in plants are often transmitted from plant to plant by insects that feed on plant sap, such as aphids; viruses in animals can be carried by blood-sucking insects. These disease-bearing organisms are known as vectors. Influenza viruses are spread by coughing and sneezing. Norovirus and rotavirus, common causes of viral gastroenteritis, are transmitted by the faecal–oral route and are passed from person to person by contact, entering the body in food or water. HIV is one of several viruses transmitted through sexual contact and by exposure to infected blood. The range of host cells that a virus can infect is called its "host range". This can be narrow, meaning a virus is capable of infecting few species, or broad, meaning it is capable of infecting many.

Viral infections in animals provoke an immune response that usually eliminates the infecting virus. Immune responses can also be produced by vaccines, which confer an artificially acquired immunity to the specific viral infection. However, some viruses including those that cause AIDS and viral hepatitis evade these immune responses and result in chronic infections. Antibiotics have no effect on viruses, but several antiviral drugs have been developed.

Etymology

The word is from the Latin neuter vīrus referring to poison and other noxious liquids, from 'the same Indo-European base as Sanskrit vi'a poison, Avestan vīša poison, ancient Greek ἰός poison›, first attested in English in 1398 in John Trevisa›s translation of Bartholomeus Anglicus›s De Proprietatibus Rerum. Virulent, from Latin virulentus (poisonous), dates to c. 1400. A meaning of "agent that causes infectious disease" is first recorded in 1728, before the discovery of viruses by Dmitri Ivanovsky in 1892. The English plural is viruses (sometimes also viri or vira), whereas the Latin word is a mass noun, which has no classically attested plural (however in Neo-Latin vīra is used). The adjective viral dates to 1948. The term virion (plural virions), which dates from 1959, is also used to refer to a single, stable infective viral particle that is released from the cell and is fully capable of infecting other cells of the same type.

ORIGINS

Viruses are found wherever there is life and have probably existed since living cells first evolved. The origin of viruses is unclear because they do not form fossils, so molecular techniques have been used to compare the DNA or RNA of viruses and are a useful means of investigating how they arose. In addition, viral genetic material may occasionally integrate into the germline of the host organisms, by which they can be passed on vertically to the offspring of the host for many generations. This provides an invaluable source of information for paleovirologists to trace back ancient viruses that have existed up to millions of years ago. There are three main hypotheses that aim to explain the origins of viruses:

Regressive Hypothesis

Viruses may have once been small cells that parasitised larger cells. Over time, genes not required by their parasitism were lost. The bacteria rickettsia and chlamydia are living cells that, like viruses, can reproduce only inside host cells. They lend support to this hypothesis, as their dependence on parasitism is likely to have caused the loss of genes that enabled them to survive outside a cell. This is also called the degeneracy hypothesis, or reduction hypothesis.

Cellular Origin Hypothesis

Some viruses may have evolved from bits of DNA or RNA that "escaped" from the genes of a larger organism. The escaped DNA could have come from plasmids (pieces of naked DNA that can move between cells) or transposons (molecules of DNA that replicate and move around to different positions within the genes of the cell). Once called "jumping genes", transposons are examples of mobile genetic elements and could be the origin of some viruses. They were discovered in maize by Barbara McClintock in 1950. This is sometimes called the vagrancy hypothesis, or the escape hypothesis.

Co-Evolution Hypothesis

This is also called the virus-first hypothesis and proposes that viruses may have evolved from complex molecules of protein and nucleic acid at the same time as cells first appeared on Earth and would have been dependent on cellular life for billions of years. Viroids are molecules of RNA that are not classified as viruses because they lack a protein coat. However, they have characteristics that are common to several viruses and are often called subviral agents. Viroids are important pathogens of plants. They do not code for proteins but interact with the host cell and use the host machinery for their replication. The hepatitis delta virus of humans has an RNA genome similar to viroids but has a protein coat derived from hepatitis B virus and cannot produce one of its own. It is, therefore, a defective virus. Although hepatitis delta virus genome may replicate independently once inside a host cell, it requires the help of hepatitis B virus to provide a protein coat so that it can be transmitted to new cells. In similar manner, the sputnik virophage is dependent on mimivirus, which infects the protozoan Acanthamoeba castellanii. These viruses, which are dependent on the presence of other virus species in the host cell, are called satellites and may represent evolutionary intermediates of viroids and viruses.

In the past, there were problems with all of these hypotheses: the regressive hypothesis did not explain why even the smallest of cellular parasites do not resemble viruses in any way. The escape hypothesis did not explain the complex capsids and other structures on virus particles. The virus-first hypothesis contravened the definition of viruses in that they require host cells. Viruses are now recognized as ancient and as having origins that pre-date the divergence of life into the three domains. This discovery has led modern virologists to reconsider and re-evaluate these three classical hypotheses.

The evidence for an ancestral world of RNA cells and computer analysis of viral and host DNA sequences are giving a better understanding of the evolutionary relationships between different viruses and may help identify the ancestors of modern viruses. To date, such analyses have not proved which of these hypotheses is correct. However, it seems unlikely that all currently known viruses have a common ancestor, and viruses have probably arisen numerous times in the past by one or more mechanisms.

Prions are infectious protein molecules that do not contain DNA or RNA. They can cause infections such as scrapie in sheep, bovine spongiform encephalopathy ("mad cow" disease) in cattle, and chronic wasting disease in deer; in humans, prionic diseases include Kuru, Creutzfeldt–Jakob disease, and Gerstmann–Sträussler–Scheinker syndrome. Although prions are fundamentally different from viruses and viroids, their discovery gives credence to the theory that viruses could have evolved from self-replicating molecules.

Microbiology

Life Properties

Opinions differ on whether viruses are a form of life, or organic structures that interact with living organisms. They have been described as "organisms at the edge of life", since they resemble organisms in that they possess genes, evolve by natural selection, and reproduce by creating multiple copies of themselves through self-assembly. Although they have genes, they do not have a cellular structure, which is often seen as the basic unit of life. Viruses do not have their own metabolism, and require a host cell to make new products. They therefore cannot naturally reproduce outside a host cell – although bacterial species such as rickettsia and chlamydia are considered living organisms despite the same limitation. Accepted forms of life use cell division to reproduce, whereas viruses spontaneously assemble within cells. They differ from autonomous growth of crystals as they inherit genetic mutations while being subject to natural selection. Virus self-assembly within host cells has implications for the study of the origin of life, as it lends further credence to the hypothesis that life could have started as self-assembling organic molecules.

Structure

Viruses display a wide diversity of shapes and sizes, called morphologies. In general, viruses are much smaller than bacteria. Most viruses that have been studied have a diameter between 20 and 300 nanometres. Some filoviruses have a total length of up to 1400 nm; their diameters are only about 80 nm. Most viruses cannot be seen with an optical microscope so scanning and transmission electron microscopes are used to visualise virions. To increase the contrast between viruses and the background, electron-dense "stains" are used. These are solutions of salts of heavy metals, such as tungsten, that scatter the electrons from regions covered with the stain. When virions are coated with stain (positive staining), fine detail is obscured. Negative staining overcomes this problem by staining the background only.

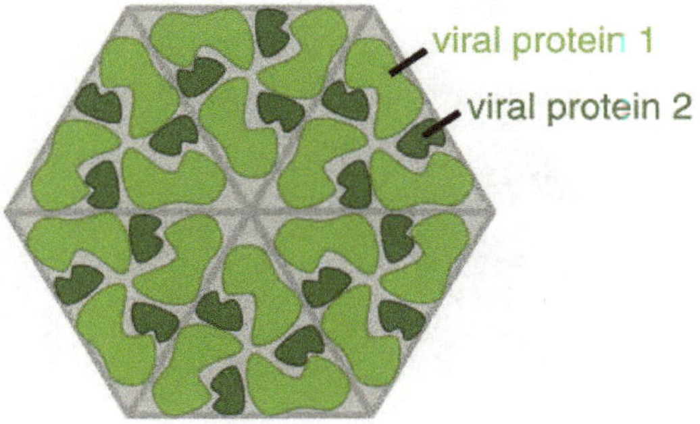

Diagram of how a virus capsid can be constructed using multiple copies of just two protein molecules.

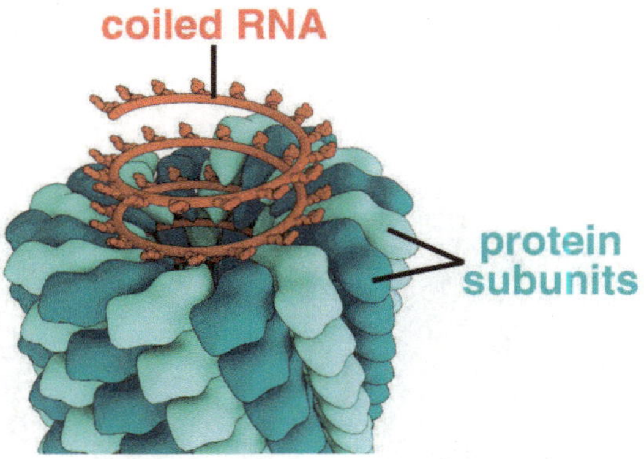

Structure of tobacco mosaic virus: RNA coiled in a helix of repeating protein sub-units.

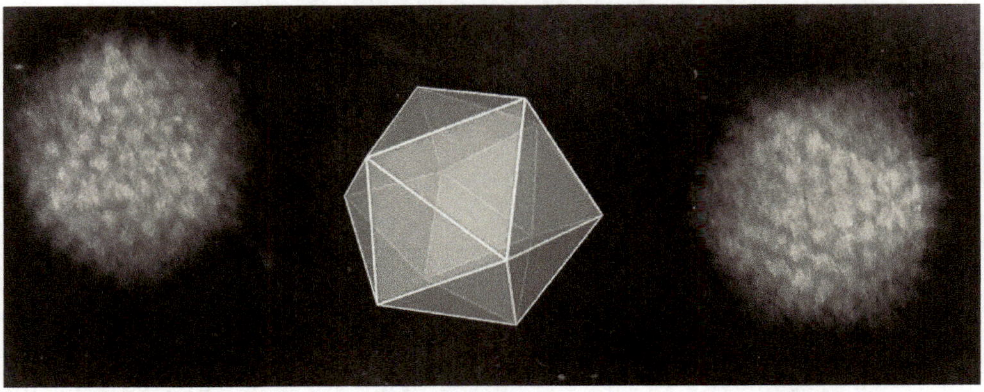

Structure of icosahedral adenovirus. Electron micrograph of with a cartoon to show shape.

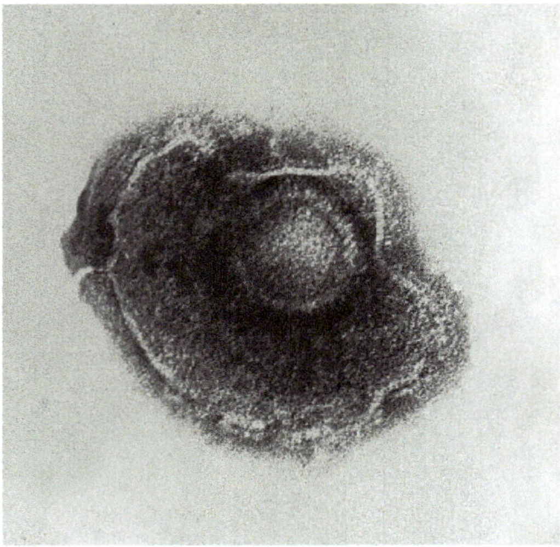

Structure of chickenpox virus. They have a lipid envelope.

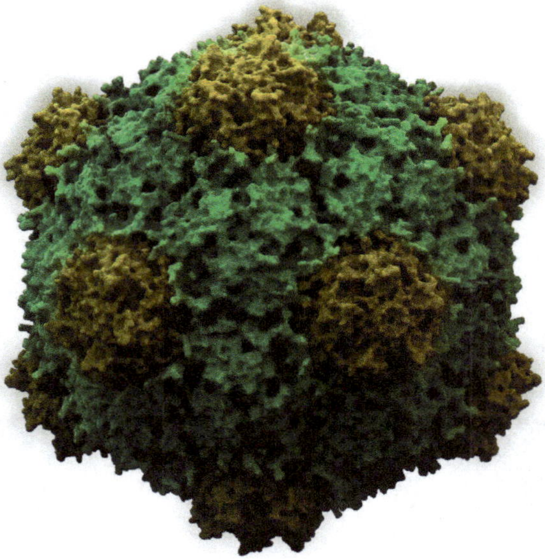

Structure of an icosahedral cowpea mosaic virus.

A complete virus particle, known as a virion, consists of nucleic acid surrounded by a protective coat of protein called a capsid. These are formed from identical protein subunits called capsomeres. Viruses can have a lipid "envelope" derived from the host cell membrane. The capsid is made from proteins encoded by the viral genome and its shape serves as the basis for morphological distinction. Virally coded protein subunits will self-assemble to form a capsid, in general requiring the presence of the virus genome.

Complex viruses code for proteins that assist in the construction of their capsid. Proteins associated with nucleic acid are known as nucleoproteins, and the association of viral capsid proteins with viral nucleic acid is called a nucleocapsid. The capsid and entire virus structure can be mechanically (physically) probed through atomic force microscopy. In general, there are four main morphological virus types:

Helical

These viruses are composed of a single type of capsomere stacked around a central axis to form a helical structure, which may have a central cavity, or tube. This arrangement results in rod-shaped or filamentous virions: These can be short and highly rigid, or long and very flexible. The genetic material, in general, single-stranded RNA, but ssDNA in some cases, is bound into the protein helix by interactions between the negatively charged nucleic acid and positive charges on the protein. Overall, the length of a helical capsid is related to the length of the nucleic acid contained within it and the diameter is dependent on the size and arrangement of capsomeres. The well-studied tobacco mosaic virus is an example of a helical virus.

Icosahedral

Most animal viruses are icosahedral or near-spherical with chiral icosahedral symmetry. A regular icosahedron is the optimum way of forming a closed shell from identical sub-units. The minimum number of identical capsomeres required is twelve, each composed of five identical sub-units. Many viruses, such as rotavirus, have more than twelve capsomers and appear spherical but they retain this symmetry. Capsomeres at the apices are surrounded by five other capsomeres and are called pentons. Capsomeres on the triangular faces are surrounded by six others and are called hexons. Hexons are in essence flat and pentons, which form the 12 vertices, are curved. The same protein may act as the subunit of both the pentamers and hexamers or they may be composed of different proteins.

Prolate

This is an icosahedron elongated along the fivefold axis and is a common arrangement of the heads of bacteriophages. This structure is composed of a cylinder with a cap at either end.

Envelope

Some species of virus envelop themselves in a modified form of one of the cell membranes, either the outer membrane surrounding an infected host cell or internal membranes such as nuclear membrane or endoplasmic reticulum, thus gaining an outer lipid bilayer known as a viral envelope. This membrane is studded with proteins coded for by the viral genome and host genome; the lipid membrane itself and any carbohydrates present originate entirely from the host. The influenza virus and HIV use this strategy. Most enveloped viruses are dependent on the envelope for their infectivity.

Complex

These viruses possess a capsid that is neither purely helical nor purely icosahedral, and that may possess extra structures such as protein tails or a complex outer wall. Some bacteriophages, such as Enterobacteria phage T4, have a complex structure consisting of an icosahedral head bound to a helical tail, which may have a hexagonal base plate with protruding protein tail fibres. This tail structure acts like a molecular syringe, attaching to the bacterial host and then injecting the viral genome into the cell.

The poxviruses are large, complex viruses that have an unusual morphology. The viral genome is associated with proteins within a central disc structure known as a nucleoid. The nucleoid is surrounded by a membrane and two lateral bodies of unknown function. The virus has an outer envelope with a thick layer of protein studded over its surface. The whole virion is slightly pleiomorphic, ranging from ovoid to brick shape. Mimivirus is one of the largest characterised viruses, with a capsid diameter of 400 nm. Protein filaments measuring 100 nm project from the surface. The capsid appears hexagonal under an electron microscope, therefore the capsid is probably icosahedral. In 2011, researchers discovered the largest then known virus in samples of water collected from the ocean floor off the coast of Las Cruces, Chile. Provisionally named Megavirus chilensis, it can be seen with a basic optical microscope. In 2013, the Pandoravirus genus was discovered in Chile and Australia, and has genomes about twice as large as Megavirus and Mimivirus.

Some viruses that infect Archaea have complex structures that are unrelated to any other form of virus, with a wide variety of unusual shapes, ranging from spindle-shaped structures, to viruses that resemble hooked rods, teardrops or even bottles. Other archaeal viruses resemble the tailed bacteriophages, and can have multiple tail structures.

Genome

Genomic diversity among viruses	
Property	**Parameters**
Nucleic acid	• DNA • RNA • Both DNA and RNA (at different stages in the life cycle)
Shape	• Linear • Circular • Segmented

Strandedness	• Single-stranded • Double-stranded • Double-stranded with regions of single-strandedness
Sense	• Positive sense (+) • Negative sense (−) • Ambisense (+/−)

An enormous variety of genomic structures can be seen among viral species; as a group, they contain more structural genomic diversity than plants, animals, archaea, or bacteria. There are millions of different types of viruses, although only about 5,000 types have been described in detail. As of September 2015, the NCBI Virus genome database has more than 75,000 complete genome sequences. but there are doubtlessly many more to be discovered.

A virus has either a **DNA** or an **RNA** genome and is called a DNA virus or an RNA virus, respectively. The vast majority of viruses have RNA genomes. Plant viruses tend to have single-stranded RNA genomes and bacteriophages tend to have double-stranded DNA genomes.

Viral genomes are circular, as in the polyomaviruses, or linear, as in the adenoviruses. The type of nucleic acid is irrelevant to the shape of the genome. Among RNA viruses and certain DNA viruses, the genome is often divided up into separate parts, in which case it is called segmented. For RNA viruses, each segment often codes for only one protein and they are usually found together in one capsid. However, all segments are not required to be in the same virion for the virus to be infectious, as demonstrated by brome mosaic virus and several other plant viruses.

A viral genome, irrespective of nucleic acid type, is almost always either single-stranded or double-stranded. Single-stranded genomes consist of an unpaired nucleic acid, analogous to one-half of a ladder split down the middle. Double-stranded genomes consist of two complementary paired nucleic acids, analogous to a ladder. The virus particles of some virus families, such as those belonging to the Hepadnaviridae, contain a genome that is partially double-stranded and partially single-stranded.

For most viruses with RNA genomes and some with single-stranded DNA genomes, the single strands are said to be either positive-sense (called the plus-strand) or negative-sense (called the minus-strand), depending on if they are complementary to the viral messenger RNA (mRNA). Positive-sense viral RNA is in the same sense as viral mRNA and thus at least a part of it can be immediately translated by the host cell. Negative-sense viral RNA is complementary to mRNA and thus must be converted to positive-sense RNA by an RNA-dependent RNA polymerase before translation. DNA nomenclature for viruses with single-sense genomic ssDNA is similar to RNA nomenclature, in that the template strand for the viral mRNA is complementary to it (−), and the coding strand is a copy of it (+). However, several types of ssDNA and ssRNA viruses have genomes that are ambisense in that transcription can occur off both strands in a double-stranded replicative intermediate. Examples include geminiviruses, which are ssDNA plant viruses and arenaviruses, which are ssRNA viruses of animals.

Genome size varies greatly between species. The smallest viral genomes – the ssDNA circoviruses, family Circoviridae – code for only two proteins and have a genome size of only two kilobases; the largest–the pandoraviruses–have genome sizes of around two megabases which code for about 2500 proteins. Virus genes rarely have introns and often are arranged in the genome so that they overlap.

In general, RNA viruses have smaller genome sizes than DNA viruses because of a higher error-rate when replicating, and have a maximum upper size limit. Beyond this limit, errors in the genome when replicating render the virus useless or uncompetitive. To compensate for this, RNA viruses often have segmented genomes – the genome is split into smaller molecules – thus reducing the chance that an error in a single-component genome will incapacitate the entire genome. In contrast, DNA viruses generally have larger genomes because of the high fidelity of their replication enzymes. Single-strand DNA viruses are an exception to this rule, however, as mutation rates for these genomes can approach the extreme of the ssRNA virus case.

Genetic Mutation

Viruses undergo genetic change by several mechanisms. These include a process called antigenic drift where individual bases in the DNA or RNA mutate to other bases. Most of these point mutations are "silent" – they do not change the protein that the gene encodes – but others can confer evolutionary advantages such as resistance to antiviral drugs. Antigenic shift occurs when there is a major change in the genome of the virus. This can be a result of recombination or reassortment. When this happens with influenza viruses, pandemics might result. RNA viruses often exist as quasispecies or swarms of viruses of the same species but with slightly different genome nucleoside sequences. Such quasispecies are a prime target for natural selection.

Segmented genomes confer evolutionary advantages; different strains of a virus with a segmented genome can shuffle and combine genes and produce progeny viruses or (offspring) that have unique characteristics. This is called reassortment or viral sex.

Genetic recombination is the process by which a strand of DNA is broken and then joined to the end of a different DNA molecule. This can occur when viruses infect cells simultaneously and studies of viral evolution have shown that recombination has been rampant in the species studied. Recombination is common to both RNA and DNA viruses.

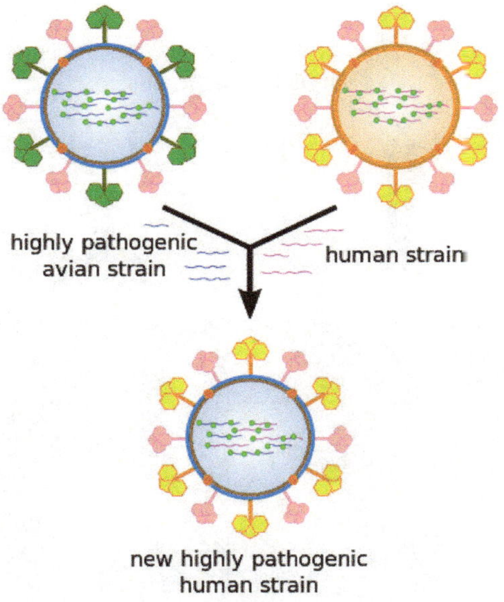

How antigenic shift, or reassortment, can result in novel and highly pathogenic strains of human flu.

Replication Cycle

Viral populations do not grow through cell division, because they are acellular. Instead, they use the machinery and metabolism of a host cell to produce multiple copies of themselves, and they assemble in the cell.

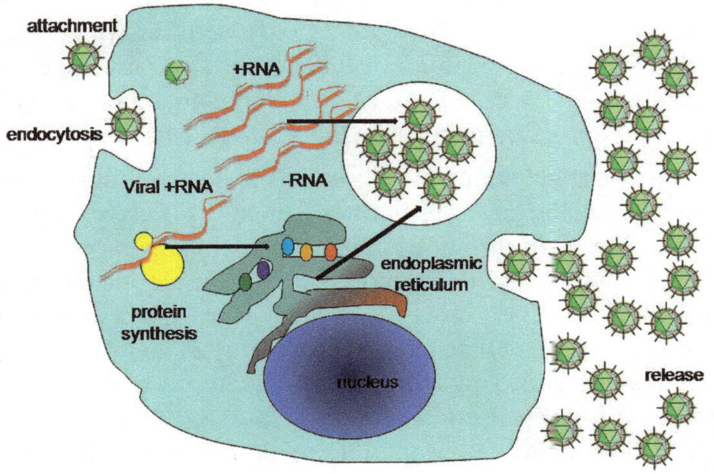

A typical virus replication cycle.

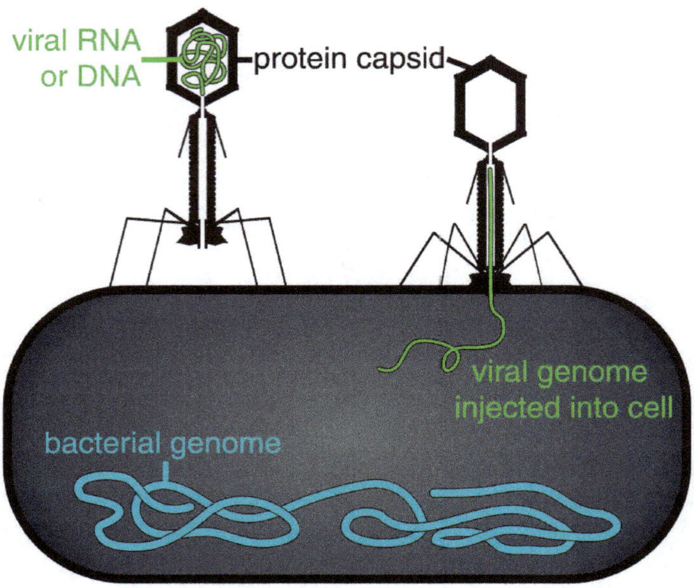

Some bacteriophages inject their genomes into bacterial cells (not to scale).

The life cycle of viruses differs greatly between species but there are six basic stages in the life cycle of viruses:

Attachment is a specific binding between viral capsid proteins and specific receptors on the host cellular surface. This specificity determines the host range of a virus. For example, HIV infects a limited range of human leucocytes. This is because its surface protein, gp120, specifically interacts with the CD4 molecule – a chemokine receptor – which is most commonly found on the surface of CD4+ T-Cells. This mechanism has evolved to favour those viruses that infect only cells in which they are capable of replication. Attachment to the receptor can induce the viral envelope protein to undergo changes that results in the fusion of viral and cellular membranes, or changes of non-enveloped virus surface proteins that allow the virus to enter.

Penetration follows attachment: Virions enter the host cell through receptor-mediated endocytosis or membrane fusion. This is often called viral entry. The infection of plant and fungal cells is different from that of animal cells. Plants have a rigid cell wall made of cellulose, and fungi one of chitin, so most viruses can get inside these cells only after trauma to the cell wall. However, nearly all plant viruses (such as tobacco mosaic virus) can also move directly from cell to cell, in the form of single-stranded nucleoprotein complexes, through pores called plasmodesmata. Bacteria, like plants, have strong cell walls that a virus must breach to infect the cell. However, given that bacterial cell walls are much less thick than plant cell walls due to their much smaller size, some viruses have evolved mechanisms that inject their genome into the bacterial cell across the cell wall, while the viral capsid remains outside.

Uncoating is a process in which the viral capsid is removed: This may be by degradation by viral enzymes or host enzymes or by simple dissociation; the end-result is the releasing of the viral genomic nucleic acid.

Replication of viruses involves primarily multiplication of the genome. Replication involves synthesis of viral messenger RNA (mRNA) from "early" genes (with exceptions for positive sense RNA viruses), viral protein synthesis, possible assembly of viral proteins, then viral genome replication mediated by early or regulatory protein expression. This may be followed, for complex viruses with larger genomes, by one or more further rounds of mRNA synthesis: "late" gene expression is, in general, of structural or virion proteins.

Assembly – Following the structure-mediated self-assembly of the virus particles, some modification of the proteins often occurs. In viruses such as HIV, this modification (sometimes called maturation) occurs after the virus has been released from the host cell.

Release – Viruses can be released from the host cell by lysis, a process that kills the cell by bursting its membrane and cell wall if present: This is a feature of many bacterial and some animal viruses. Some viruses undergo a lysogenic cycle where the viral genome is incorporated by genetic recombination into a specific place in the host's chromosome. The viral genome is then known as a "provirus" or, in the case of bacteriophages a "prophage". Whenever the host divides, the viral genome is also replicated. The viral genome is mostly silent within the host. However, at some point, the provirus or prophage may give rise to active virus, which may lyse the host cells. Enveloped viruses (e.g., HIV) typically are released from the host cell by budding. During this process the virus acquires its envelope, which is a modified piece of the host's plasma or other, internal membrane.

Genome Replication

The genetic material within virus particles, and the method by which the material is replicated, varies considerably between different types of viruses.

DNA Viruses

The genome replication of most DNA viruses takes place in the cell's nucleus. If the cell has the appropriate receptor on its surface, these viruses enter the cell sometimes by direct fusion with the cell membrane (e.g., herpesviruses) or – more usually – by receptor-mediated endocytosis. Most DNA viruses are entirely dependent on the host cell's DNA and RNA synthesizing machinery, and RNA processing machinery. However, viruses with larger genomes may encode much of this machinery themselves. In eukaryotes the viral genome must cross the cell's nuclear membrane to access this machinery, while in bacteria it need only enter the cell.

RNA Viruses

Replication usually takes place in the cytoplasm. RNA viruses can be placed into four different groups depending on their modes of replication. The polarity (whether or not it can be used directly by ribosomes to make proteins) of single-stranded RNA viruses largely determines the replicative mechanism; the other major criterion is whether the genetic material is single-stranded or double-stranded. All RNA viruses use their own RNA replicase enzymes to create copies of their genomes.

Reverse Transcribing Viruses

These have ssRNA (Retroviridae, Metaviridae, Pseudoviridae) or dsDNA (Caulimoviridae, and Hepadnaviridae) in their particles. Reverse transcribing viruses with RNA genomes (retroviruses), use a DNA intermediate to replicate, whereas those with DNA genomes (pararetroviruses) use an RNA intermediate during genome replication. Both types use a reverse transcriptase, or RNA-dependent DNA polymerase enzyme, to carry out the nucleic acid conversion. Retroviruses integrate the DNA produced by reverse transcription into the host genome as a provirus as a part of the replication process; pararetroviruses do not, although integrated genome copies of especially plant pararetroviruses can give rise to infectious virus. They are susceptible to antiviral drugs that inhibit the reverse transcriptase enzyme, e.g. zidovudine and lamivudine. An example of the first type is HIV, which is a retrovirus. Examples of the second type are the Hepadnaviridae, which includes Hepatitis B virus.

Effects on the Host Cell

The range of structural and biochemical effects that viruses have on the host cell is extensive. These are called cytopathic effects. Most virus infections eventually result in the death of the host cell. The causes of death include cell lysis, alterations to the cell's surface membrane and apoptosis. Often cell death is caused by cessation of its normal activities because of suppression by virus-specific proteins, not all of which are components of the virus particle.

Some viruses cause no apparent changes to the infected cell. Cells in which the virus is latent and inactive show few signs of infection and often function normally. This causes persistent infections and the virus is often dormant for many months or years. This is often the case with herpes viruses. Some viruses, such as Epstein–Barr virus, can cause cells to proliferate without causing malignancy, while others, such as papillomaviruses, are established causes of cancer.

Host Range

Viruses are by far the most abundant biological entities on Earth and they outnumber all the others put together. They infect all types of cellular life including animals, plants, bacteria and fungi. However, different types of viruses can infect only a limited range of hosts and many are species-specific. Some, such as smallpox virus for example, can infect only one species – in this case humans, and are said to have a narrow host range. Other viruses, such as rabies virus, can infect different species of mammals and are said to have a broad range. The viruses that infect plants are harmless to animals, and most viruses that infect other animals are harmless to humans. The host range of some bacteriophages is limited to a single strain of bacteria and they can be used to trace the source of outbreaks of infections by a method called phage typing.

CLASSIFICATION

Classification seeks to describe the diversity of viruses by naming and grouping them on the basis of similarities. In 1962, André Lwoff, Robert Horne, and Paul Tournier were the first to develop a means of virus classification, based on the Linnaean hierarchical system. This system bases classification on phylum, class, order, family, genus, and species. Viruses were grouped according to their shared properties (not those of their hosts) and the type of nucleic acid forming their genomes. Later the International Committee on Taxonomy of Viruses was formed. However, viruses are not classified on the basis of phylum or class, as their small genome size and high rate of mutation makes it difficult to determine their ancestry beyond order. As such, the Baltimore classification is used to supplement the more traditional hierarchy.

ICTV Classification

The International Committee on Taxonomy of Viruses (ICTV) developed the current classification system and wrote guidelines that put a greater weight on certain virus properties to maintain family uniformity. A unified taxonomy (a universal system for classifying viruses) has been established. The 9th ICTV Report defines the concept of the virus species as the lowest taxon (group) in a branching hierarchy of viral taxa. However, at present only a small part of the total diversity of viruses has been studied, with analyses of samples from humans finding that about 20% of the virus sequences recovered have not been seen before, and samples from the environment, such as from seawater and ocean sediments, finding that the large majority of sequences are completely novel.

The general taxonomic structure is as follows:

Order (-virales)

Family (-viridae)

Subfamily (-virinae)

Genus (-virus)

Species (-virus)

In the current (2013) ICTV taxonomy, 7 orders have been established, the Caudovirales, Herpesvirales, Ligamenvirales, Mononegavirales, Nidovirales, Picornavirales, and Tymovirales. The committee does not formally distinguish between subspecies, strains, and isolates. In total there are 7 orders, 103 families, 22 subfamilies, 455 genera, about 2,827 species and over 4,000 types yet unclassified.

Baltimore Classification

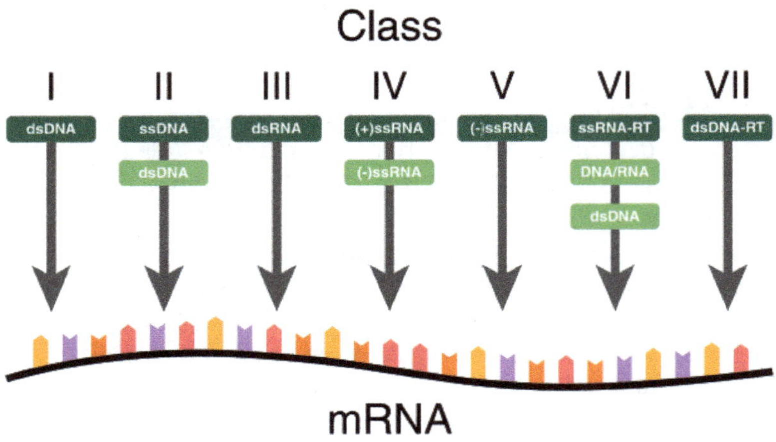

The Baltimore Classification of viruses is based on the method of viral mRNA synthesis.

The Nobel Prize-winning biologist David Baltimore devised the Baltimore classification system. The ICTV classification system is used in conjunction with the Baltimore classification system in modern virus classification.

The Baltimore classification of viruses is based on the mechanism of mRNA production. Viruses must generate mRNAs from their genomes to produce proteins and replicate themselves, but different mechanisms are used to achieve this in each virus family. Viral genomes may be single-stranded (ss) or double-stranded (ds), RNA or DNA, and may or may not use reverse transcriptase (RT). In addition, ssRNA viruses may be either sense (+) or antisense (−). This classification places viruses into seven groups:

- I: dsDNA viruses (e.g. Adenoviruses, Herpesviruses, Poxviruses)
- II: ssDNA viruses (+ strand or "sense") DNA (e.g. Parvoviruses)
- III: dsRNA viruses (e.g. Reoviruses)
- IV: (+)ssRNA viruses (+ strand or sense) RNA (e.g. Picornaviruses, Togaviruses)
- V: (−)ssRNA viruses (− strand or antisense) RNA (e.g. Orthomyxoviruses, Rhabdoviruses)
- VI: ssRNA-RT viruses (+ strand or sense) RNA with DNA intermediate in life-cycle (e.g. Retroviruses)
- VII: dsDNA-RT viruses (e.g. Hepadnaviruses)

As an example of viral classification, the chicken pox virus, varicella zoster (VZV), belongs to the order Herpesvirales, family Herpesviridae, subfamily Alphaherpesvirinae, and genus Varicellovirus. VZV is in Group I of the Baltimore Classification because it is a dsDNA virus that does not use reverse transcriptase.

The complete set of viruses in an organism or habitat is called the virome; for example, all human viruses constitute the human virome.

Role in Human Disease

Examples of common human diseases caused by viruses include the common cold, influenza, chickenpox, and cold sores. Many serious diseases such as Ebola virus disease, AIDS, avian influenza, and SARS are caused by viruses. The relative ability of viruses to cause disease is described in terms of virulence. Other diseases are under investigation to discover if they have a virus as the causative agent, such as the possible connection between human herpesvirus 6 (HHV6) and neurological diseases such as multiple sclerosis and chronic fatigue syndrome. There is controversy over whether the bornavirus, previously thought to cause neurological diseases in horses, could be responsible for psychiatric illnesses in humans.

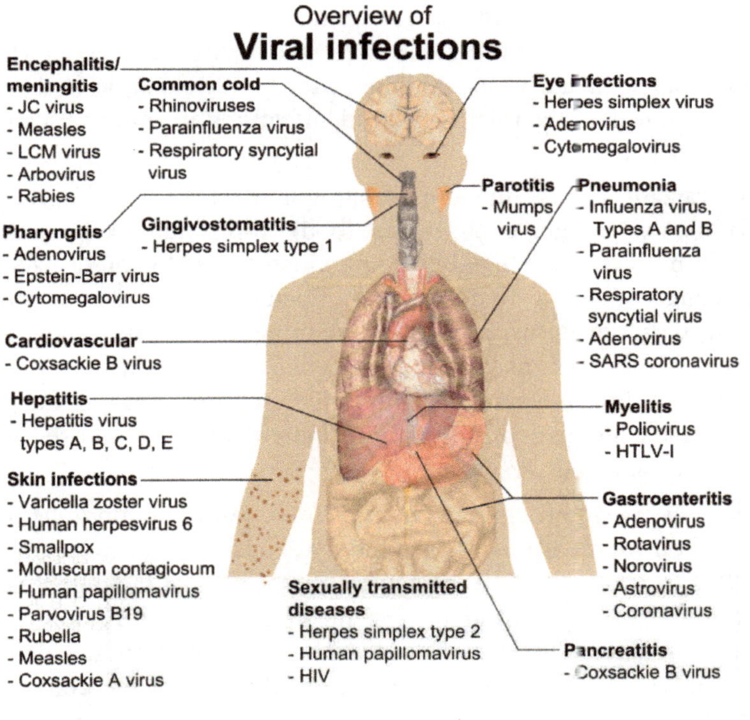

Overview of the main types of viral infection and the most notable species involved.

Viruses have different mechanisms by which they produce disease in an organism, which depends largely on the viral species. Mechanisms at the cellular level primarily include cell lysis, the breaking open and subsequent death of the cell. In multicellular organisms, if enough cells die, the whole organism will start to suffer the effects. Although viruses cause disruption of healthy homeostasis, resulting in disease, they may exist relatively harmlessly within an organism. An example would include the ability of the herpes simplex virus, which causes cold sores, to remain in a dormant state within the human body. This is called latency and is a characteristic of the herpes viruses, including Epstein–Barr virus, which causes glandular fever, and varicella zoster virus, which causes chickenpox and shingles. Most people have been infected with at least one of these types of herpes virus. However, these latent viruses might sometimes be beneficial, as the presence of the virus can increase immunity against bacterial pathogens, such as Yersinia pestis.

Some viruses can cause lifelong or chronic infections, where the viruses continue to replicate in the body despite the host's defence mechanisms. This is common in hepatitis B virus and hepatitis C virus infections. People chronically infected are known as carriers, as they serve as reservoirs of infectious virus. In populations with a high proportion of carriers, the disease is said to be endemic.

Epidemiology

Viral epidemiology is the branch of medical science that deals with the transmission and control of virus infections in humans. Transmission of viruses can be vertical, which means from mother to child, or horizontal, which means from person to person. Examples of vertical transmission include hepatitis B virus and HIV, where the baby is born already infected with the virus. Another, more rare, example is the varicella zoster virus, which, although causing relatively mild infections in humans, can be fatal to the foetus and newborn baby.

Horizontal transmission is the most common mechanism of spread of viruses in populations. Transmission can occur when: body fluids are exchanged during sexual activity, e.g., HIV; blood is exchanged by contaminated transfusion or needle sharing, e.g., hepatitis C; exchange of saliva by mouth, e.g., Epstein–Barr virus; contaminated food or water is ingested, e.g., norovirus; aerosols containing virions are inhaled, e.g., influenza virus; and insect vectors such as mosquitoes penetrate the skin of a host, e.g., dengue. The rate or speed of transmission of viral infections depends on factors that include population density, the number of susceptible individuals, (i.e., those not immune), the quality of healthcare and the weather.

Epidemiology is used to break the chain of infection in populations during outbreaks of viral diseases. Control measures are used that are based on knowledge of how the virus is transmitted. It is important to find the source, or sources, of the outbreak and to identify the virus. Once the virus has been identified, the chain of transmission can sometimes be broken by vaccines. When vaccines are not available, sanitation and disinfection can be effective. Often, infected people are isolated from the rest of the community, and those that have been exposed to the virus are placed in quarantine. To control the outbreak of foot-and-mouth disease in cattle in Britain in 2001, thousands of cattle were slaughtered. Most viral infections of humans and other animals have incubation periods during which the infection causes no signs or symptoms. Incubation periods for viral diseases range from a few days to weeks, but are known for most infections. Somewhat overlapping, but mainly following the incubation period, there is a period of communicability — a time when an infected individual or animal is contagious and can infect another person or animal. This, too, is known for many viral infections, and knowledge of the length of both periods is important in the control of outbreaks. When outbreaks cause an unusually high proportion of cases in a population, community, or region, they are called epidemics. If outbreaks spread worldwide, they are called pandemics.

Epidemics and Pandemics

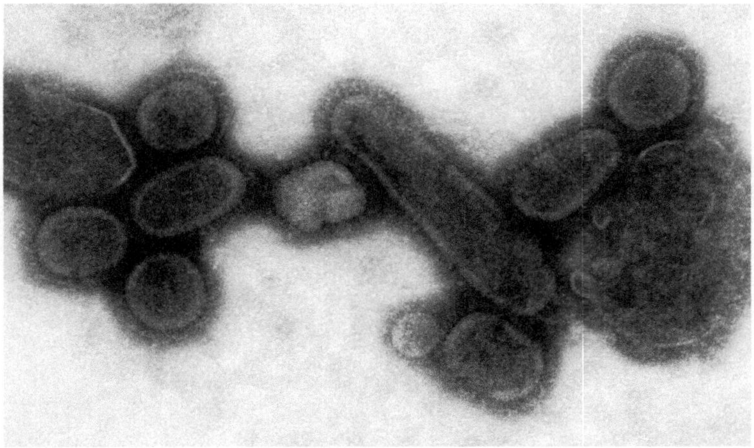

Transmission electron microscope image of a recreated 1918 influenza virus.

Native American populations were devastated by contagious diseases, in particular, smallpox, brought to the Americas by European colonists. It is unclear how many Native Americans were killed by foreign diseases after the arrival of Columbus in the Americas, but the numbers have been estimated to be close to 70% of the indigenous population. The damage done by this disease significantly aided European attempts to displace and conquer the native population.

A pandemic is a worldwide epidemic. The 1918 flu pandemic, which lasted until 1919, was a category 5 influenza pandemic caused by an unusually severe and deadly influenza A virus. The victims were often healthy young adults, in contrast to most influenza outbreaks, which predominantly affect juvenile, elderly, or otherwise-weakened patients. Older estimates say it killed 40–50 million people, while more recent research suggests that it may have killed as many as 100 million people, or 5% of the world's population in 1918.

Most researchers believe that HIV originated in sub-Saharan Africa during the 20th century; it is now a pandemic, with an estimated 38.6 million people now living with the disease worldwide. The Joint United Nations Programme on HIV/AIDS (UNAIDS) and the World Health Organization (WHO) estimate that AIDS has killed more than 25 million people since it was first recognised on 5 June 1981, making it one of the most destructive epidemics in recorded history. In 2007 there were 2.7 million new HIV infections and 2 million HIV-related deaths.

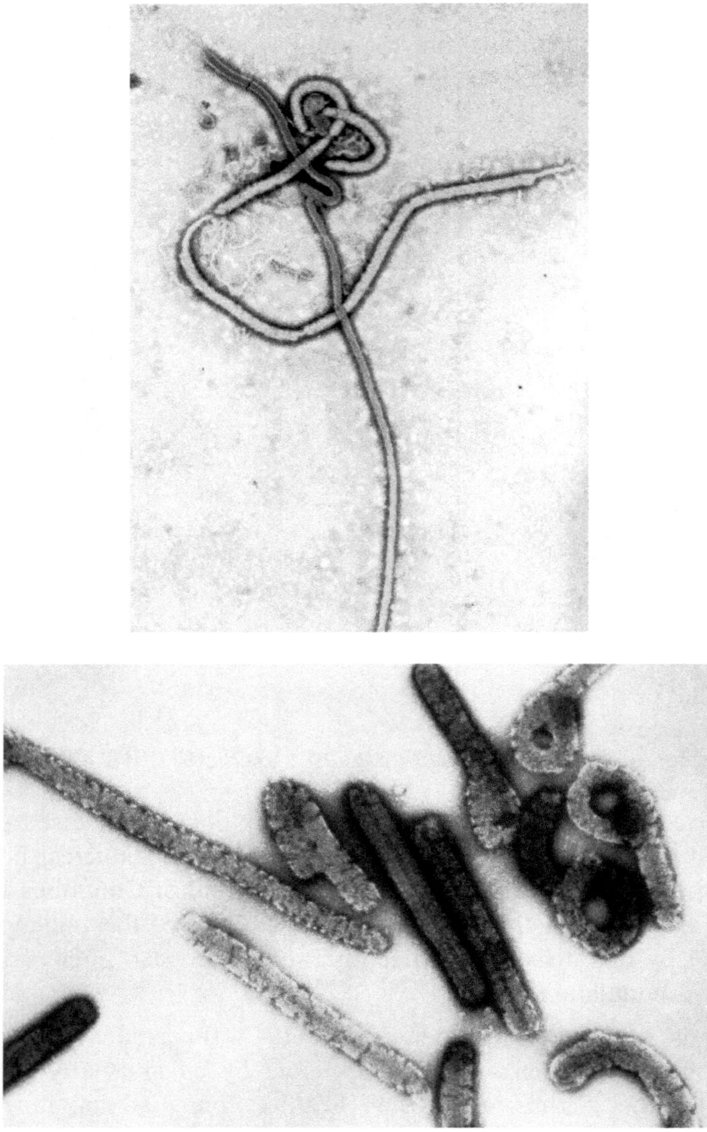

Ebola (top) and Marburg viruses (bottom).

Several highly lethal viral pathogens are members of the Filoviridae. Filoviruses are filament-like viruses that cause viral hemorrhagic fever, and include ebolaviruses and marburgviruses. Marburg virus, first discovered in 1967, attracted widespread press attention in April 2005 for an outbreak in Angola.Ebola Virus Disease has also caused intermittent outbreaks with high mortality rates since 1976 when it was first identified. The worst and most recent one is the West Africa epidemic.

Cancer

Viruses are an established cause of cancer in humans and other species. Viral cancers occur only in a minority of infected persons (or animals). Cancer viruses come from a range of virus families, including both RNA and DNA viruses, and so there is no single type of "oncovirus" (an obsolete term originally used for acutely transforming retroviruses). The development of cancer is determined by a variety of factors such as host immunity and mutations in the host.Viruses accepted to cause human cancers include some genotypes of human papillomavirus, hepatitis B virus, hepatitis C virus, Epstein–Barr virus, Kaposi's sarcoma-associated herpesvirus and human T-lymphotropic virus. The most recently discovered human cancer virus is a polyomavirus (Merkel cell polyomavirus) that causes most cases of a rare form of skin cancer called Merkel cell carcinoma. Hepatitis viruses can develop into a chronic viral infection that leads to liver cancer. Infection by human T-lymphotropic virus can lead to tropical spastic paraparesis and adult T-cell leukaemia. Human papillomaviruses are an established cause of cancers of cervix, skin, anus, and penis. Within the Herpesviridae, Kaposi's sarcoma-associated herpesvirus causes Kaposi's sarcoma and body-cavity lymphoma, and Epstein–Barr virus causes Burkitt's lymphoma, Hodgkin's lymphoma, B lymphoproliferative disorder, and nasopharyngeal carcinoma. Merkel cell polyomavirus closely related to SV40 and mouse polyomaviruses that have been used as animal models for cancer viruses for over 50 years.

Host Defence Mechanisms

The body's first line of defence against viruses is the innate immune system. This comprises cells and other mechanisms that defend the host from infection in a non-specific manner. This means that the cells of the innate system recognize, and respond to, pathogens in a generic way, but, unlike the adaptive immune system, it does not confer long-lasting or protective immunity to the host.

RNA interference is an important innate defence against viruses. Many viruses have a replication strategy that involves double-stranded RNA (dsRNA). When such a virus infects a cell, it releases its RNA molecule or molecules, which immediately bind to a protein complex called a dicer that cuts the RNA into smaller pieces. A biochemical pathway – the RISC complex, is activated, which ensures cell survival by degrading the viral mRNA. Rotaviruses have evolved to avoid this defence mechanism by not uncoating fully inside the cell, and releasing newly produced mRNA through pores in the particle's inner capsid. Their genomic dsRNA remains protected inside the core of the virion.

When the adaptive immune system of a vertebrate encounters a virus, it produces specific antibodies that bind to the virus and often render it non-infectious. This is called humoral immunity. Two types of antibodies are important. The first, called IgM, is highly effective at neutralizing viruses but is produced by the cells of the immune system only for a few weeks. The second, called IgG, is produced indefinitely. The presence of IgM in the blood of the host is used to test for acute infection, whereas IgG indicates an infection sometime in the past. IgG antibody is measured when tests for immunity are carried out.

Antibodies can continue to be an effective defence mechanism even after viruses have managed to gain entry to the host cell. A protein that is in cells, called TRIM21, can attach to the antibodies on the surface of the virus particle. This primes the subsequent destruction of the virus by the enzymes of the cell's proteosome system.

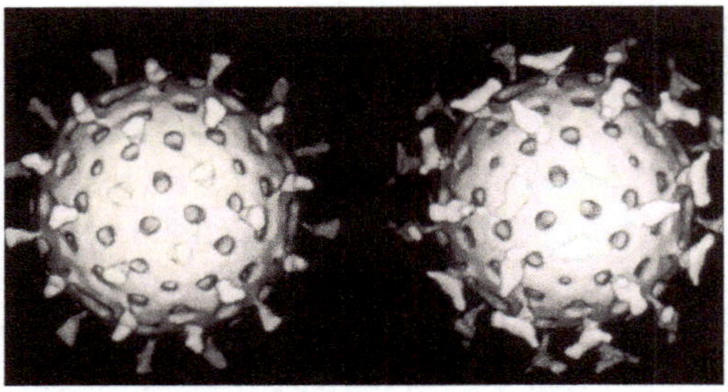

Two rotaviruses: the one on the right is coated with antibodies that stop its attaching to cells and infecting them.

A second defence of vertebrates against viruses is called cell-mediated immunity and involves immune cells known as T cells. The body's cells constantly display short fragments of their proteins on the cell's surface, and, if a T cell recognises a suspicious viral fragment there, the host cell is destroyed by killer T cells and the virus-specific T-cells proliferate. Cells such as the macrophage are specialists at this antigen presentation. The production of interferon is an important host defence mechanism. This is a hormone produced by the body when viruses are present. Its role in immunity is complex; it eventually stops the viruses from reproducing by killing the infected cell and its close neighbours.

Not all virus infections produce a protective immune response in this way. HIV evades the immune system by constantly changing the amino acid sequence of the proteins on the surface of the virion. This is known as "escape mutation" as the viral epitopes escape recognition by the host immune response. These persistent viruses evade immune control by sequestration, blockade of antigen presentation, cytokine resistance, evasion of natural killer cell activities, escape from apoptosis, and antigenic shift. Other viruses, called neurotropic viruses, are disseminated by neural spread where the immune system may be unable to reach them.

Prevention and Treatment

Because viruses use vital metabolic pathways within host cells to replicate, they are difficult to eliminate without using drugs that cause toxic effects to host cells in general. The most effective medical approaches to viral diseases are vaccinations to provide immunity to infection, and antiviral drugs that selectively interfere with viral replication.

Vaccines

Vaccination is a cheap and effective way of preventing infections by viruses. Vaccines were used to prevent viral infections long before the discovery of the actual viruses. Their use has resulted in a dramatic decline in morbidity (illness) and mortality (death) associated with viral infections such as polio, measles, mumps and rubella. Smallpox infections have been eradicated. Vaccines are available to prevent over thirteen viral infections of humans, and more are used to prevent viral infections of animals. Vaccines can consist of live-attenuated or killed viruses, or viral proteins (antigens). Live vaccines contain weakened forms of the virus, which do not cause the disease but, nonetheless, confer immunity. Such viruses are called attenuated. Live vaccines can be dangerous when given to people with a weak immunity (who are described as immunocompromised), because in these people, the weakened virus can cause the original disease. Biotechnology and genetic engineering techniques are used to produce subunit vaccines. These vaccines use only the capsid proteins of the virus. Hepatitis B vaccine is an example of this type of vaccine. Subunit vaccines are safe for immunocompromised patients because they cannot cause the disease. The yellow fever virus vaccine, a live-attenuated strain called 17D, is probably the safest and most effective vaccine ever generated.

Antiviral Drugs

Antiviral drugs are often nucleoside analogues (fake DNA building-blocks), which viruses mistakenly incorporate into their genomes during replication The life-cycle of the virus is then halted because the newly synthesised DNA is inactive. This is because these analogues lack the hydroxyl groups, which, along with phosphorus atoms, link together to form the strong "backbone" of the DNA molecule. This is called DNA chain termination. Examples of nucleoside analogues are aciclovir for Herpes simplex virus infections and lamivudine for HIV and Hepatitis B virus infections. Aciclovir is one of the oldest and most frequently prescribed antiviral drugs. Other antiviral drugs in use target different stages of the viral life cycle. HIV is dependent on a proteolytic enzyme called the HIV-1 protease for it to become fully infectious. There is a large class of drugs called protease inhibitors that inactivate this enzyme.

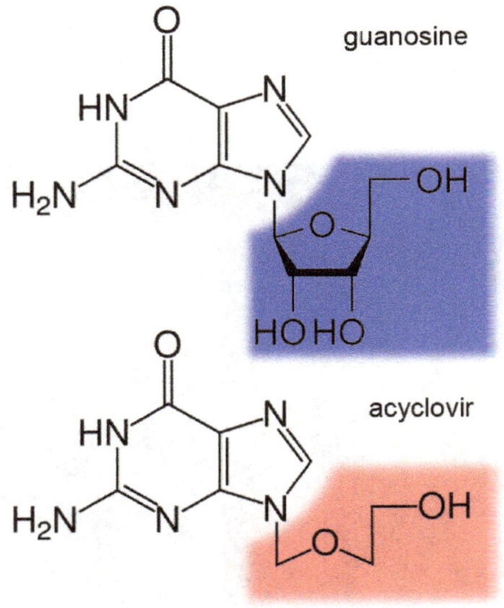

The structure of the DNA base guanosine and the antiviral drug acyclovir.

Hepatitis C is caused by an RNA virus. In 80% of people infected, the disease is chronic, and without treatment, they are infected for the remainder of their lives. However, there is now an effective treatment that uses the nucleoside analogue drug ribavirin combined with interferon. The treatment of chronic carriers of the hepatitis B virus by using a similar strategy using lamivudine has been developed.

Infection in other species

Viruses infect all cellular life and, although viruses occur universally, each cellular species has its own specific range that often infect only that species. Some viruses, called satellites, can replicate only within cells that have already been infected by another virus.

Animal Viruses

Viruses are important pathogens of livestock. Diseases such as foot-and-mouth disease and bluetongue are caused by viruses. Companion animals such as cats, dogs, and horses, if not vaccinated, are susceptible to serious viral infections. Canine parvovirus is caused by a small DNA virus and infections are often fatal in pups. Like all invertebrates, the honey bee is susceptible to many viral infections. However, most viruses co-exist harmlessly in their host and cause no signs or symptoms of disease.

Plant Viruses

There are many types of plant virus, but often they cause only a loss of yield, and it is not economically viable to try to control them. Plant viruses are often spread from plant to plant by organisms, known as vectors. These are normally insects, but some fungi, nematode worms, and single-celled organisms have been shown to be vectors. When control of plant virus infections is considered economical, for perennial fruits, for example, efforts are concentrated on killing the vectors and removing alternate hosts such as weeds. Plant viruses cannot infect humans and other animals because they can reproduce only in living plant cells.

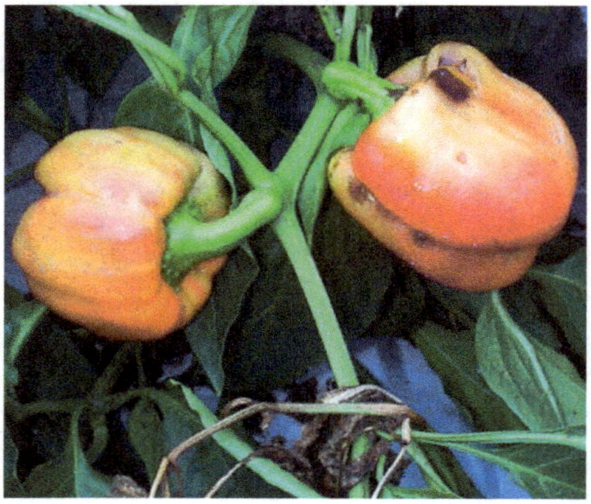

Peppers infected by mild mottle virus.

Plants have elaborate and effective defence mechanisms against viruses. One of the most effective is the presence of so-called resistance (R) genes. Each R gene confers resistance to a particular virus by triggering localised areas of cell death around the infected cell, which can often be seen with the unaided eye as large spots. This stops the infection from spreading. RNA interference is also an effective defence in plants. When they are infected, plants often produce natural disinfectants that kill viruses, such as salicylic acid, nitric oxide, and reactive oxygen molecules.

Plant virus particles or virus-like particles (VLPs) have applications in both biotechnology and nanotechnology. The capsids of most plant viruses are simple and robust structures and can be produced in large quantities either by the infection of plants or by expression in a variety of heterologous systems. Plant virus particles can be modified genetically and chemically to encapsulate foreign material and can be incorporated into supramolecular structures for use in biotechnology.

Bacterial Viruses

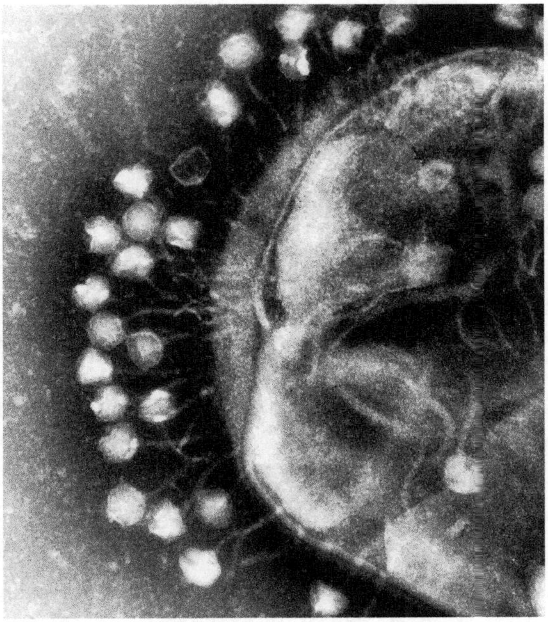

Transmission electron micrograph of multiple bacteriophages attached to a bacterial cell wall.

Bacteriophages are a common and diverse group of viruses and are the most abundant form of biological entity in aquatic environments – there are up to ten times more of these viruses in the oceans than there are bacteria, reaching levels of 250,000,000 bacteriophages per millilitre of seawater.These viruses infect specific bacteria by binding to surface receptor molecules and then entering the cell. Within a short amount of time, in some cases just minutes, bacterial polymerase starts translating viral mRNA into protein. These proteins go on to become either new virions within the cell, helper proteins, which help assembly of new virions, or proteins involved in cell lysis. Viral enzymes aid in the breakdown of the cell membrane, and, in the case of the T4 phage, in just over twenty minutes after injection over three hundred phages could be released.

The major way bacteria defend themselves from bacteriophages is by producing enzymes that destroy foreign DNA. These enzymes, called restriction endonucleases, cut up the viral DNA that bacteriophages inject into bacterial cells. Bacteria also contain a system that uses CRISPR sequences to retain fragments of the genomes of viruses that the bacteria have come into contact with in the past, which allows them to block the virus's replication through a form of RNA interference. This genetic system provides bacteria with acquired immunity to infection.

Archaean Viruses

Some viruses replicate within archaea: these are double-stranded DNA viruses with unusual and sometimes unique shapes. These viruses have been studied in most detail in the thermophilic archaea, particularly the orders Sulfolobales and Thermoproteales. Defences against these viruses involve RNA interference from repetitive DNA sequences within archaean genomes that are related to the genes of the viruses. Most archaea have CRISPR–Cas systems as an adaptive defence against viruses. These enable archaea to retain sections of viral DNA, which are then used to target and eliminate subsequent infections by the virus using a process similar to RNA interference.

Role in Aquatic Ecosystems

A teaspoon of seawater contains about one million viruses. Most of these are bacteriophages, which are harmless to plants and animals, and are in fact essential to the regulation of saltwater and freshwater ecosystems. They infect and destroy bacteria in aquatic microbial communities, and are the most important mechanism of recycling carbon in the marine environment. The organic molecules released from the dead bacterial cells stimulate fresh bacterial and algal growth. Viral activity may also contribute to the biological pump, the process whereby carbon is sequestered in the deep ocean.

Microorganisms constitute more than 90% of the biomass in the sea. It is estimated that viruses kill approximately 20% of this biomass each day and that there are 15 times as many viruses in the oceans as there are bacteria and archaea. Viruses are the main agents responsible for the rapid destruction of harmful algal blooms, which often kill other marine life. The number of viruses in the oceans decreases further offshore and deeper into the water, where there are fewer host organisms.

Like any organism, marine mammals are susceptible to viral infections. In 1988 and 2002, thousands of harbour seals were killed in Europe by phocine distemper virus. Many other viruses, including caliciviruses, herpesviruses, adenoviruses and parvoviruses, circulate in marine mammal populations.

Role in Evolution

Viruses are an important natural means of transferring genes between different species, which increases genetic diversity and drives evolution. It is thought that viruses played a central role in the early evolution, before the diversification of bacteria, archaea and eukaryotes, at the time of the last universal common ancestor of life on Earth. Viruses are still one of the largest reservoirs of unexplored genetic diversity on Earth.

APPLICATIONS

Life Sciences and Medicine

Viruses are important to the study of molecular and cell biology as they provide simple systems that can be used to manipulate and investigate the functions of cells. The study and use of viruses have provided valuable information about aspects of cell biology. For example, viruses have been useful in the study of genetics and helped our understanding of the basic mechanisms of molecular genetics, such as DNA replication, transcription, RNA processing, translation, protein transport, and immunology.

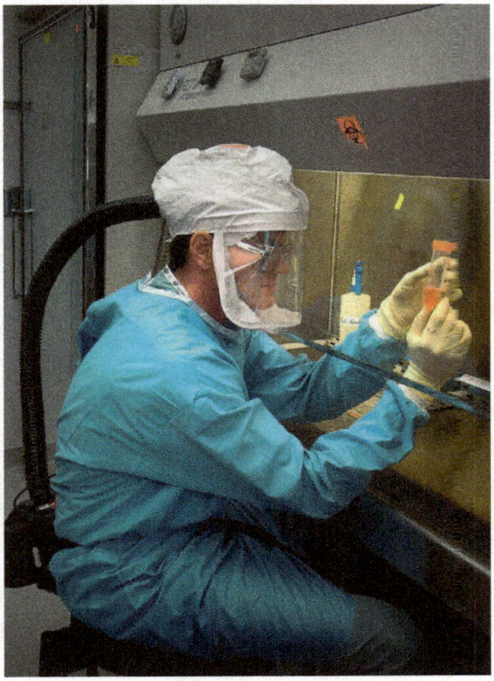

Scientist studying the H5N1 influenza virus.

Geneticists often use viruses as vectors to introduce genes into cells that they are studying. This is useful for making the cell produce a foreign substance, or to study the effect of introducing a new gene into the genome. In similar fashion, virotherapy uses viruses as vectors to treat various diseases, as they can specifically target cells and DNA. It shows promising use in the treatment of cancer and in gene therapy. Eastern European scientists have used phage therapy as an alternative to antibiotics for some time, and interest in this approach is increasing, because of the high level of antibiotic resistance now found in some pathogenic bacteria. Expression of heterologous proteins by viruses is the basis of several manufacturing processes that are currently being used for the production of various proteins such as vaccine antigens and antibodies. Industrial processes have been recently developed using viral vectors and a number of pharmaceutical proteins are currently in pre-clinical and clinical trials.

Virotherapy

Virotherapy involves the use of genetically modified viruses to treat diseases. Viruses have been modified by scientists to reproduce in cancer cells and destroy them but not infect healthy cells. Talimogene laherparepvec (T-VEC), for example, is a modified herpes simplex virus that has had a gene, which is required for viruses to replicate in healthy cells, deleted and replaced with a human gene (GM-CSF) that stimulates immunity. When this virus infects cancer cells, it destroys them and in doing so the presence the GM-CSF gene attracts dendritic cells from the surrounding tissues of the body. The dendritic cells process the dead cancer cells and present components of them to other cells of the immune system. Having completed successful clinical trials, this virus is expected to gain approval for the treatment of a skin cancer called melanoma in late 2015. Viruses that have been reprogrammed to kill cancer cells are called oncolytic viruses.

Materials Science and Nanotechnology

Current trends in nanotechnology promise to make much more versatile use of viruses. From the viewpoint of a materials scientist, viruses can be regarded as organic nanoparticles. Their surface carries specific tools designed to cross the barriers of their host cells. The size and shape of viruses, and the number and nature of the functional groups on their surface, is precisely defined. As such, viruses are commonly used in materials science as scaffolds for covalently linked surface modifications. A particular quality of viruses is that they can be tailored by directed evolution. The powerful techniques developed by life sciences are becoming the basis of engineering approaches towards nanomaterials, opening a wide range of applications far beyond biology and medicine.

Because of their size, shape, and well-defined chemical structures, viruses have been used as templates for organising materials on the nanoscale. Recent examples include work at the Naval Research Laboratory in Washington, D.C., using Cowpea mosaic virus (CPMV) particles to amplify signals in DNA microarray based sensors. In this application, the virus particles separate the fluorescent dyes used for signalling to prevent the formation of non-fluorescent dimers that act as quenchers. Another example is the use of CPMV as a nanoscale breadboard for molecular electronics.

Synthetic Viruses

Many viruses can be synthesised de novo ("from scratch") and the first synthetic virus was created in 2002. Although somewhat of a misconception, it is not the actual virus that is synthesised, but rather its DNA genome (in case of a DNA virus), or a cDNA copy of its genome (in case of RNA viruses). For many virus families the naked synthetic DNA or RNA (once enzymatically converted back from the synthetic cDNA) is infectious when introduced into a cell. That is, they contain all the necessary information to produce new viruses. This technology is now being used to investigate novel vaccine strategies. The ability to synthesise viruses has far-reaching consequences, since viruses can no longer be regarded as extinct, as long as the information of their genome sequence is known and permissive cells are available. As of March 2014, the full-length genome sequences of 3843 different viruses, including smallpox, are publicly available in an online database maintained by the National Institutes of Health.

Weapons

The ability of viruses to cause devastating epidemics in human societies has led to the concern that viruses could be weaponised for biological warfare. Further concern was raised by the successful recreation of the infamous 1918 influenza virus in a laboratory. Smallpox virus devastated numerous societies throughout history before its eradication. There are only two centers in the world that are authorized by the WHO to keep stocks of smallpox virus: the Vector Institute in Russia and the Centers for Disease Control and Prevention in the United States. Fears that it may be used as a weapon may not be totally unfounded. As the vaccine for smallpox sometimes had severe side-effects, it is no longer used routinely in any country. Thus, much of the modern human population has almost no established resistance to smallpox, and would be vulnerable to the virus.

REFERENCES

1. Crawford, Dorothy (2011). Viruses: A Very Short Introduction. New York, NY: Oxford University Press. p. 4. ISBN 0199574855.
2. Cann, Alan (2011). Principles of Molecular Virology (5 ed.). London: Academic Press. ISBN 978-0123849397.
3. "Prion Diseases". CDC. Retrieved 2016-03-25.
4. Evans, Alfred (1982). Viral Infections of Humans. New York, NY: Plenum Publishing Corporation. p. xxv-xxxi. ISBN 0306406764.
5. Lövheim H, Gilthorpe J, Adolfsson R, Nilsson LG, Elgh F (July 2014). "Reactivated herpes simplex infection increases the risk of Alzheimer's disease.". Alzheimer's & Dementia. 11 (6): 593–9. doi:10.1016/j.jalz.2014.04.522. PMID 25043910.
6. 1 Moved | Prion Diseases | CDC

7. Dimmock NJ, Easton AJ, Leppard K, Introduction to Modern Virology, (Oxford: Blackwell Publishers, 2007), ch 23 "Horizons in human virology", subch 23.3 "Subtle and insidious virus-host interactions", sec "Virus infections can give their host an evolutionary advantage", p 432.
8. Stanley Maloy. "Horizontal Gene Transfer". Retrieved 2016-03-25.
9. Viruses: The new cancer hunters, IsraCast, 1 March 2006
10. "Virus", Merriam-Webster, Inc, 2011.
11. Sussman, Max; Topley, W. W. C.; Wilson, Graham K.; Collier, L. H.; Balows, Albert (1998). Topley & Wilson's microbiology and microbial infections. London: Arnold. p. 3. ISBN 0-340-66316-2.
12. Iwanowski, D. (1892). "Über die Mosaikkrankheit der Tabakspflanze". Bulletin Scientifique publié par l'Académie Impériale des Sciences de Saint-Pétersbourg / Nouvelle Serie III (in German and Russian). St. Petersburg. 35: 67—70. Translated into English in Johnson, J., Ed. (1942) Phytopathological classics (St. Paul, Minnesota: American Phytopathological Society) No. 7, pp. 27—30.
13. Iwanowski, D. (1903). "Über die Mosaikkrankheit der Tabakspflanze". Zeitschrift für Pflanzenkrankheiten und Pflanzenschutz (in German). 13: 1–41.
14. Pennazio S (2007). "Genetics and virology: Two interdisciplinary branches of biology". Rivista di Biologia. 100 (1): 119–46. PMID 17592822.
15. Van Epps HL (2005). "Peyton Rous: Father of the tumor virus" (PDF). Journal of Experimental Medicine. 201 (3): 320. doi:10.1084/jem.2013fta. PMC 2213042Freely accessible. PMID 15756727.
16. The Medical and Scientific Conceptions of Influenza, Human Virology at Stanford
17. Skloot, Rebecca (2010). The Immortal Life of Henrietta Lacks. New York: Broadway Paperbacks. p. 128.
18. Montagnier L (2002). "Historical essay. A History of HIV Discovery". Science. 298 (5599): 1727–8. doi:10.1126/science.1079027. PMID 12459575.
19. Gallo RC (2002). "Historical essay. The Early Years of HIV/AIDS". Science. 298 (5599): 1728–30. doi:10.1126/science.1078050. PMID 12459576.
20. Gallo RC, Montagnier L (2002). "Historical essay. Prospects for the Future". Science. 298 (5599): 1730–1. doi:10.1126/science.1079864. PMID 12459577.
21. 2000 Albert Lasker Award for Clinical Medical Research Archived October 28, 2007, at the Wayback Machine., The Lasker Foundation. Accessed 20 February 2008
22. Debyser Zeger (2003). "A Short Course on Virology / Vectorology / Gene Therapy" (PDF). Current Gene Therapy. 3: 495–499.
23. Kolata, Gina (2005-10-06). "Experts Unlock Clues to Spread of 1918 Flu Virus". The New York Times. ISSN 0362-4331. Retrieved 2008-02-03.
24. Stem Cells—This Time without the Cancer, Scientific American News, 30 November 2007

25. "Biggest Known Virus Yields First-Ever Virophage". Microbe Magazine. November 2008. Archived from the original on July 22, 2011.

26. "Virus hiding in our genome protects early human embryos". New Scientist. 20 April 2015.

CHAPTER 5

Parasitology the Study of Parasites

Chapter Contents

- **Introduction**
- **Fields**
- **Conservation Biology of Parasites**
- **Taxonomy and Phylogenetics**
- **History**

Parasitology is the study of parasites, organisms that live, grow, and feed on or in other organisms. The prevention of parasite-infested consumption of raw (or undercooked) meat, fish, seafood, vegetables, and dairy products, as well as contaminated water, is a matter of public health. The United States Food and Drug Administration (FDA), the Centers for Disease Control (CDC), and several other local and state sanitary agencies are responsible for regulatory food safety measures and regular inspections of food and water quality to prevent the outbreak of epidemics caused by parasites and other pathogens .

INTRODUCTION

Parasitology is the study of parasites, their hosts, and the relationship between them. As a biological discipline, the scope of parasitology is not determined by the organism or environment in question, but by their way of life. This means it forms a synthesis of other disciplines, and draws on techniques from fields such as cell biology, bioinformatics, biochemistry, molecular biology, immunology, genetics, evolution and ecology.

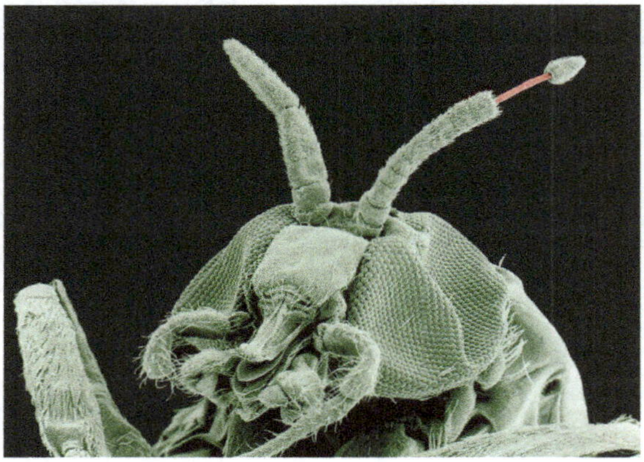

Adult black fly (*Simulium yahense*) with (*Onchocerca volvulus*) emerging from the insect's antenna. The parasite is responsible for the disease known as river blindness in Africa. Sample was chemically fixed and critical point dried, then observed using conventional scanning electron microscopy. Magnified 100×.

FIELDS

The study of these diverse organisms means that the subject is often broken up into simpler, more focused units, which use common techniques, even if they are not studying the same organisms or diseases. Much research in parasitology falls somewhere between two or more of these definitions. In general, the study of prokaryotes falls under the field of bacteriology rather than parasitology.

Medical Parasitology

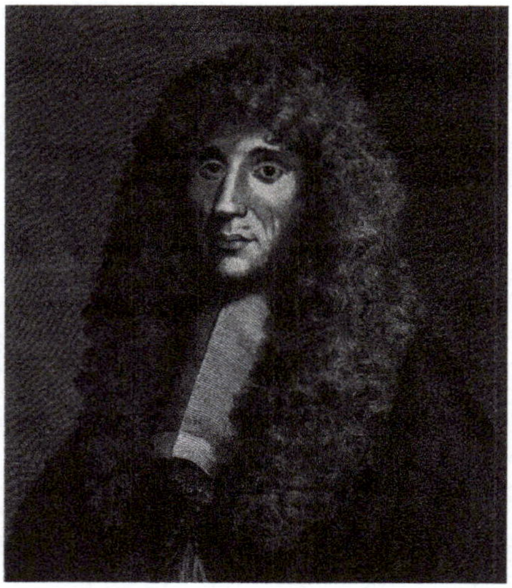

The Italian Francesco Redi, considered to be the father of modern parasitology, he was the first to recognize and correctly describe details of many important parasites.

"Humans are hosts to nearly 300 species of parasitic worms and over 70 species of protozoa, some derived from our primate ancestors and some acquired from the animals we have domesticated or come in contact with during our relatively short history on Earth".

One of the largest fields in parasitology, medical parasitology is the subject which deals with the parasites that infect humans, the diseases caused by them, clinical picture and the response generated by humans against them. It is also concerned with the various methods of their diagnosis, treatment and finally their prevention & control. A parasite is an organism that live on or within another organism called the host . These include organisms such as:

- *Plasmodium* spp., the protozoan parasite which causes malaria. The four species of malaria parasites infective to humans are *Plasmodium falciparum*,*Plasmodium malariae*, *Plasmodium vivax* & *Plasmodium ovale*.
- *Leishmania donovani*, the unicellular organism which causes leishmaniasis
- *Entamoeba* and *Giardia*, which cause intestinal infections (dysentery and diarrhoea)
- Multicellular organisms and intestinal worms (helminths) such as *Schistosoma* spp., *Wuchereria bancrofti*, *Necator americanus* (hookworm) and *Taenia* spp. (tapeworm)
- Ectoparasites such as ticks, scabies and lice

Medical parasitology can involve drug development, epidemiological studies and study of zoonoses.

Veterinary Parasitology

Veterinary parasitology is the study of animal parasites, especially relationships between parasites and animal hosts. Parasites of domestic animals, (livestock and pet animals), as well as wildlife animals are considered. Veterinary parasitologists study the genesis and development of parasitoses in animal hosts, as well as the taxonomy and systematics of parasites, including the morphology, life cycles, and living needs of parasites in the environment and in animal hosts. Using a variety of research methods, they diagnose, treat, and prevent animal parasitoses. Data obtained from parasitological research in animals helps in veterinary practice and improves animal breeding. The major goal of veterinary parasitology is to protect animals and improve their health, but because a number of animal parasites are transmitted to humans, veterinary parasitology is also important for public health.

Diagnostic Methods

Various methods are used to identify parasites in animals, using feces, blood, and tissue samples from the host animal.

Coprological

Coprological examinations involve examining the feces of animals to identify and count parasite eggs. Some common methods include fecal flotation and sedimentation to separate eggs from fecal matter. Others include the McMaster method, which uses a special two-chamber slide that allows parasite eggs to be more clearly visible and easily counted. It is most commonly used to monitor parasites in horses and other grazing and livestock animals. The Baermann method is similar but requires more specialized equipment and more time and is typically used to diagnose lungworm and threadworm.

Haematological

Haematological examinations involve examining the blood of animals to determine the presence of parasites. Blood parasites tend to inhabit the erythrocytes or white blood cells and are most likely to be detected during the acute phase of infection. Veterinary parasitologists use blood smears, which involve placing a drop of blood onto a slide and spreading it over the surface in a thin film in order to examine it under a microscope. The blood is stained with a dye in order for the cells to be easily distinguished.

Histopathological

Histopathological examinations involve examining tissue samples from animals. A small slice of the organ suspected of being infected by parasites is mounted on a slide, stained, and examined under a microscope.

Though not technically considered a histopathological technique, skin scraping – which involves taking a small sample of the epidermal cells of a dog, cat, or other household pet – is commonly used to detect the presence of mites.

Immunological

Immunological examinations, such as indirect immunofluorescence, ELISA, Immunoblotting (Western blot), and Complement fixation test are methods of identifying different kinds of parasites by detecting the presence of their antigens on or within the parasite itself. These diagnostic methods are used in conjunction with coprological examinations for more specific identification of different parasite species in fecal samples.

Molecular Biological

Molecular biological methods involve studying the DNA of the parasite in order to identify it. PCR and RFLP are used to detect and amplify parasite DNA found in the feces, blood, or tissue of the host. These techniques are very sensitive, which is useful for diagnosing parasites even when they are present in very low numbers; they are also useful for identifying parasites not only in large animal hosts but smaller insect vectors.

Structural Parasitology

Structural parasitology is the study of the structures of proteins of parasites. It applies the techniques of structural biology (such as X-ray crystallography or NMR) to determine the 3-D structures of protein molecules involved in a parasitic relationship. One goal is to distinguish the workings of functional pathways in these organisms in comparison to humans. More importantly, it is hoped that structures of parasite proteins will lead to faster discovery of drugs for diseases neglected by pharmaceutical companies.

This is a challenging field because parasite proteins are often more difficult to express using a heterologous system. The challenge is particularly great for proteins from eukaryotic parasites.

Parasites of interest include Plasmodium, Trypanosoma, Leishmania, Giardia, Entamoeba, Cryptosporidium, Helminth and Toxoplasma, many of which are agents for Neglected Diseases.

Many academic labs around the world study structural parasitology. Two groups in particular have contributed many parasite structures: the SGPP (Structural Genomnics of Pathogenic Protozoa) and the SGC (Structural Genomics Consortium).

Quantitative Parasitology

In parasitology, the quantitative study of parasitism in a host population involves the use of statistics to draw meaningful conclusions from observations of the prevalence and intensity of parasitic infection.

Counting Parasites

Quantifying parasites in a sample of hosts or comparing measures of infection across two or more samples can be challenging.

The parasitic infection of a sample of hosts inherently exhibits a complex pattern that cannot be adequately quantified by a single statistical measure. As the use of two or more separate indices is advisable, only two or more separate statistical tests can reliably compare infections different samples of hosts.

A few of the available statistical measures have markedly different biological interpretations, while others have more-or-less overlapping interpretations or no interpretations at all. Therefore, one should apply measures that have clear and separate biological interpretations thus do not predict each other.

Parasite individuals typically exhibit an aggregated (right-skewed) distribution among host individuals; most hosts harbour few if any parasites and a few hosts harbour many of them. This quantitative feature of parasitism makes the application of many traditional statistical methods inappropriate by violating assumptions about the underlying data distribution, requiring the use of more advanced computationally-intensive methods.

Describing the Parasitic Infection of a Sample of Hosts

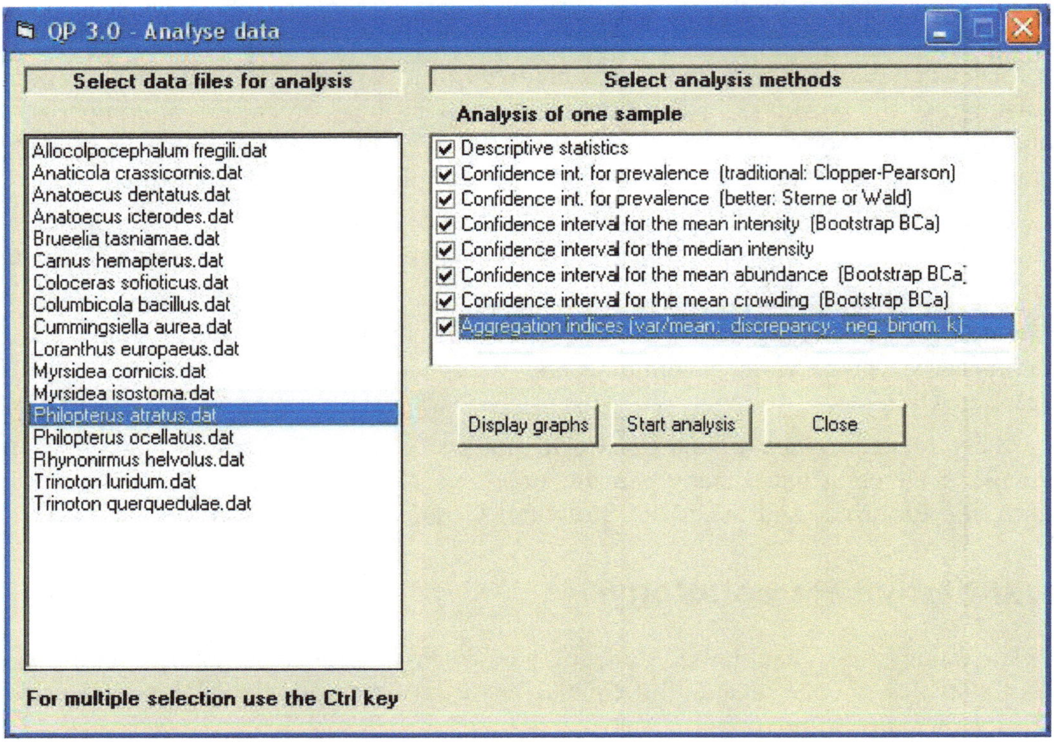

Statistical procedures to characterize the infection/infestation of a sample of hosts.

Always give the host sample size. In most cases, this is expressed as the number of hosts individuals examined. (Exceptionally, other units may also be used for special cases.)

Describe prevalence. This is the proportion of infected hosts among all the hosts examined. Give the confidence interval (CI) of prevalence (either as a Clopper-Pearson interval or as adjusted Wald/Sterne's interval) to indicate the accuracy of the estimation (use of the confidence intervals belonging to the 95% probability is advisable).

Describe mean intensity. This is the mean number of parasites found in the infected hosts (the zeros of uninfected hosts are excluded). Since sample size and prevalence are known, mean intensity defines the quantity of parasites found in the sample of hosts. Given the typical aggregated (right-skewed) distribution of parasites, its actual value is highly dependent on a few extremely infected hosts. Also give CI to indicate the accuracy of the estimation. Use bias-corrected and accelerated bootstrap (BCa Bootstrap) to get this confidence interval.

Describe median intensity. This is the median number of parasites found in infected hosts (the zeros of uninfected hosts are excluded). Median intensity shows a typical level of infection among the infected hosts. Use exact CI to indicate the accuracy of the estimation.

In certain cases one may prefer to use mean abundance instead of mean intensity. This is the mean number of parasites found in all hosts (involves the zero values of uninfected hosts). Give BCa Bootstrap confidence interval to indicate the accuracy of this estimation. This measure unifies two of the former ones: prevalence and mean intensity. Do not use it, unless you have a clearly specified a reason why to prefer it.

Describing mean crowding (intensity values averaged across parasite individuals) and its confidence interval is essential only for those who study density-dependent characters of parasites. BCa Bootstrap CI can be used to indicate the accuracy of the estimation.

Finally, quantify levels of skewness of the parasites' distribution among hosts. There are 3 indices widely used for this purpose, but their interpretation is quite similar. They predict each other rather well, thus it is not necessary to use all the 3 of them.

Comparing Parasite Burdens across two or More Samples

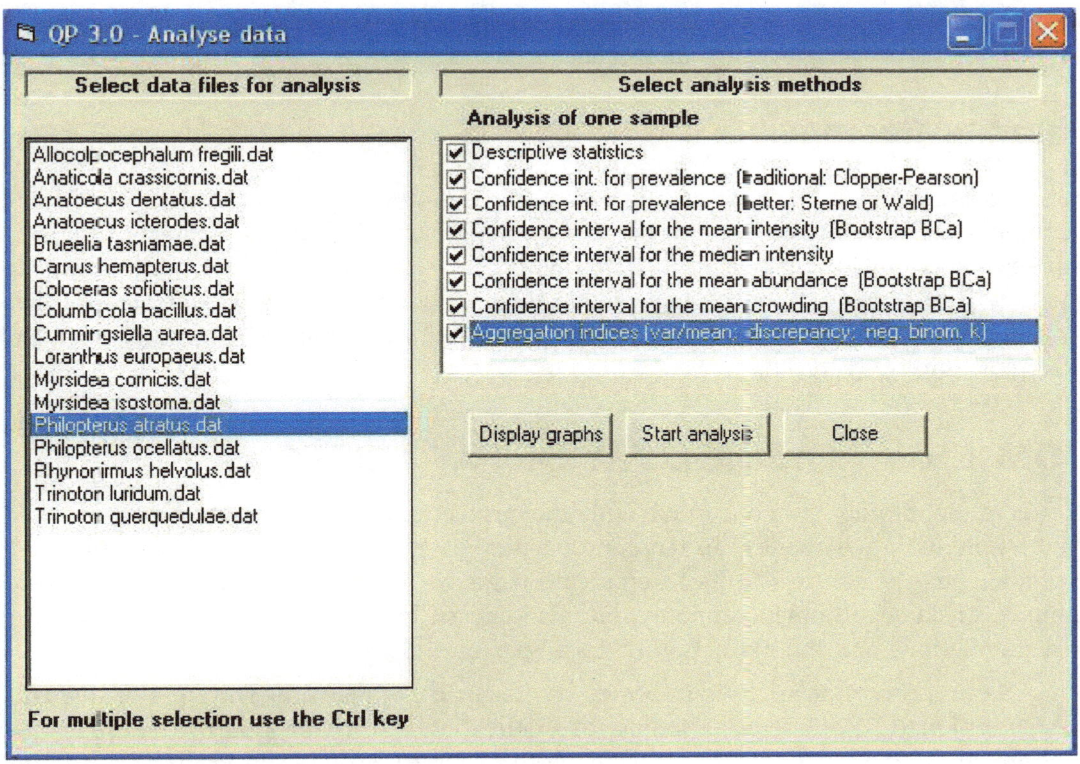

Statistical procedures to compare levels of infection/infestation across two or more samples of hosts.

Compare prevalences by Fisher's exact test. This will show whether the proportion of infected individuals differs significantly between the two (or more) samples. The time need of this test may increase dramatically when several samples are involved. Using Chi-squared test for the same purpose may be advisable in such cases.

Compare mean intensities by a Bootstrap t-test. This will show whether parasite quantities differ significantly between the infected proportions of the two samples.

Compare median intensities by Mood's median test. This will show whether the typical level of infection differs significantly between the infected proportions of the two samples.

One can also compare the frequency distributions of intensities by a Stochastic equality test. It compares several random pairs of individual values taken from the two samples to test whether or not there is a significant tendency to get higher values from one sample than from the other.

In certain cases, one may also decide to compare mean abundances by a Bootstrap t-test. This will show whether parasite quantities differ significantly between two samples. This comparison unifies two of the former ones: the comparison of prevalences and the comparison of mean intensities.

Finally, mean crowding can be compared across samples by a simple method: provided that the two 97.5% confidence intervals do not overlap, we conclude that the two values are different at a 95% level of significance.

Parasite Ecology

Parasites can provide information about host population ecology. In fisheries biology, for example, parasite communities can be used to distinguish distinct populations of the same fish species co-inhabiting a region. Additionally, parasites possess a variety of specialized traits and life-history strategies that enable them to colonize hosts. Understanding these aspects of parasite ecology, of interest in their own right, can illuminate parasite-avoidance strategies employed by hosts.

CONSERVATION BIOLOGY OF PARASITES

Conservation biology is concerned with the protection and preservation of vulnerable species, including parasites. A large proportion of parasite species are threatened by extinction, partly due to efforts to eradicate parasites which infect humans or domestic animals, or damage human economy, but also caused by the decline or fragmentation of host populations and the extinction of host species.

A large proportion of living species on Earth live a parasitic way of life. Parasites have traditionally been seen as targets of eradication efforts, and they have often been overlooked in conservation efforts. In the case of parasites living in the wild – and thus harmless to humans and domesticated animals – this view is changing.

Endangered Parasite Species

A note published in 1990 pointed out that the captive breeding and reintroduction program to save the black-footed ferret would cause the loss of its specific parasites and demanded *"equal rights for parasites!"*. Then a paper in 1992 has warned that not only the loss of certain host species from the wild, but even host population bottlenecks or the fragmentation of host populations would predictably lead to the extinction of several host specific parasite species. It also noted that parasites are not only components of biodiversity by definition, but they also exert selective pressures upon their host populations that increase host genetic diversity. Firstly, this view met with open scepticism. Soon after, it became clear that the co-extinction of hosts and their specific parasites is likely to increase the current estimates of extinction rates significantly. A decade later, a study focusing on some highly host-specific groups (such as fig wasps, parasites, butterflies, and myrmecophil butterflies) estimated the number of co-endangered species (i.e. endangered by the endangered status of the host) at about 6300. Other authors argued that host specific parasite faunae have an unexpected advantage for conservation scientists. Their genealogies and population genetic patterns may help to illuminate their hosts' evolutionary and demographic history. Recently, scientists suggested that rich parasite faunae are inevitably needed for healthy ecosystem functioning and also that parasites and mutualists are the most endangered species on Earth. Even vets have started to argue about the conservational values of parasite species.

A recent study on parasites of coral reef fish suggested that extinction of a coral reef fish species would eventually result in the coextinction of at least ten species of parasites. Although this number might seem high, the study included only large parasites such as parasitic worms and crustaceans, but not microparasites such as Myxosporea and Microsporidia.

Example: Extinct Avian Lice

The list below follows that of Mey (2005)

- *Acutifrons caracarensis* parasite of the extinct Guadalupe caracara (*Caracara lutosa*), Guadelupe Island, Mexico;
- *Longimenopon dominicanum* parasite of the extinct Guadalupe storm petrel, *Oceanodroma macrodactyla*, Guadelupe Island, Mexico;
- *Rallicola piageti* parasite of the extinct New Caledonian rail (*Gallirallus lafresnayanus*), New-Caledonia;
- *Coloceras hemiphagae* parasite of the extinct Norfolk Island pigeon (*Hemiphaga novaeseelandiae spadicea*), Norfolk Island, New-Zealand;
- *Coloceras restinctus* parasite of the extinct Norfolk Island pigeon (*Hemiphaga novaeseelandiae spadicea*), Norfolk Island, New-Zealand;
- *Rallicola extinctus* parasite of the extinct huia (*Heteralocha acutirostris*), New-Zealand;
- *Philopteroides xenicus* parasite of the extinct bushwren (*Xenicus longipes*), New-Zealand;
- *Psittacobrosus bechsteini* parasite of the extinct Cuban red macaw (*Ara tricolor*), Cuba;

- *Colpocephalum californici*, parasite of the California condor (*Gymnogyps californianus*). The host have been saved by captive breeding and repatriation programs, however, the parasite have been lost, either spontaneously or perhaps exterminated by wildlife vets.

Additionally, *Columbicola extinctus* is a parasite of the extinct passenger pigeon (*Ectopistes migratorius*). However, recent taxonomic studies show that it is conspecific with the lice living on band-tailed pigeon (*Columba fasciata*), thus it is not extinct.

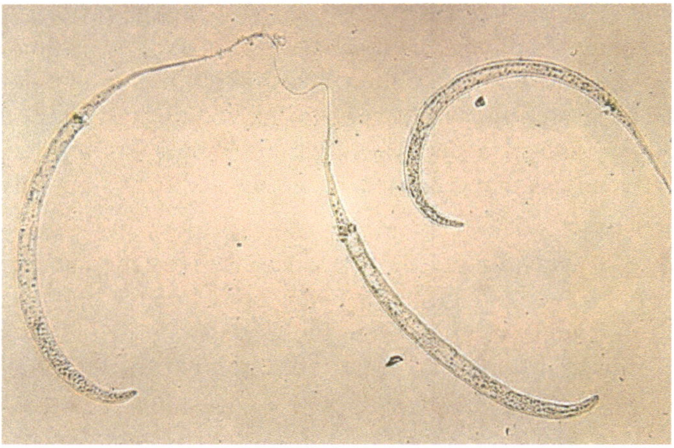

Larvae of the guinea worm: probably the next species to exterminate.

Extermination by Purpose

Naturally, medical (and veterinary) science and practice aim to exterminate parasites and pathogens living in humans (and in domesticated animals). In case of the few highly host-specific pathogens, this equals the extinction of the pathogen species. Throughout human history, however, only a single one species, i.e. smallpox virus, was eradicated from the Globe. The last cases of smallpox occurred 1978. However, secured stocks still exist in the United States and Russia for defensive purposes such as developing new vaccines, antiviral drugs, and diagnostic tests. It is not known whether or not these superpowers have shared their stocks with some of their allies during the Cold War.

A second candidate for purposeful extermination is the *Dracunculus medinensis* (guinea worm). Once widespread across some 20 nations of Africa and Asia, the parasite nowadays is much withdrawn occurring only in four countries in Sub-Saharan Africa with only a few hundred known cases of infection in 2011. Prevalent civil wars in the region, such as the War in Darfur have ensured the survival of this species up to the present.

TAXONOMY AND PHYLOGENETICS

The huge diversity between parasitic organisms creates a challenge for biologists who wish to describe and catalogue them. Recent developments in using DNA to identify separate species and to investigate the relationship between groups at various taxonomic scales has been enormously useful to parasitologists, as many parasites are highly degenerate, disguising relationships between species.

HISTORY

"Our knowledge of parasitic infections extends into antiquity, and descriptions of parasites and parasitic infections are found in the earliest writings and have been confirmed by the finding of parasites in archaeological material".

REFERENCES

1. Roncalli Amici R (2001). "The history of Italian parasitology" (PDF). Veterinary Parasitology. 98 (1–3): 3–10. doi:10.1016/S0304-4017(01)00420-4. PMID 11516576.
2. Cox F.E.G. 2002. "History of human parasitology"
3. Jurášek, V., Dubinský, P., 1993. Veterinárna parazitológia. Príroda a.s., Bratislava, 382 pp.
4. Kaufmann, J., 1996. Parasitic infections of domestic animals: a diagnostic manual. Birkhauser, Berlin, 423 pp.
5. Elsheikha, HM; Khan, NA (editor) (2011). Essentials of Veterinary Parasitology. Caister Academic Press. ISBN 978-1-904455-79-0.
6. Leland S. Shapiro; Patricia Mandel (22 May 2009). Pathology & Parasitology for Veterinary Technicians. Cengage Learning. pp. 237–239. ISBN 978-1-4354-3855-2. Retrieved 11 September 2011.
7. A. Zajac; Gary A. Conboy; American Association of Veterinary Parasitologists (24 March 2006). Veterinary clinical parasitology. Wiley-Blackwell. p. 162. ISBN 978-0-8138-1734-7. Retrieved 11 September 2011.
8. John E. Hyde (1993). Protocols in molecular parasitology. Humana Press. pp. 213–214. ISBN 978-0-89603-239-2. Retrieved 11 September 2011.
9. Windsor DA (1998). "Most of the species on Earth are parasites". International Journal for Parasitology. 28 (12): 1939–1941. doi:10.1016/S0020-7519(98)00153-2. PMID 9925276.
10. Windsor DA (1990). "Heavenly hosts". Nature. 348 (6297): 104. doi:10.1038/348104c0.
11. Rózsa L (1992). "Endangered parasite species" (PDF). International Journal for Parasitology. 22 (3): 265–266. doi:10.1016/S0020-7519(05)80002-5. PMID 1639560.

12. Bush AO, Kennedy CR (1994). "Host fragmentation and helminth parasites: Hedging your bets against extinction". International Journal for Parasitology. 24 (8): 1333–1343. doi:10.1016/0020-7519(94)90199-6. PMID 7729985.
13. Stork NE, Lyal CH (1993). "Extinction or 'co-extinction' rates?". Nature. 366 (6453): 307–8. doi:10.1038/366307a0.
14. Koh LP, Dunn RR, Sodhi NS, Colwell RK, Proctor HC, Smith VS (2004). "Species Coextinctions and the Biodiversity Crisis" (PDF). Science. 305 (5690): 1632–1634. doi:10.1126/science.1101101. PMID 15361627.
15. Whiteman NK, Parker PG (2005). "Using parasites to infer host population history: a new rationale for parasite conservation" (PDF). Animal Conservation. 8 (2): 175–181. doi:10.1017/S1367943005001915.
16. Hudson PJ, Dobson AP, Lafferty KD (2006). "Is a healthy ecosystem one that is rich in parasites?". Trends in Ecology & Evolution. 21 (7): 381–385. CiteSeerX 10.1.1.79.9080Freely accessible. doi:10.1016/j.tree.2006.04.007.
17. Dunn RR, Harris NC, Colwell RK, Koh LP, Sodhi NS (2009). "The sixth mass coextinction: are most endangered species parasites and mutualists?" (PDF). Proceedings of the Royal Society B. 276 (1670): 3037–3045. doi:10.1098/rspb.2009.0413. PMC 2817118Freely accessible. PMID 19474041.
18. Pizzi R (2009). "Veterinarians and Taxonomic Chauvinism: The Dilemma of Parasite Conservation". Journal of Exotic Pet Medicine. 18 (4): 279–282. doi:10.1053/j.jepm.2009.09.005.
19. Justine, J.-L., Beveridge, I., Boxshall, G. A., Bray, R. A., Miller, T. L., Moravec, F., Trilles, J.-P. & Whittington, I. D. 2012: An annotated list of fish parasites (Isopoda, Copepoda, Monogenea, Digenea, Cestoda, Nematoda) collected from Snappers and Bream (Lutjanidae, Nemipteridae, Caesionidae) in New Caledonia confirms high parasite biodiversity on coral reef fish. Aquatic Biosystems, 8, 22. doi:10.1186/2046-9063-8-22
20. Mey E (2005). "Psittacobrosus bechsteini: a new extinct chewing louse (Insecta, Phthiraptera, Amblycera) off the Cuban Macaw Ara tricolor (Psittaciiformes), with an annotated review of fossil and recently extinct animal lice" (PDF). Anzeiger des Vereins Thüringer Ornithologen. 5: 201–217.
21. Mey E (1992). "Eine neue ausgestorbene Vogel-Ischnozere von Neuseeland, Huiacola extinctus (Insecta, Phthiraptera)" (PDF). Zoologischer Anzeiger. 224: 49–73.
22. Clayton, Dale H.; Roger D. Price (1999). "Taxonomy of New World Columbicola (Phthiraptera: Philopteridae) from the Columbiformes (Aves), with Descriptions of Five New Species" (PDF). Annals of the Entomological Society of America. Entomological Society of America. 92 (5): 675–85.
23. Connor, Steve (2002-01-03). "How terrorism prevented smallpox being wiped off the face of the planet for ever". The Independent. Retrieved 2009-12-13.
24. Hammond, Edward (2007). "Should the US and Russia destroy their stocks of smallpox virus?". BMJ. 334 (7597): 774. doi:10.1136/bmj.39155.695255.94. PMC 1851992Freely accessible. PMID 17431261.

25. Agwunobi, John O. (2007). "Should the US and Russia destroy their stocks of smallpox virus?". BMJ. 334 (7597): 775. doi:10.1136/bmj.39156.490799.BE. PMC 1851995Freely accessible. PMID 17431262.

26. Rózsa L, Nixdorff K 2006. Biological weapons in non-Soviet Warsaw Pact countries. In: Wheelis M et al. (eds.) Deadly cultures: biological weapons since 1945. Cambridge, US: Harvard University Press.

27. "The Carter Center Guinea Worm Disease Eradication".

CHAPTER 6

Protozoology: The study of Protozoa

Chapter Contents

- **Introduction**
- **Protozoa**
- **History and Terminology**
- **Characteristics**
- **Classification**
- **Ecological Role**

Protozoa are unicellular, heterotrophic eukaryotes that have been studied for more than 300 years, at first as microscopic curiosities, later as organisms causing disease and more recently as important components of ecosystems. In addition to being of intrinsic interest in their own right, protozoa are important in a number of fields of study, including: (1) as model organisms for investigations of cell biology, physiology and biochemistry; (2) ecological processes, such as predation and competition, and how these might affect the evolution of life history traits; (3) nutrient cycling, food webs and soil fertility; (4) reconstructing past climate change and (5) locating oil deposits. In addition, protozoa cause a number of important diseases of humans and animals, including malaria, sleeping sickness, Chagas disease, amoebic dysentery, coccidiosis, leishmaniasis and toxoplasmosis. Consequently, protozoology – the study of protozoa – is a discipline with a substantial following throughout the world.

INTRODUCTION

Protozoology is the study of protozoa, the "animal-like" (i.e., motile and heterotrophic) protists.

This term has become dated as understanding of the evolutionary relationships of the eukaryotes has improved. For example, the Society of Protozoloogists, founded in 1947, was renamed International Society of Protistologists in 2005. However, the term persists in some cases (e.g., the Polish journal *Acta Protozoologica*).

PROTOZOA

In 21st-century systems of biological classification, the Protozoa are defined as a diverse group of unicellular eukaryotic organisms. Historically, protozoa were defined as single-celled animals or organisms with animal-like behaviors, such as motility and predation. The group was regarded as the zoological counterpart to the "protophyta", which were considered to be plant-like, as they are capable of photosynthesis.

The terms *protozoa* and *protozoans* are now mostly used informally to designate single-celled, non-photosynthetic protists, such as the ciliates, amoebae and flagellates.

The term Protozoa was introduced in 1818 for a taxonomic class, but in later classification schemes the group was elevated to higher ranks, including phylum, subkingdom and kingdom. In several classification systems proposed by Thomas Cavalier-Smith and his collaborators since 1981, Protozoa is ranked as a kingdom. The seven-kingdom scheme proposed by Ruggiero et al. in 2015, places eight phyla under Protozoa: Euglenozoa, Amoebozoa, Metamonada, Choanozoa, Loukozoa, Percolozoa, Microsporidia and Sulcozoa. This kingdom does not form a clade, but an evolutionary grade or paraphyletic group, from which the fungi and animals are specifically excluded.

The use of Protozoa as a formal taxon has been discouraged by some recent researchers, mainly because the term, which is formed from the Greek *protos* "first" + *zoia*, plural of *zoion*, "animal", implies kinship with animals (metazoa) and promotes a separation of "animal-like" from "plant-like" organisms, neither of which they encourage. Modern ultrastructural, biochemical, and genetic techniques have shown that protozoa, as traditionally defined, belong to widely divergent lineages, and can no longer be regarded as "primitive animals." For this reason, the terms "protists," "Protista" or "Protoctista" are sometimes preferred for the high-level classification of eukaryotic microbes. In 2005, members of the Society of Protozoologists voted to change the name of that organization to the International Society of Protistologists.

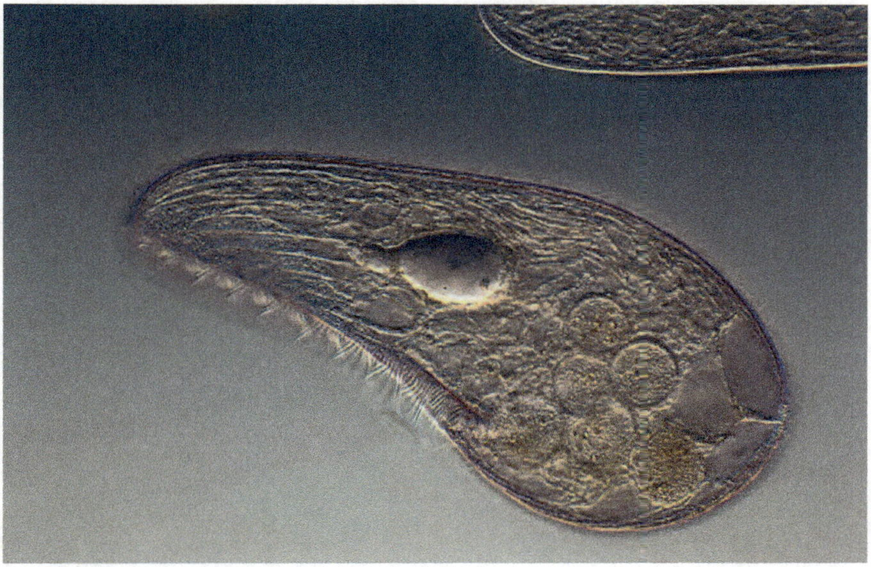

Blepharisma japonicum, a free-living ciliated protozoan.

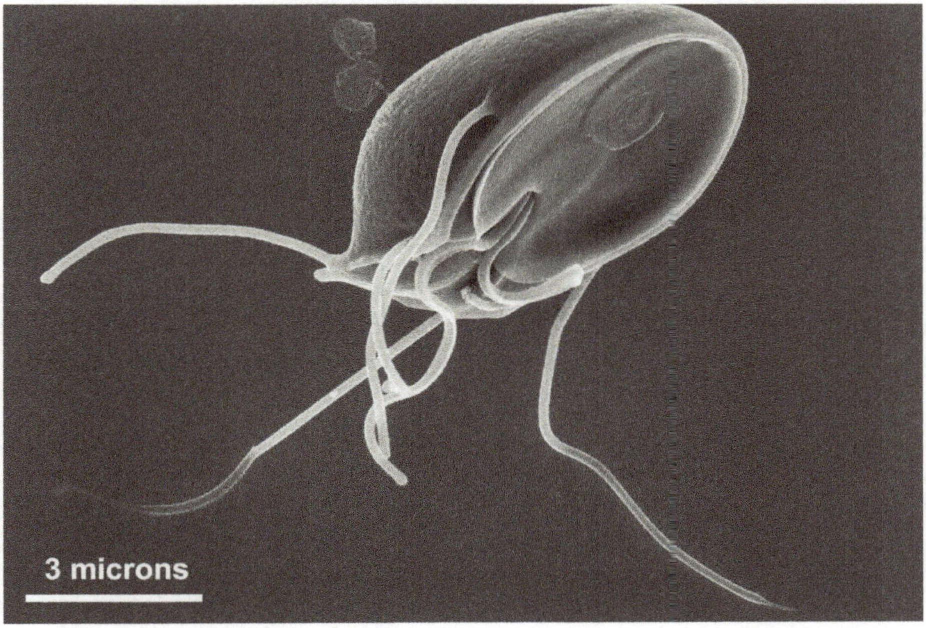

Giardia muris, a flagellate protozoan, is an intestinal parasite found in rodents, birds and reptiles.

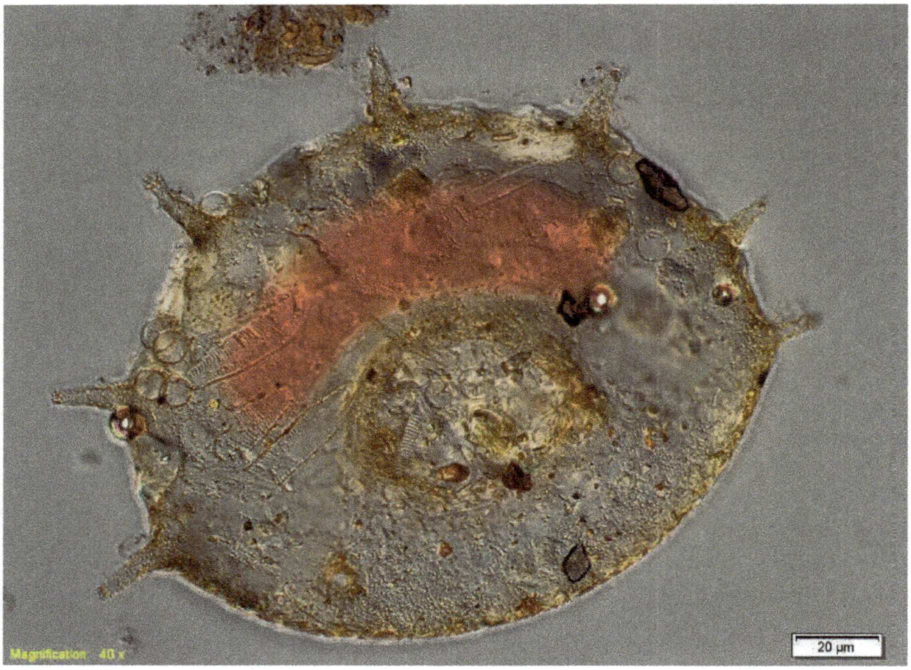

Centropyxis aculeata, a testate (shelled) amoeba.

HISTORY AND TERMINOLOGY

The word "protozoa" (singular *protozoon* or *protozoan*) was coined in 1818 by zoologist Georg August Goldfuss, as the Greek equivalent of the German *Urthiere*, meaning „primitive, or original animals" (*ur-* 'proto-' + *Thier* 'animal'). Goldfuss erected Protozoa as a class containing what he believed to be the simplest animals. Originally, the group included not only microbes, but also some „lower" multicellular animals, such as rotifers, corals, sponges, jellyfish, bryozoa and polychaete worms.

In 1848, in light of advancements in cell theory pioneered by Theodore Schwann and Matthias Schleiden, the anatomist and zoologist C.T. von Siebold proposed that the bodies of microbial organisms such as ciliates and amoebae were made up of single cells, similar to those from which the multicellular tissues of plants and animals were constructed. Von Siebold redefined Protozoa to include only such unicellular forms, to the exclusion of all metazoa. At the same time, he raised the group to the level of a phylum containing two broad classes of microbes: Infusoria (mostly ciliates and flagellated algae), and Rhizopoda (amoeboid organisms). The definition of Protozoa as a phylum or sub-kingdom made up of „unicellular animals" was adopted by the zoologist Otto Bütschli—celebrated at his centenary as the „architect of protozoology"—and the term came into wide use.

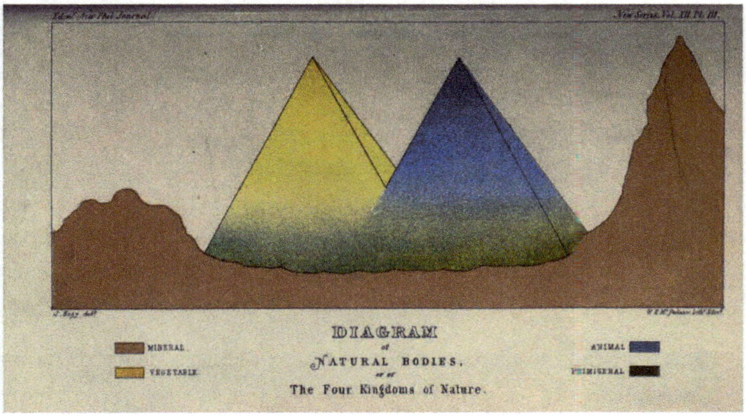

John Hogg's illustration of the Four Kingdoms of Nature, showing "Primigenal" as a greenish haze at the base of the Animals and Plants, 1860.

As a phylum under Animalia, the Protozoa were firmly rooted in the old "two-kingdom" classification of life, according to which all living beings were classified as either animals or plants. As long as this scheme remained dominant, the protozoa were understood to be animals and studied in departments of Zoology, while photosynthetic microbes and microscopic fungi—the so-called Protophyta—were assigned to the Plants, and studied in departments of Botany.

Criticism of this system began in the latter half of the 19th century, with the realization that many organisms met the criteria for inclusion among both plants and animals. For example, the algae *Euglena* and *Dinobryon* have chloroplasts for photosynthesis, but can also feed on organic matter and are motile. In 1860, John Hogg argued against the use of "protozoa", on the grounds that "naturalists are divided in opinion—and probably some will ever continue so—whether many of these organisms, or living beings, are animals or plants." As an alternative, he proposed a new kingdom called Primigenum, consisting of both the protozoa and unicellular algae (protophyta), which he combined together under the name "Protoctista". In Hoggs's conception, the animal and plant kingdoms were likened to two great "pyramids" blending at their bases in the Kingdom Primigenum.

Six years later, Ernst Haeckel also proposed a third kingdom of life, which he named Protista. At first, Haeckel included a few multicellular organisms in this kingdom, but in later work he restricted the Protista to single-celled organisms, or simple colonies whose individual cells are not differentiated into different kinds of tissues.

Despite these proposals, Protozoa emerged as the preferred taxonomic placement for heterotrophic microbes such as amoebae and ciliates, and remained so for more than a century. In the course of the 20th century, however, the old "two kingdom" system began to weaken, with the growing awareness that fungi did not belong among the plants, and that most of the unicellular protozoa were no more closely related to the animals than they were to the plants. By mid-century, some biologists, such as Herbert Copeland, Robert H. Whittaker and Lynn Margulis, advocated the revival of Haeckel's Protista or Hogg's Protoctista as a kingdom-level eukaryotic group, alongside Plants, Animals and

Fungi. A variety of multi-kingdom systems were proposed, and Kingdoms Protista and Protoctista became well established in biology texts and curricula.

While many taxonomists have abandoned Protozoa as a high-level group, Thomas Cavalier-Smith has retained it as a kingdom in the various classifications he has proposed. As of 2015, Cavalier-Smith's Protozoa excludes several major groups of organisms traditionally placed among the protozoa, including the ciliates, dinoflagellates and foraminifera (all members of the SAR supergroup). In its current form, his kingdom Protozoa is a paraphyletic group which includes a common ancestor and most of its descendents, but excludes two important clades that branch within it: the animals and fungi.

CHARACTERISTICS

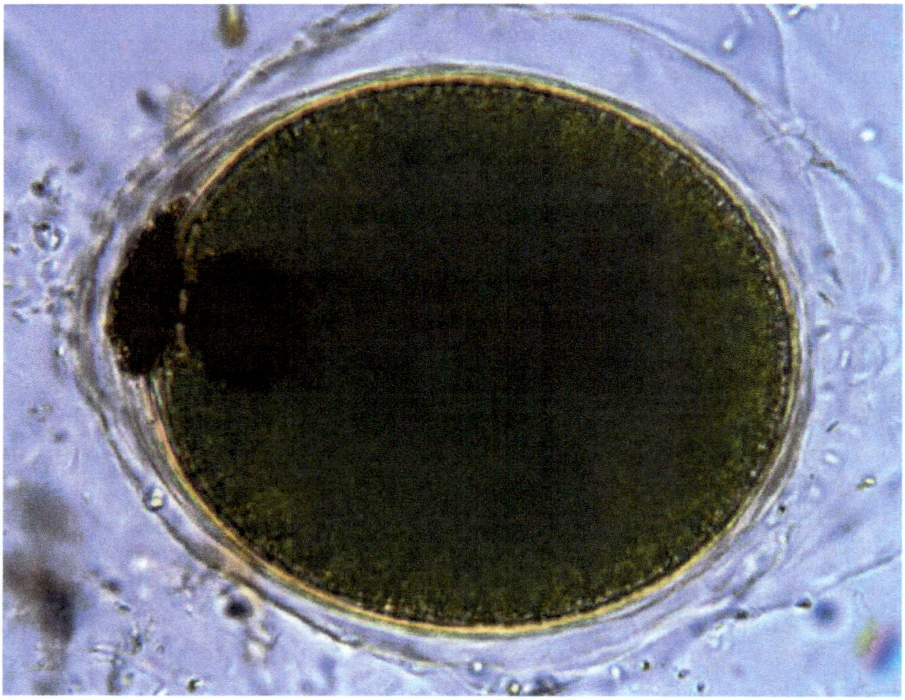

Resting cyst of ciliated protozoan *Dileptus viridis*.

Protozoa, as traditionally defined, are mainly microscopic organisms, ranging in size from 10 to 52 micrometers. Some, however, are significantly larger. Among the largest are the deep-sea–dwelling xenophyophores, single-celled foraminifera whose shells can reach 20 cm in diameter. Free-living forms are restricted to moist environments, such as soils, mosses and aquatic habitats, although many form resting cysts which enable them to survive drying. Many protozoan species are symbionts, some are parasites, and some are predators of bacteria, algae and other protists.

Motility and Feeding

Organisms traditionally classified as protozoa are abundant in aqueous environments and soil, occupying a range of trophic levels. The group includes flagellates (which move with the help of whip-like structures called flagella), ciliates (which move by using hair-like structures called cilia) and amoebae (which move by the use of foot-like structures called pseudopodia). Some protozoa are sessile, and do not move at all.

Protozoa may take in food by osmotrophy, absorbing nutrients through their cell membranes; or they may feed by phagocytosis, either by engulfing particles of food with pseudopodia (as amoebae do), or taking in food through a mouth-like aperture called a cytostome. All protozoa digest their food in stomach-like compartments called vacuoles.

Pellicle

The pellicle is a thin layer supporting the cell membrane in various protozoa, such as ciliates, protecting them and allowing them to retain their shape, especially during locomotion, allowing the organism to be more hydrodynamic. The pellicle varies from flexible and elastic to rigid. Although somewhat stiff, the pellicle is also flexible and allows the protist to fit into tighter spaces. In ciliates and Apicomplexa, it is formed from closely packed vesicles called alveoli. In euglenids, it is formed from protein strips arranged spirally along the length of the body. Familiar examples of protists with a pellicle are the euglenoids and the ciliate *Paramecium*. In some protozoa, the pellicle hosts epibiotic bacteria that adhere to the surface by their fimbriae (attachment pili).

Life Cycle

Some protozoa have life phases alternating between proliferative stages (e.g., trophozoites) and dormant cysts. As cysts, protozoa can survive harsh conditions, such as exposure to extreme temperatures or harmful chemicals, or long periods without access to nutrients, water, or oxygen for periods of time. Being a cyst enables parasitic species to survive outside of a host, and allows their transmission from one host to another. When protozoa are in the form of trophozoites (Greek *tropho* = to nourish), they actively feed. The conversion of a trophozoite to cyst form is known as encystation, while the process of transforming back into a trophozoite is known as excystation. Protozoa reproduce asexually by binary fission or multiple fission. Many protozoan species exchange genetic material by sexual means (typically, through conjugation); however, sexuality is generally decoupled from the process of reproduction, and does not immediately result in increased population.

CLASSIFICATION

The classification of protozoa has been and remains a problematic area of taxonomy. Where they are available, DNA sequences are used as the basis for classification; however, for the majority of described protozoa, such material is not available. Protozoa have been and still are organized mostly on the basis of their morphology, means of locomotion, and for the parasitic species their hosts.

- Flagellates (e.g., *Giardia lamblia*)
- Amoeboids (e.g., *Entamoeba histolytica*)
- Sporozoans (e.g., *Plasmodium knowlesi*)
  - Apicomplexa (now in Alveolata)
  - Microsporidia (now in Fungi)
  - Ascetosporea (now in Rhizaria)
  - Myxosporidia (now in Cnidaria)
- Ciliates (e.g., *Balantidium coli*)

As a phylum the Protozoa were, historically, divided into four subphyla reflecting the means of locomotion:

- Subphylum Sarcomastigophora
  - Superclass Mastigophora (includes flagellates)
  - Superclass Sarcodina
  - Superclass Opalinata
- Subphylum Sporozoa (includes apicomplexans)
- Subphylum Cnidospora
  - Class Microsporidea
- Subphylum Ciliophora (includes ciliates)

These systems are no longer considered to be valid.

ECOLOGICAL ROLE

As components of the micro- and meiofauna, protozoa are an important food source for microinvertebrates. Thus, the ecological role of protozoa in the transfer of bacterial and algal production to successive trophic levels is important. As predators, they prey upon unicellular or filamentous algae, bacteria, and microfungi. Protozoan species include both herbivores and consumers in the decomposer link of the food chain. They also control bacteria populations and biomass to some extent. On average, protozoa eat ~ 100 to 1,000 bacteria per hour. Protozoa can stimulate decomposition of organic matter, digest cellulose in the rumen of cows and termite guts, and can play a role in nutrient mobilization.

Diseases

In Humans

A number of protozoan pathogens are human parasites, causing diseases such as malaria (by *Plasmodium*), amoebiasis, giardiasis, toxoplasmosis, cryptosporidiosis, trichomoniasis, Chagas disease, leishmaniasis, African trypanosomiasis (sleeping sickness), amoebic dysentery, acanthamoeba keratitis, and primary amoebic meningoencephalitis (naegleriasis).

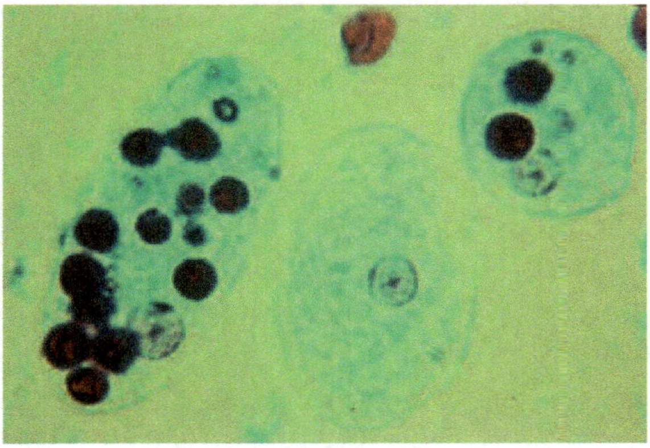

Trophozoites of the amoebic dysentery pathogen *Entamoeba histolytica* with ingested human red blood cells (dark circles).

In Other Animals

The protozoan *Ophryocystis elektroscirrha* is a parasite of butterfly larvae, passed from female to caterpillar. Severely infected individuals are weak, unable to expand their wings, or unable to eclose, and have shortened lifespans, but parasite levels vary in populations. Infection creates a culling effect, whereby infected migrating animals are less likely to complete the migration. This results in populations with lower parasite loads at the end of the migration. This is not the case in laboratory or commercial rearing, where after a few generations, all individuals can be infected.

REFERENCES

1. Edward Alcamo; Jennifer M. Warner (28 August 2009). Schaum's Outline of Microbiology. McGraw Hill Professional. pp. 144– ISBN 978-0-07-162326-1. Retrieved 14 November 2010.
2. Ruggiero, Michael A.; Gordon, Dennis P.; Orrell, Thomas M.; Bailly, Nicolas; Bourgoin, Thierry; Brusca, Richard C.; Cavalier-Smith, Thomas; Guiry, Michael D.; Kirk, Paul M. (April 29, 2015). "A Higher Level Classification of All Living Organisms". PLoS ONE. 10 (4): e0119248. doi:10.1371/journal.pone.0119248. PMC 4418965Freely accessible. PMID 25923521. Retrieved 2015-05-01.
3. Goldfuss, Georg August (1820). Handbuch der Zoologie. Nuremberg: J. L. Schrag. pp. 11–16.
4. Cavalier-Smith, T. (1981). "Eukaryote kingdoms: seven or nine?". Bio Systems. 14 (3-4): 461–481. doi:10.1016/0303-2647(81)90050-2. ISSN 0303-2647. PMID 7337818.
5. Cavalier-Smith, T. (Dec 1993). "Kingdom protozoa and its 18 phyla". Microbiological Reviews. 57 (4): 953–994. ISSN 0146-0749. PMC 372943Freely accessible. PMID 8302218.

6. Cavalier-Smith, Thomas (2010-06-23). "Kingdoms Protozoa and Chromista and the eozoan root of the eukaryotic tree". Biology Letters. 6 (3): 342–345. doi:10.1098/rsbl.2009.0948. ISSN 1744-9561. PMC 2880060Freely accessible. PMID 20031978.
7. Hogg, John (1860). "On the distinctions of a plant and an animal and on a fourth kingdom of Nature". Edinb N Phil J (N Ser). 12: 216–225.
8. Scamardella, J. M. (Dec 1999). "Not plants or animals: a brief history of the origin of Kingdoms Protozoa, Protista and Protoctista". International Microbiology. 2 (4): 207–216. ISSN 1139-6709. PMID 10943416.
9. Copeland, Herbert F. (1947). "Progress Report on Basic Classification". The American Naturalist. 81: 340–361. doi:10.1086/281531. JSTOR 2458229.
10. "New President's Address". protozoa.uga.edu. Retrieved 2015-05-01.
11. "Details - Lehrbuch der vergleichenden Anatomie der Wirbellosen Thiere / von C. Th. v. Siebold. - Biodiversity Heritage Library". www.biodiversitylibrary.org. Retrieved 2015-05-20.
12. Dobell, C. (Apr 1951). "In memoriam Otto Bütschli (1848-1920) "architect of protozoology"". Isis; an International Review Devoted to the History of Science and Its Cultural Influences. 42 (127): 20–22. ISSN 0021-1753. PMID 14831973.
13. Taylor, F. J. R. 'Max' (11 January 2003). "The collapse of the two-kingdom system, the rise of protistology and the founding of the International Society for Evolutionary Protistology (ISEP)". International Journal of Systematic and Evolutionary Microbiology. 53 (6): 1707–1714. doi:10.1099/ijs.0.02587-0. ISSN 1466-5026. PMID 14657097.
14. Hogg, John (1860). "On the distinctions of a plant and an animal, and on a fourth kingdom of nature". Edinburgh New Philosophical Journal.
15. Whittaker, R. H. (Jan 10, 1969). "New concepts of kingdoms or organisms. Evolutionary relations are better represented by new classifications than by the traditional two kingdoms". Science. 163 (3863): 150–160. doi:10.1126/science.163.3863.150. ISSN 0036-8075. PMID 5762760.
16. Margulis, Lynn (1974). Dobzhansky, Theodosius; Hecht, Max K.; Steere, William C., eds. Five-Kingdom Classification and the Origin and Evolution of Cells. Springer US. pp. 45–78. ISBN 978-1-4615-6946-6.
17. Cavalier-Smith T (August 1998). "A revised six-kingdom system of life". Biological Reviews. 73: 203–266. doi:10.1111/j.1469-185X.1998.tb00030.x. PMID 9809012. Retrieved 2015-06-09.
18. Ruggiero, Michael A.; Gordon, Dennis P.; Orrell, Thomas M.; Bailly, Nicolas; Bourgoin, Thierry; Brusca, Richard C.; Cavalier-Smith, Thomas; Guiry, Michael D.; Kirk, Paul M. (April 29, 2015). "A Higher Level Classification of All Living Organisms". PLoS ONE. 10 (4): e0119248. doi:10.1371/journal.pone.0119248. PMC 4418965Freely accessible. PMID 25923521. Retrieved 2015-05-01.

19. "Xenophyophores (Rhizaria, Foraminifera) from the Nazaré Canyon (Portuguese margin, NE Atlantic)". Deep-Sea Research Part II: Topical Studies in Oceanography. 58: 2401–2419. doi:10.1016/j.dsr2.2011.04.005. Retrieved 2015-06-09.
20. "Protozoa". MicrobeWorld. American Society for Chemistry. 2006. Archived from the original on 19 May 2008. Retrieved 15 June 2008.
21. Protozoa in biological research
22. "Sex and Death in Protozoa". Cambridge University Press. Retrieved 2015-06-09.
23. Honigberg, B. M.; W. Balamuth; E. C. Bovee; J. C. Corliss; M. Gojdics; R. P. Hall; R. R. Kudo; N. D. Levine; A. R. Lobblich; J. Weiser (1964). "A Revised Classification of the Phylum Protozoa". Journal of Eukaryotic Microbiology. 11 (1): 7–20. doi:10.1111/j.1550-7408.1964.tb01715.x.
24. Bartel, Rebecca; Oberhauser, Karen; De Roode, Jacob; Atizer, Sonya (February 2011). "Monarch butterfly migration and parasite transmission in eastern North America". Ecology. 92 (2): 342–351. doi:10.1890/10-0489.1. PMID 21618914.
25. Leong, K. L. H.; M. A. Yoshimura; H. K. Kaya; H. Williams (1997). "Instar Susceptibility of the Monarch Butterfly (Danaus plexippus) to the Neogregarine Parasite, Ophryocystis elektroscirrha". Journal of Invertebrate Pathology. 69 (1): 79–83. doi:10.1006/jipa.1996.4634. PMID 9028932. Lay summary.

CHAPTER 7

Nematolgy: Sudy of Nematodes

Chapter Contents

INTRODUCTION

Nematology is the scientific discipline concerned with the study of nematodes, or roundworms. Although nematological investigation dates back to the days of Aristotle or even earlier, nematology as an independent discipline has its recognizable beginnings in the mid to late 19th century.

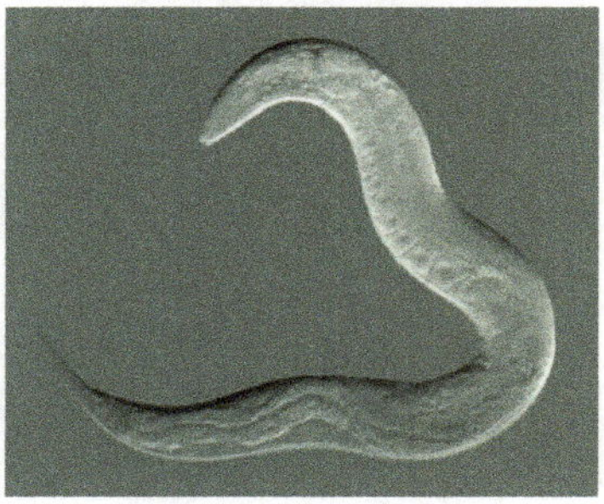

C. elegans

HISTORY

Pre-1850

Nematology research, like most fields of science, has its foundations in observations and the recording of these observations. The earliest written account of a nematode "sighting," as it were, may be found in the Pentateuch of the Old Testament in the Bible, in the Fourth Book of Moses called Numbers: "And the Lord sent fiery serpents among the people, and they bit the people; and much people of Israel died". Although no empirical data exists to test the hypothesis, many nematologists assume and circumstantial evidence suggests the "fiery serpents" to be the Guinea worm, *Dracunculus medinensis*, as this nematode is known to inhabit the region near the Red Sea.

Before 1750, a large number of nematode observations were recorded, many by the notable great minds of ancient civilization. Hippocrates (ca. 420 B.C.), Aristotle (ca. 350 B.C.), Celsus (ca 10 B.C.), Galen (ca. 180 A.D.) and Redi (1684) all described nematodes parasitizing humans or other large animals and birds. Borellus (1653) was the first to observe and describe a free-living nematode, which he dubbed the "vinegar eel;" and Tyson (1683) used a crude microscope to describe the rough anatomy of the human intestinal roundworm, *Ascaris lumbricoides*.

Other well-known microscopists spent time observing and describing free-living and animal-parasitic nematodes: Hooke (1683), Leeuwenhoek (1722), Needham (1743), and Spallanzani (1769) are among these. Observations and descriptions of plant parasitic nematodes, which were less conspicuous to ancient scientists, didn't receive as much or as early attention as did animal parasites. The earliest allusion to a plant parasitic nematode is, however, preserved in famous writ. "Sowed cockle, reap'd no corn," a line by William Shakespeare penned in 1594 in *Love's Labour's Lost*, Act IV, Scene 3, most certainly has reference to blighted wheat caused by the plant parasite, *Anguina tritici*.

Needham (1743) solved the "riddle of cockle" when he crushed one of the diseased wheat grains and observed "Aquatic Animals...denominated Worms, Eels, or Serpents, which they very much resemble." It is likely that few or no other recorded observations of plant parasitic nematodes or their effects are to be found in ancient literature.

From 1750 to the early 1900s, nematology research continued to be descriptive and taxonomic, focusing primarily on free-living nematodes and plant and animal parasites. During this period a number of productive researchers contributed to the field of nematology in the United States and abroad. Beginning with Needham and continuing to Cobb, nematologists compiled and continuously revised a broad descriptive morphological taxonomy of nematodes.

1850 to the Present

Kuhn (1874) is thought to be the first to use soil fumigation to control nematodes, applying carbon disulfide treatments in sugar beet fields in Germany. In Europe from 1870 to 1910, nematological research focused heavily on controlling the sugar beet nematode as sugar beet production became an important economy during this time in the Old World.

Although 18th and 19th century scientists yielded a considerable amount of important fundamental and applied knowledge about nematode biology, nematology research really began to advance in quality and quantity near the turn of the 20th century. In 1918, the first permanent nematology field station was constructed in the U.S. Post Office in Salt Lake City, Utah under the direction of Harry B. Shaw, after scientists observed the sugar beet nematode in a field south of the city. In this same year, Nathan Cobb (1918) published his Contributions to a Science of Nematology and his lab manual "Estimating the Nema Population of Soil." These two publications provide definitive resources for many methods and apparatus used in nematology even to this day.

Of Cobb's far-reaching influence on nematology research, Jenkins and Taylor write:

Although many workers have played important roles in development of plant nematology, none have had a greater impact, particularly in the United States, than N.A. Cobb. In 1913 Cobb published his first paper on nematology in the United States. From [1913] to 1932 he was the undisputed leader in [nematology] in this country. Through his efforts the widely renowned [USDA] nematology research program was initiated and developed. Many of his students and colleagues developed into the leaders in plant nematology in the 1930s, 1940's, and 1950's. In addition, during his productive career he contributed major discoveries in the areas of nematode taxonomy, morphology, and in methodology. Many of his techniques are still unsurpassed!

Perhaps no one person has had as favorable an impact on the field of nematology as has Nathan Augustus Cobb.

From 1900–1925 various state-run agricultural experimental stations investigated important problems relating to agro-economy, though few stations devoted much attention to plant-parasitic nematodes. Accounts of the history of nematology (the few that exist) mention three major events occurring between 1926 and 1950 that affected the relative importance of nematodes in the eyes of farmers, legislators and the U.S. public in general. These same events had profound worldwide effects on the course of nematology research over the next fifty to seventy-five years

First, the discovery of the golden nematode in the potato fields of Long Island led to a trip by U.S. quarantine officials to the potato fields of Europe, where the devastating effects of this parasite had been known for many years. This excursion allayed all skepticism about the seriousness of this agricultural pest. Second, the introduction of the soil fumigants, D-D and EDB made available for the first time nematicides that could be used effectively and practically on a field scale. Third, the development of nematode-resistant crop cultivars brought substantial government funding to applied nematology research.

These events contributed to a shift from broad taxonomy-based nematology research to deep, yet focused investigations of plant parasitic nematodes, especially the control of agricultural pests. From the early 1930s until recently, the bulk of researchers studying nematodes have been plant pathologists by training. Consequently, nematological research leaned heavily toward answering plant pathological and agro-economical questions for the last three-quarters of the 20th century.

NEMATODE

The nematodes or roundworms constitute the phylum Nematoda. They are a diverse animal phylum inhabiting a broad range of environments. Nematode species can be difficult to distinguish, and although over 25,000 have been described, of which more than half are parasitic, the total number of nematode species has been estimated to be about 1 million. Nematodes are classified along with insects and other moulting animals in the clade Ecdysozoa, and, unlike flatworms, have tubular digestive systems with openings at both ends.

Nematodes have successfully adapted to nearly every ecosystem from marine (salt water) to fresh water, to soils, and from the polar regions to the tropics, as well as the highest to the lowest of elevations. They are ubiquitous in freshwater, marine, and terrestrial environments, where they often outnumber other animals in both individual and species counts, and are found in locations as diverse as mountains, deserts and oceanic trenches. They are found in every part of the earth's lithosphere, even at great depths (0.9–3.6 km) below the surface of the Earth in gold mines in South Africa. They represent 90% of all animals on the ocean floor. Their numerical dominance, often exceeding a million individuals per square meter and accounting for about 80% of all individual animals on earth, their diversity of life cycles, and their presence at various trophic levels point at an important role in many ecosystems. The many parasitic forms include pathogens in most plants and animals (including humans). Some nematodes can undergo cryptobiosis.

Nathan Cobb, a nematologist, described the ubiquity of nematodes on Earth thus:

In short, if all the matter in the universe except the nematodes were swept away, our world would still be dimly recognizable, and if, as disembodied spirits, we could then investigate it, we should find its mountains, hills, vales, rivers, lakes, and oceans represented by a film of nematodes. The location of towns would be decipherable, since for every massing of human beings there would be a corresponding massing of certain nematodes. Trees would still stand in ghostly rows representing our streets and highways. The location of the various plants and animals would still be decipherable, and, had we sufficient knowledge, in many cases even their species could be determined by an examination of their erstwhile nematode parasites."

TAXONOMY AND SYSTEMATICS

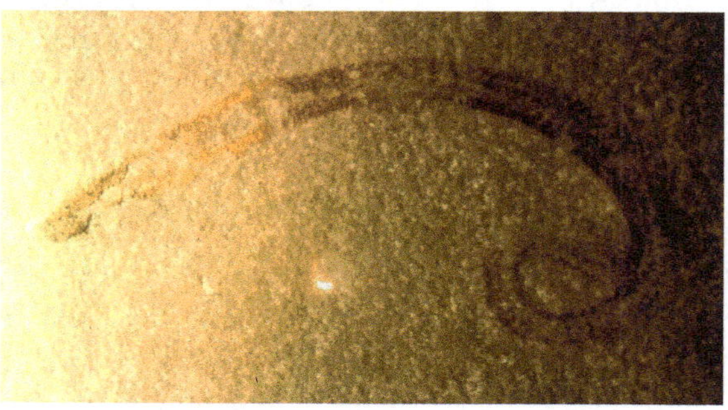

Eophasma jurasicum, a fossilized nematode.

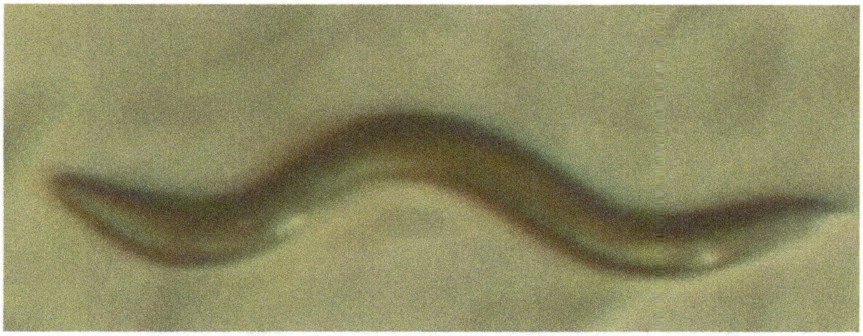

Caenorhabditis elegans.

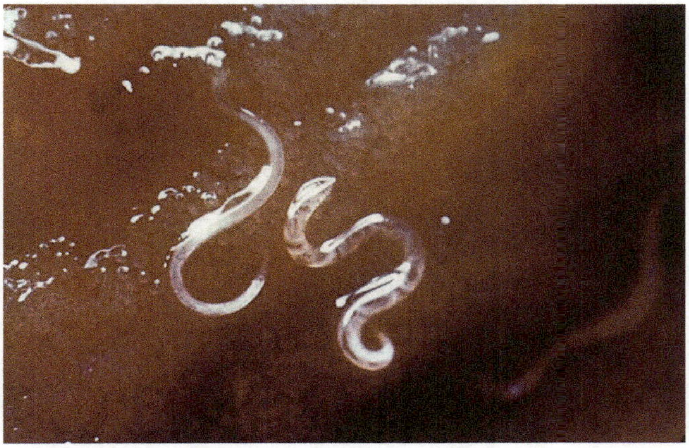

Rhabditia.

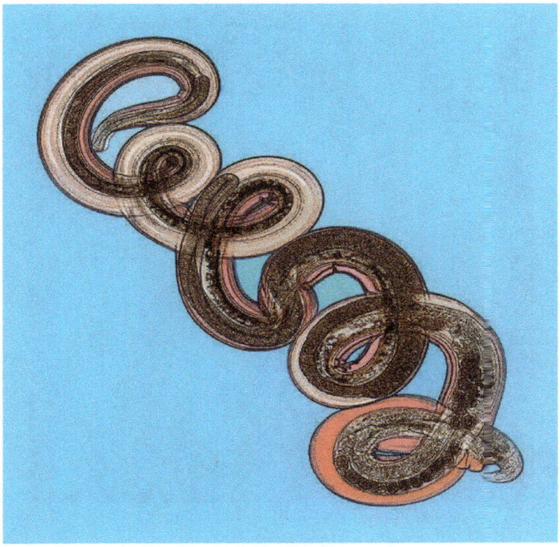

Nippostrongylus brasiliensis.

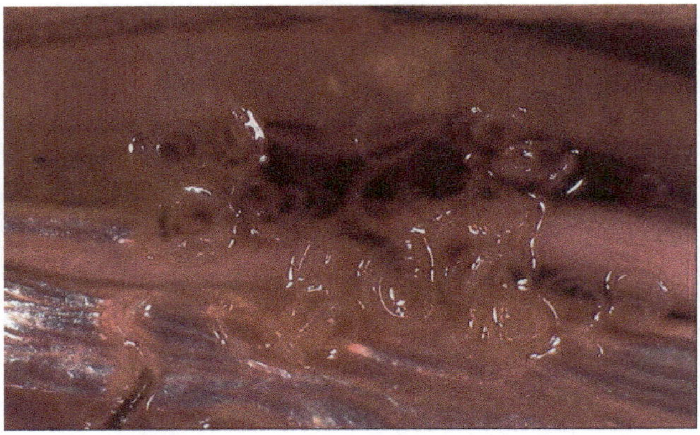

Unidentified Anisakidae (Ascaridina: Ascaridoidea).

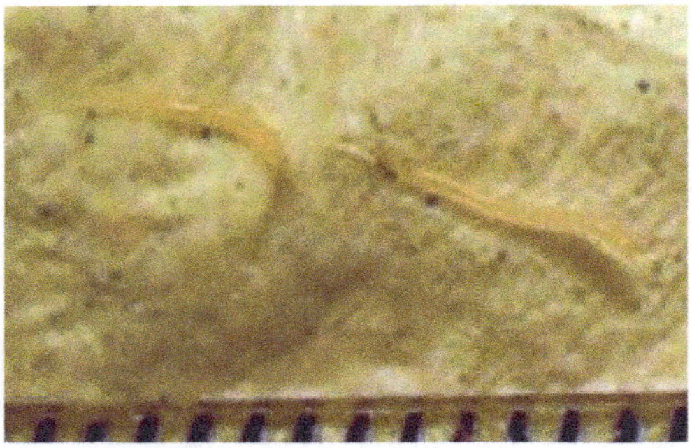

Oxyuridae Threadworm.

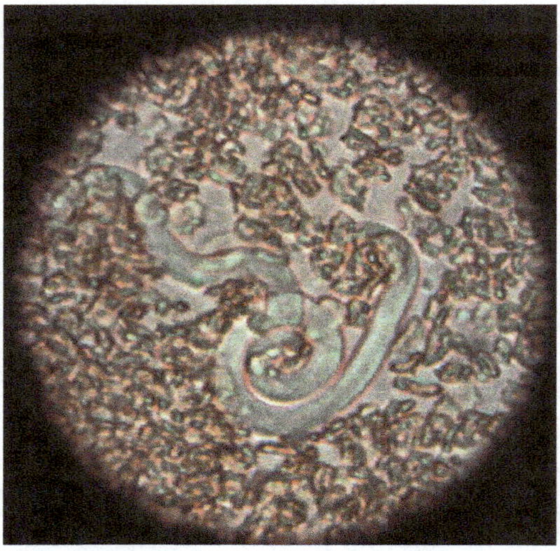

Spiruridae *Dirofilaria immitis*.

Phylogeny

The phylogenetic relationships of the nematodes and their close relatives among the protostomian Metazoa are unresolved. Traditionally, they were held to be a lineage of their own but in the 1990s, they were proposed to form the group Ecdysozoa together with moulting animals, such as arthropods. The identity of the closest living relatives of the Nematoda has always been considered to be well resolved. Morphological characters and molecular phylogenies agree with placement of the roundworms as a sister taxon to the parasitic Nematomorpha; together they make up the Nematoida. Together with the Scalidophora (formerly Cephalorhyncha), the Nematoida form the clade Cycloneuralia, but much disagreement occurs both between and among the available morphological and molecular data. The Cycloneuralia or the Introverta—depending on the validity of the former—are often ranked as a superphylum.

Nematode Systematics

Due to the lack of knowledge regarding many nematodes, their systematics is contentious. An earliest and influential classification was proposed by Chitwood and Chitwood—later revised by Chitwood—who divided the phylum into two—the Aphasmidia and the Phasmidia. These were later renamed Adenophorea (gland bearers) and Secernentea (secretors), respectively. The Secernentea share several characteristics, including the presence of phasmids, a pair of sensory organs located in the lateral posterior region, and this was used as the basis for this division. This scheme was adhered to in many later classifications, though the Adenophorea were not a uniform group.

Initial studies of incomplete DNA sequences suggested the existence of five clades:

- Dorylaimida
- Enoplia
- Spirurina
- Tylenchina
- Rhabditina

As it seems, the Secernentea are indeed a natural group of closest relatives. But the "Adenophorea" appear to be a paraphyletic assemblage of roundworms simply retaining a good number of ancestral traits. The old Enoplia do not seem to be monophyletic either, but to contain two distinct lineages. The old group "Chromadoria" seem to be another paraphyletic assemblage, with the Monhysterida representing a very ancient minor group of nematodes. Among the Secernentea, the Diplogasteria may need to be united with the Rhabditia, while the Tylenchia might be paraphyletic with the Rhabditia.

The understanding of roundworm systematics and phylogeny as of 2002 is summarised below:

Phylum Nematoda

- Basal order Monhysterida

- Class Dorylaimida
- Class Enoplea
- Class Secernentea
    - Subclass Diplogasteria (disputed)
    - Subclass Rhabditia (paraphyletic?)
    - Subclass Spiruria
    - Subclass Tylenchia (disputed)
- "Chromadorea" assemblage

Later work has suggested the presence of 12 clades. The Secernentea—a group that includes virtually all major animal and plant 'nematode' parasites—apparently arose from within the Adenophorea.

A major effort to improve the systematics of this phylum is in progress and being organised by the 959 Nematode Genomes.

A complete checklist of the World's nematode species can be found in the World Species Index:Nematoda.

An analysis of the mitochondrial DNA suggests that the following groupings are valid

- subclass Dorylaimia
- orders Rhabditida, Trichinellida and Mermithida
- suborder Rhabditina
- infraorders Spiruromorpha and Oxyuridomorpha

The Ascaridomorpha, Rhabditomorpha and Diplogasteromorpha appear to be related.

The suborders Spirurina and Tylenchina and the infraorders Rhabditomorpha, Panagrolaimomorpha and Tylenchomorpha are paraphytic.

The monophyly of the Ascaridomorph is uncertain.

ANATOMY

Nematodes are slender worms: typically approximately 5 to 100 μm thick, and at least 0.1 mm (0.0039 in) but less than 2.5mm long.The smallest nematodes are microscopic, while free-living species can reach as much as 5 cm (2.0 in), and some parasitic species are larger still, reaching over a meter in length.:[271] The body is often ornamented with ridges, rings, bristles, or other distinctive structures.

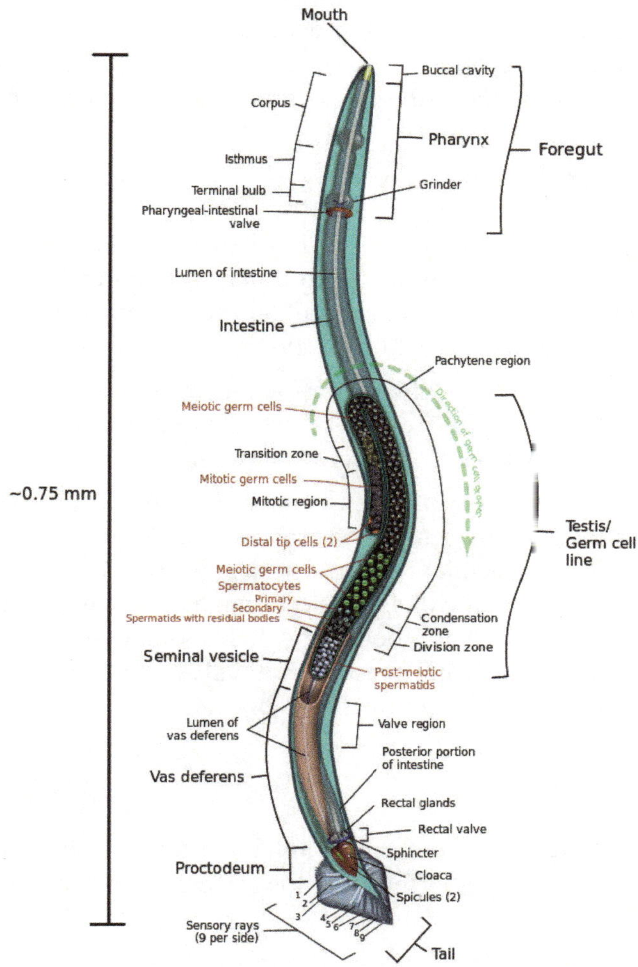

Internal anatomy of a male *C. elegans* nematode.

The head of a nematode is relatively distinct. Whereas the rest of the body is bilaterally symmetrical, the head is radially symmetrical, with sensory bristles and, in many cases, solid 'head-shields' radiating outwards around the mouth. The mouth has either three or six lips, which often bear a series of teeth on their inner edges. An adhesive 'caudal gland' is often found at the tip of the tail.

The epidermis is either a syncytium or a single layer of cells, and is covered by a thick collagenous cuticle. The cuticle is often of complex structure, and may have two or three distinct layers. Underneath the epidermis lies a layer of longitudinal muscle cells. The relatively rigid cuticle works with the muscles to create a hydroskeleton as nematodes lack circumferential muscles. Projections run from the inner surface of muscle cells towards the nerve cords; this is a unique arrangement in the animal kingdom, in which nerve cells normally extend fibres into the muscles rather than *vice versa*.

Digestive System

The oral cavity is lined with cuticle, which is often strengthened with ridges or other structures, and, especially in carnivorous species, may bear a number of teeth. The mouth often includes a sharp stylet, which the animal can thrust into its prey. In some species, the stylet is hollow, and can be used to suck liquids from plants or animals.

The oral cavity opens into a muscular, sucking pharynx, also lined with cuticle. Digestive glands are found in this region of the gut, producing enzymes that start to break down the food. In stylet-bearing species, these may even be injected into the prey.

There is no stomach, with the pharynx connecting directly to a muscleless intestine that forms the main length of the gut. This produces further enzymes, and also absorbs nutrients through its single cell thick lining. The last portion of the intestine is lined by cuticle, forming a rectum, which expels waste through the anus just below and in front of the tip of the tail. Movement of food through the digestive system is the result of body movements of the worm. The intestine has valves or sphincters at either end to help control the movement of food through the body.

Excretory System

Nitrogenous waste is excreted in the form of ammonia through the body wall, and is not associated with any specific organs. However, the structures for excreting salt to maintain osmoregulation are typically more complex.

In many marine nematodes, one or two unicellular 'renette glands' excrete salt through a pore on the underside of the animal, close to the pharynx. In most other nematodes, these specialized cells have been replaced by an organ consisting of two parallel ducts connected by a single transverse duct. This transverse duct opens into a common canal that runs to the excretory pore.

Nervous System

Four peripheral nerves run the length of the body on the dorsal, ventral, and lateral surfaces. Each nerve lies within a cord of connective tissue lying beneath the cuticle and between the muscle cells. The ventral nerve is the largest, and has a double structure forward of the excretory pore. The dorsal nerve is responsible for motor control, while the lateral nerves are sensory, and the ventral combines both functions.

The nervous system is also the only place in the nematode body that contains cilia, which are all non-motile and with a sensory function.

At the anterior end of the animal, the nerves branch from a dense, circular nerve (nerve ring) round surrounding the pharynx, and serving as the brain. Smaller nerves run forward from the ring to supply the sensory organs of the head.

The bodies of nematodes are covered in numerous sensory bristles and papillae that together provide a sense of touch. Behind the sensory bristles on the head lie two small pits, or 'amphids'. These are well supplied with nerve cells, and are probably chemoreception organs. A few aquatic nematodes possess what appear to be pigmented eye-spots, but is unclear whether or not these are actually sensory in nature.

REPRODUCTION

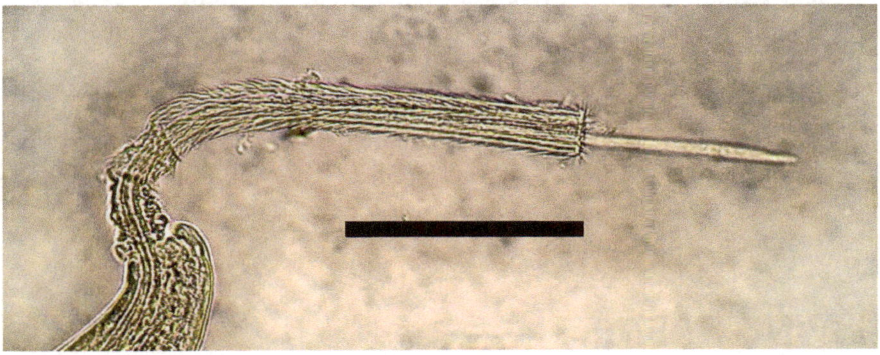

Extremity of a male nematode showing the spicule, used for copulation. Bar = 100 µm.

Most nematode species are dioecious, with separate male and female individuals, though some, such as *Caenorhabditis elegans*, are androdioecious, consisting of hermaphrodites and rare males. Both sexes possess one or two tubular gonads. In males, the sperm are produced at the end of the gonad and migrate along its length as they mature. The testis opens into a relatively wide seminal vesicle and then during intercourse into a glandular and muscular ejaculatory duct associated with the vas deferens and cloaca. In females, the ovaries each open into an oviduct (in hermaphrodites, the eggs enter a spermatheca first) and then a glandular uterus. The uteri both open into a common vulva/ vagina, usually located in the middle of the morphologically ventral surface.

Reproduction is usually sexual, though hermaphrodites are capable of self-fertilization. Males are usually smaller than females/ hermaphrodites (often much smaller) and often have a characteristically bent or fan-shaped tail for holding the other intercourse. During copulation, one or more chitinized spicules move out of the cloaca and are inserted into the genital pore of the female. Amoeboid sperm crawl along the spicule into the female worm. Nematode sperm is thought to be the only eukaryotic cell without the globular protein G-actin.

Eggs may be embryonated or unembryonated when passed by the female, meaning their fertilized eggs may not yet be developed. A few species are known to be ovoviviparous. The eggs are protected by an outer shell, secreted by the uterus. In free-living roundworms, the eggs hatch into larvae, which appear essentially identical to the adults, except for an underdeveloped reproductive system; in parasitic roundworms, the life cycle is often much more complicated.

Nematodes as a whole possess a wide range of modes of reproduction. Some nematodes, such as *Heterorhabditis* spp., undergo a process called *endotokia matricida*: intrauterine birth causing maternal death. Some nematodes are hermaphroditic, and keep their self-fertilized eggs inside the uterus until they hatch. The juvenile nematodes will then ingest the parent nematode. This process is significantly promoted in environments with a low food supply.

The nematode model species *Caenorhabditis elegans* and *C. briggsae* exhibit androdioecy, which is very rare among animals. The single genus *Meloidogyne* (root-knot nematodes) exhibit a range of reproductive modes, including sexual reproduction, facultative sexuality (in which most, but not all, generations reproduce asexually), and both meiotic and mitoticparthenogenesis.

The genus *Mesorhabditis* exhibits an unusual form of parthenogenesis, in which sperm-producing males copulate with females, but the sperm do not fuse with the ovum. Contact with the sperm is essential for the ovum to begin dividing, but because there is no fusion of the cells, the male contributes no genetic material to the offspring, which are essentially clones of the female.

FREE-LIVING SPECIES

In free-living species, development usually consists of four molts of the cuticle during growth. Different species feed on materials as varied as algae, fungi, small animals, fecal matter, dead organisms and living tissues. Free-living marine nematodes are important and abundant members of the meiobenthos. They play an important role in the decomposition process, aid in recycling of nutrients in marine environments, and are sensitive to changes in the environment caused by pollution. One roundworm of note, *Caenorhabditis elegans*, lives in the soil and has found much use as a model organism. *C. elegans* has had its entire genome sequenced, as well as the developmental fate of every cell determined, and every neuron mapped.

PARASITIC SPECIES

Nematodes commonly parasitic on humans include ascarids (*Ascaris*), filarias, hookworms, pinworms (*Enterobius*) and whipworms (*Trichuris trichiura*). The species *Trichinella spiralis*, commonly known as the 'trichina worm', occurs in rats, pigs, and humans, and is responsible for the disease trichinosis. *Baylisascaris* usually infests wild animals, but can be deadly to humans, as well. *Dirofilaria immitis* are known for causing heartworm disease by inhabiting the hearts, arteries, and lungs of dogs and some cats. *Haemonchus contortus* is one of the most abundant infectious agents in sheep around the world, causing great economic damage to sheep. In contrast, entomopathogenic nematodes parasitize insects and are mostly considered beneficial by humans, but some attack beneficial insects.

One form of nematode is entirely dependent upon fig wasps, which are the sole source of fig fertilization. They prey upon the wasps, riding them from the ripe fig of the wasp's birth to the fig flower of its death, where they kill the wasp, and their offspring await the birth of the next generation of wasps as the fig ripens.

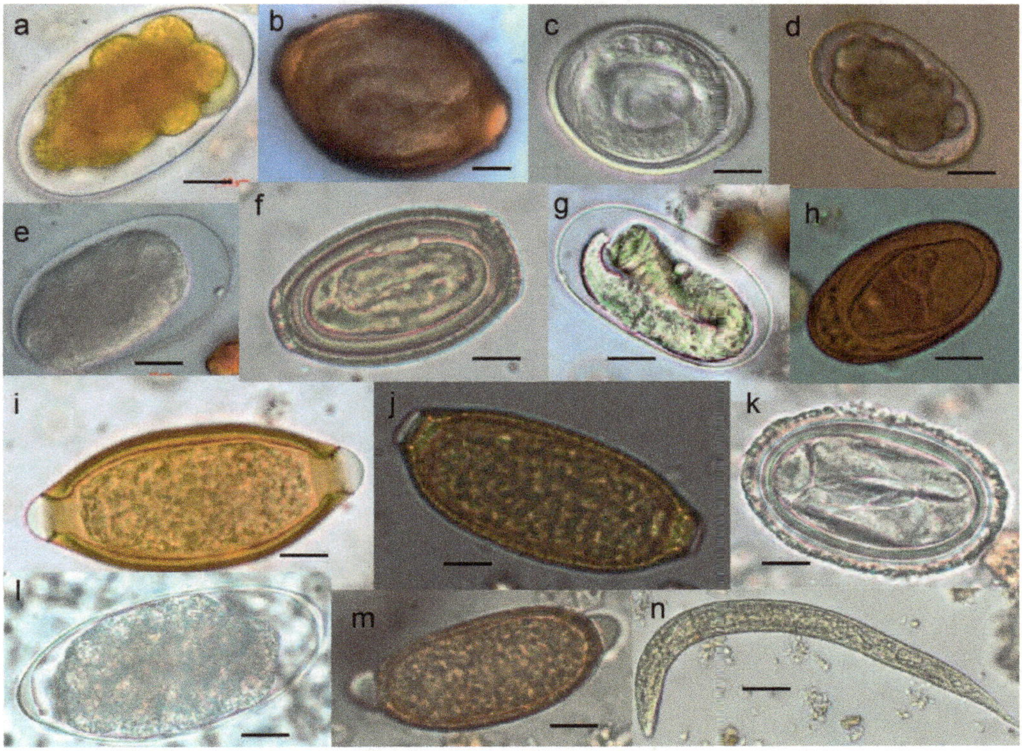

Eggs (mostly nematodes) from stools of wild primates.

A newly discovered parasitic tetradonematid nematode, *Myrmeconema neotropicum*, apparently induces fruit mimicry in the tropical ant *Cephalotes atratus*. Infected ants develop bright red gasters (abdomens), tend to be more sluggish, and walk with their gasters in a conspicuous elevated position. It is likely that these changes cause frugivorous birds to confuse the infected ants for berries, and eat them. Parasite eggs passed in the bird's feces are subsequently collected by foraging *Cephalotes atratus* and are fed to their larvae, thus completing the life cycle of *M. neotropicum*.

Similarly, multiple varieties of nematodes have been found in the abdominal cavities of the primitively social sweat bee, *Lasioglossum zephyrum*. Inside the female body, the nematode hinders ovarian development and renders the bee less active and thus less effective in pollen collection.

Plant-parasitic nematodes include several groups causing severe crop losses. The most common genera are *Aphelenchoides* (foliar nematodes), *Ditylenchus*, *Globodera* (potato cyst nematodes), *Heterodera* (soybean cyst nematodes), *Longidorus*, *Meloidogyne* (root-knot nematodes), *Nacobbus*, *Pratylenchus* (lesion nematodes), *Trichodorus* and *Xiphinema* (dagger nematodes). Several phytoparasitic nematode species cause histological damages to roots, including the formation of visible galls (e.g. by root-knot nematodes), which are useful characters for their diagnostic in the field. Some nematode species transmit plant viruses through their feeding activity on roots. One of them is *Xiphinema index*, vector of grapevine fanleaf virus, an important disease of grapes, another one is *Xiphinema diversicaudatum*, vector of arabis mosaic virus.

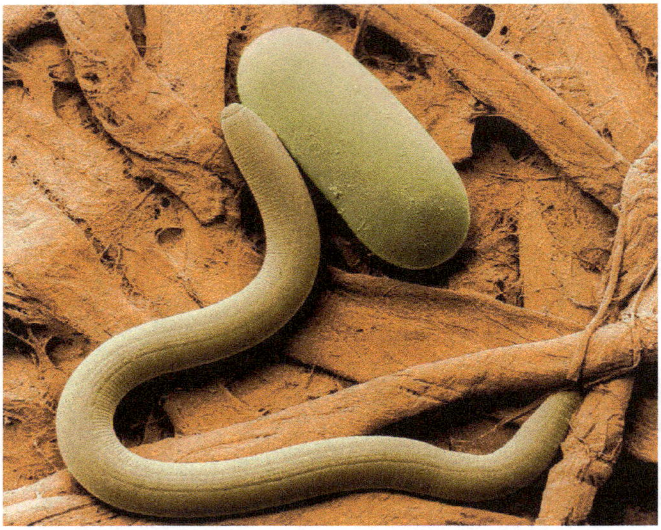

Colorized electron micrograph of soybean cyst nematode (*Heterodera* sp.) and egg

Other nematodes attack bark and forest trees. The most important representative of this group is *Bursaphelenchus xylophilus*, the pine wood nematode, present in Asia and America and recently discovered in Europe.

Agriculture and Horticulture

Depending on the species, a nematode may be beneficial or detrimental to plant health. From agricultural and horticulture perspectives, the two categories of nematodes are the predatory ones, which will kill garden pests like cutworms and corn earworm moths, and the pest nematodes, like the root-knot nematode, which attack plants, and those that act as vectors spreading plant viruses between crop plants. Predatory nematodes can be bred by soaking a specific recipe of leaves and other detritus in water, in a dark, cool place, and can even be purchased as an organic form of pest control.

Rotations of plants with nematode-resistant species or varieties is one means of managing parasitic nematode infestations. For example, marigolds, grown over one or more seasons (the effect is cumulative), can be used to control nematodes. Another is treatment with natural antagonists such as the fungus *Gliocladium roseum*. Chitosan, a natural biocontrol, elicits plant defense responses to destroy parasitic cyst nematodes on roots of soybean, corn, sugar beet, potato and tomato crops without harming beneficial nematodes in the soil. Soil steaming is an efficient method to kill nematodes before planting a crop, but indiscriminately eliminates both harmful and beneficial soil fauna.

The Golden Nematode (Globodera rostochiensis) is a particularly harmful variety of nematode pest that has resulted in quarantines and crop failures worldwide. CSIRO has found a 13- to 14-fold reduction of nematode population densities in plots having Indian mustard (*Brassica juncea*) green manure or seed meal in the soil.

Epidemiology

A number of intestinal nematodes cause diseases affecting human beings, including ascariasis, trichuriasis and hookworm disease. Filarial nematodes cause filariasis.

Soil Ecosystems

90 percent of nematodes reside in the top 15 cm of soil. Nematodes do not decompose organic matter, but, instead, are parasitic and free-living organisms that feed on living material. Nematodes can effectively regulate bacterial population and community composition - they may eat up to 5,000 bacteria per minute Also, Nematodes can play an important role in the nitrogen cycle by way of nitrogen mineralization.

One group of carnivorous fungi, the nematophagous fungi, are predators of soil nematodes. They set enticements for the nematodes in the form of lassos or adhesive structures.

Society and Culture

Nematode worms (*C. elegans*), the focus of an ongoing research project continued on shuttle mission STS-107, survived the Space Shuttle Columbia re-entry breakup. It is believed to be the first known life-form to survive a virtually unprotected atmospheric descent to Earth's surface.

Popular Culture

In the very first episode of *Doug*, Doug is tricked into a snipe hunt attempting to catch "neematoads" in the swamp, by town bully Roger Klotz.

In the *SpongeBob SquarePants* episode "Home Sweet Pineapple", SpongeBob's house is consumed by a swarm of nematodes. They appeared again in the episode "Best Day Ever".

On the BBC2 quiz show QI, when Clive Anderson was asked, "What lives in the Dead Sea?", he answered, "There must be a nematode worm, because nematode worms live everywhere." The correct answer, generally, is "extremophile."

REFERENCES

1. Chen, Z. X., Chen, S. Y., and Dickson, D. W. (2004). "A Century of Plant Nematology", pp. 1–42 in Nematology Advances and Perspectives, Vol 1. Tsinghua University Press, Beijing, China.

2. Chitwood, B. G., and Chitwood, M. B. (1950). "An Introduction to Nematology", pp. 1–5 in Introduction to Nematology. University Park Press, Baltimore.
3. Holy Bible, King James Version. (1979) p. 227. The Church of Jesus Christ of Latter-day Saints. Salt Lake City, Utah.
4. Hippocrates (460-375 B.C.) 1849. Works of Hippocrates, translated by F. Adams. London, "Aphorisms."
5. Aristotle (384-322 B.C.) 1910. Historia animalium. Translated by D'Arcy Wentworth Thompson. In: Works. J. A. Smith and W. D. Ross, eds. Vol. IV. Garrison Morton.
6. Celsus, A. C. (53 B.C.-7 A.D.) 1657. De medicina libri octo, ex recognitione Joh. Antonidae von Linden D. & Prof. Med. Pract. Ord.
7. Galen, C. (130–200) 1552. De simplicum medicamentorum faculatibus libre xi. Lugdoni.
8. Redi, F. (1684) p. 253 in Osservazioni...intorno agli animali viventi che si trovano negli animali viventi. 26 pls. Firenze.
9. Borellus, P. (1653) p. 240 in Historiarum, et observationum medicophysicarum, centuria prima, etc. Castris.
10. Tyson, E. (1683). "Lumbricus Teres, or Some Anatomical Observations on the Round Worm Bred in Human Bodies. By Edward Tyson M. D. Col. Med. Lond. Nec Non. Reg. Societ. Soc". Philosophical Transactions of the Royal Society of London. 13 (143–154): 154. doi:10.1098/rstl.1683.0023.
11. Hooke, R. (1667). Micrographia: etc. London.
12. Leeuwenhoek, O. (1722). Opera omnia seu arcana naturae (etc.). Lugduni Batavorum.
13. Needham, T. (1742). "A Letter from Mr. Turbevil Needham, to the President; Concerning Certain Chalky Tubulous Concretions, Called Malm: With Some Microscopical Observations on the Farina of the Red Lily, and of Worms Discovered in Smutty Corn". Philosophical Transactions of the Royal Society of London. 42 (462–471): 634. doi:10.1098/rstl.1742.0101.
14. Spallanzani, L. (1769). Nouvelles recherches sur les decouvertes microscopiques, etc. Londres & Paris.
15. Thorne, G. (1961). "Introduction", pp. 1–21 in Principles of Nematology. McGraw-Hill Book Company, Inc., New York.
16. Steiner, G. (1960). "Nematology-An Outlook", pp. 3–7 in Nematology: Fundamentals and Recent Advances. J. N. Sasser and W. R. Jenkins, eds. The University of North Carolina Press, Chapel Hill.
17. Van Gundy, S. D. (1987). "Perspectives on Nematology Research", pp. 28–31 in Vistas on Nematology. J. A. Veech and D. W. Dickson, eds. Society of Nematologists, Inc. Hyattsville, Maryland.
18. Kuhn, J. (1874). "Ubers das Vorkommen von Ruben-Nematoden an den Wurzeln der Halmfruchte". Landwirts. Jahrb. 3:47–50.

19. Cobb, N. A. (1918). "Estimating the nema population of soil". U.S. Department of Agriculture, Bur. Plant. Indrusty, Agr. Tech. Cir. 1:1–48.

20. Jenkins, W. R., and Taylor, D. P. (1967). "Introduction", p. 7 in Plant Nematology. Reinhold Publishing Corporation, New York.

21. Christie, J. R. (1960). "The Role of the Nematologist", pp. 8–11 in Nematology: Fundamentals and Recent Advances. J. N. Sasser and W. R. Jenkins, eds. The University of North Carolina Press, Chapel Hill.

22. Butschli, O. (1875). "Vorlaufige Mittheilung uber Untersuchungen betreffend die ersten Entwickelungsvorgange im befruchehen Ei von Nematoden und Schnecken". Ztschr. Wiss. Zool. v. 25:201–213.

23. Beneden, E. van. (1883). Recherches sur la maturation de l'oeuf, la fecondation et la division cellulaire. Gand & Leipzig.

24. Boveri, T. (1893). "Ueber die Entstehung des Gegensatzes zwischen den Geschlectszellen und den somatischen Zellen bei Ascaris megalocephala, nebst Bemerkungen zur Entwicklungsgeschichte der Nematoden". Sitzungsb. Gesellsch. Morph. u. Physiol. in Munchen.

CHAPTER 8

Phycology

Chapter Contents

- Introduction
- History of Phycology
- Development of Public Awareness
- Evolution of Classification in the Algae
- Algae
- Etymology and Study
- Classification
- Relationship to Land Plants
- Morphology
- Physiology
- Symbiotic Algsae
- Lifecycle
- Distribution

INTRODUCTION

Phycology is the scientific study of algae. Also known as algology, phycology is a branch of life science and often is regarded as a subdiscipline of botany.

Algae are important as primary producers in aquatic ecosystems. Most algae are eukaryotic, photosynthetic organisms that live in a wet environment. They are distinguished from the higher plants by a lack of true roots, stems or leaves. They do not flower. Many species are single-celled and microscopic (including phytoplankton and other microalgae); many others are multicellular to one degree or another, some of these growing to large size (for example, seaweeds such as kelp and Sargassum).

Phycology includes the study of prokaryotic forms known as blue-green algae or cyanobacteria. A number of microscopic algae also occur as symbionts in lichens.

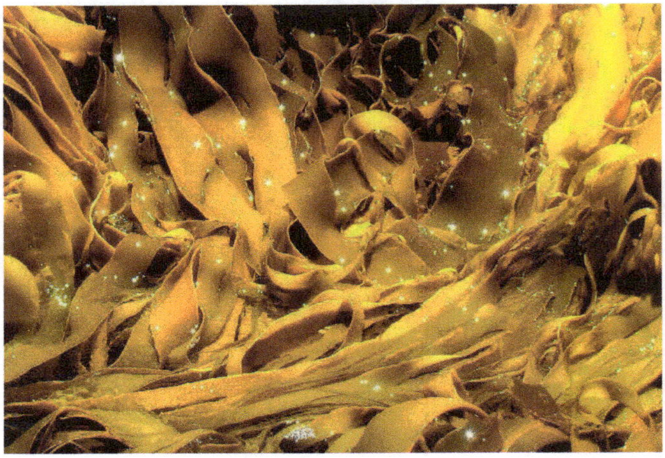

Kelp in Hazards Bay, Freycinet National Park, Tasmania, Australia.

HISTORY OF PHYCOLOGY

The history of phycology is the history of the scientific study of algae. Human interest in plants as food goes back into the origins of the species and knowledge of algae can be traced back more than two thousand years. However, only in the last three hundred years has that knowledge evolved into a rapidly developing science.

Early Days

The study of botany goes back into pre-history as plants were the food of people from the beginning of the human race. The first attempts at plant cultivation are believed to have been made shortly before 10,000 BC in Western Asia (Morton, 1981) and the first references to algae are to be found in early Chinese literature. Records as far back as 3000 BC indicate that algae were used by the emperor of China as food (Huisman, 2000 p. 13). The use of Porphyra in China dates back to at least A.D. 533–44 (Mumfard and Miura, 1988), there are also references in Roman and Greek literature. The Greek word for algae was "Phycos" whilst in Roman times the name became Fucus. There are early references to the use of algae for manure. The first coralline algae to be recognized as living organisms were probably Corallina, by Pliny the Elder in the 1st century AD (Irvine and Chamberlain, 1994 p. 11).

The classification of plants suffered many changes since Theophrastus (372–287 B.C.) and Aristotle (384–322 B.C.) grouped them as "trees", "shrubs" and "herbs" (Smith, 1955 p. 1).

Little is known of botany during the Middle Ages — it was the Dark Ages of botany.

The development of the study of phycology runs in a pattern comparable with, and parallel to, other biological fields but at a different rate. After the invention of the printing-press in the 15th century (with the publication of the first printed book: Gutenberg's Bible of 1488) education enabled people to read and knowledge to spread.

Exploration of the World and the Advance of Knowledge

Written accounts of the algae of South Africa were made by the Portuguese explorers of the 15th and 16th centuries, however it is not clear to which species reference was being made (Huisman, 2000 p. 7).

17th Century

In the 17th Century there was a great awakening of scientific interest all over Europe, and after the invention of the printing-press books on botany were published. Among them was the work of John Ray who wrote in 1660: Catalogus Plantarum circa Cantabrigiam., this initiated a new era in the study of Botany (Smith, 1975 p. 4). Ray "influenced both the theory and the practice of botany more decisively than any other single person in the latter half of the seventeenth century" (Morton, 1981).

However no real progress was made in the scientific study of algae until the invention of the microscope — in about 1600. It was Anton van Leeuwenhoek (1632–1723) who discovered bacteria and saw the cell structure of plants. His unsystematic glimpses of plant structure, reported to the Royal Society between 1678 and his death in 1723, produced no significant advances (Morton, 1981 p. 180).

As adventurers explored the world more species of all animals and plants were discovered, this demanded efforts to bring order out of this quickly accumulating knowledge.

The first Australian marine plant recorded in print was collected from Shark Bay on the Western Australian coast by William Dampier who described many new species of Australian wildlife in the 17th century (Huisman, 2000 p. 7).

18th Century

Before Carl von Linné (1707–1778) animals and plants had names, but it took him to arrange the names and group the plants of this Earth in some sort of order. Carl Linnaeus (Carl von Linné) was a Swedish botanist, the son of a pastor of the Lutheran church, a physician and zoologist. He laid the foundations of modern biological systematics and nomenclature in his Species Plantarum (1753). He adopted and popularized a binomial (or binary) system of designation (Morton, 1981) using one name as the genus and a second name as the species name both in Latin or Latinised. This specific name he referred to as a trivial name nomen triviale consisting of a single word, normally a Latin adjective, but any single word would suffice, to identify a particular species, but not intended to describe it. He developed a coherent system for naming organisms and divided the plant kingdom into 25 classes (according to Smith p. 1 and p. 24 according to Dixon, 1973) (Smith, 1955 p. 1), one of which, the Cryptogamia, included all plants with concealed reproductive organs. He divided the Cryptogamia into four orders: Filices, Musci (mosses), Algae — which included lichens and liverworts and fungi (Smith, 1955 p. 1).

Examination for the reproductive structures had already started. In 1711, R.A.F de Réaumur gave an account of Fucus in which noted the two types of external openings in the thallus: the non-sexual cryptostromata (sterile surface cavities) and the conceptacles (fertile cavities, immersed but with a surface opening) containing the sexual organs, which he thought were female flowers. With a lens he was able to see the oogonoa (the female sex organs) and the antheridia (the male sex organs) within the conceptacles, but he interpreted these as seeds (Morton, 1981 p. 245). Johann Hedwig (1730–1799) provided further evidence of the sexual process in algae, and figured conjugation in Spirogyra Hedwig in 1797. He also illustrated Chara (Charales) and identified the antheridia and oogonia as male and female sexual organs (Morton, 1981 p. 323 & 357).

Harvey commented on ...motion, apparently spontaneous, among the seeds at the period of germination. Some found it difficult...to account for these anomalous motions. ...that the seeds becomes (how is not said) a perfect nimalcule, which after enjoying an animal existence for a time ceases to live animally, and, reverting to its original nature, gives birth to a vegetable. Thus, this seed was first vegetable, then animal, and then again vegeable,... . During the 18th Century there was a stormy controversy as to whether coralline algae were plants or animals. Up to the mid-18th century coralline algae (and coral animals) were generally treated as plants. By 1768 many, but by no means all authorities, considered them animal. Five years later, Harvey concluded that they were certainly of vegetable material he noted: "The question of the vegetable nature of Corallines, among which the Melobesia take rank, may now be considered as finally set at rest, by the researches of Kützing, Phillipi and Decaisne." (Harvey,1847, pl. 73).

The first scientific species description of a South African seaweed accepted for most nomenclatural purposes is that of Ecklonia maxima, published in 1757 as Fucus maximus (Stegenga et al., 1997).

Knowledge of North American Pacific algae begins with the 1791–95 expedition of Captain George Vancouver (Papenfuss,1976 p. 21).

Archibald Menzies (1754–1842) was the appointed botanist on the expedition led by Captain George Vancouver in the ships Discovery and Chatham of 1791–1795 to the Pacific coast of North America and south-western Australia. The algae collected by Menzies were passed to Dawson Turner (1775–1858) who described and illustrated them in a four-volumed work published in 1808–1819. However Turner only referred to the taxa referable to Fucus; either Menzies collected very few or he gave only a few to Turner. Three of these species described by Turner later became the types of new genera (Papenfuss, 1976) and (Huisman, 2000) Turner also received plants from Robert Brown (1773–1858) the botanist who accompanied Captain Matthew Flinders on the Investigator (1801–1805). This collection also included many plants from Australia (Huisman, 2000).

The real awakening of interest in American algae resulted from a visit by William Henry Harvey in 1849–1850 when he visited areas from Florida to Nova Scotia and produced three volumes of Nereis Boreali-Americana. These gave an incentive to others to study algae (Taylor, 1972 p. 21).

The first collector of marine algae in Greenland waters seems to have been J.M.Vahl who lived in Greenland from 1828 to 1836. Vahl's East Greenland species were not recorded until 1893 when Rosenvinge included them in his work of 1893 together with the species collected by Sylow (Lund, 1959). F.R.Kjellman records only 12 species from East Greenland 4 of which are doubtful, these records are based on Zeller's list (Lund, 1959).

Early 19th Century

Carl Adolph Agardh was one of the most prominent algologists of all time, he was born in Sweden on 23 January 1785 and died on 28 January 1859. He was Professor of Botany at the University of Lund and later Bishop of Karlstad Diocese (Papenfuss, 1976). Many species still show his name as the authority of the scientific name. He traveled widely in Europe visiting Germany, Poland, Denmark, the Netherlands, Belgium, France and Italy and was the first to emphasize the importance of the reproductive characters of algae and use them to distinguish the different genera and families. His son, Jacob Georg Agardh (1813–1901), who became Professor of Botany at Lund in 1839, made a study of the life-histories of algae, described many new genera and species. It was to him that many workers sent specimens for determination and as donations. Because of this the herbarium at Lund is the most important algal herbaria in the world (Papenfuss, 1976).

The first records of algae from the Faroe Islands were made by Jørgen Landt in his book of 1800 where he mentions about 30 species. Following this, Hans Christian Lyngbye visited the Faroe Islands in 1817 and published his work in 1819. In this, he described several new genera and species, some 100 new species were listed. Emil Rostrup who visited the Faroe Islands in 1867 listed ten new species and a total not far from 100. In 1895, Herman G. Simmons mentioned 125 species. In that year F. Børgesen (1866–1956) started work and in 1902 published his work (Børgesen, 1902).

Jean Vincent Félix Lamouroux (1779–1825) was the first, in 1813, to separate the algae into groups on the basis of colour (Dixon and Irvine, 1977 p. 59). At this time all coralline algae were considered animals, it was R. Philippi who in 1837 published his paper in which he finally recognized that coralline algae were not animals and he proposed the generic names Lithophyllum and Lithothamnion (Irvine and Chamberlain, 1994 p. 11).

Freshwater algae are commonly treated separately from marine algae and may be considered not correctly placed in phycology. Lewis Weston Dillwyn (1778–1855) "British Confervae" (1809) was one of the earliest attempts to bring together all that was then known on the British Freshwater algae .

Specimens of Anne E. Ball (1808–1872) have been found in both the Herbarium of the Irish National Botanic Gardens, Dublin and the Ulster Museum (BEL). A.E.Ball was an Irish algologist who corresponded with W.H. Harvey and whose records appear in his Phycologia Britannica. The specimens in Dublin do not contain any unusual or rare items. However, they are well documented.

W.H. Harvey

Willian Henry Harvey (1811–1866), Keeper of the Herbarium and Professor in Botany at Trinity College, Dublin, was one of the most distinguished algologists of his time (Papenfuss, 1976 p. 26). Apart from Ireland he visited South Africa, the Atlantic seaboard of America as far south as the Florida Keys on the east coast of North America and Australia (1854–1856). Between 1853 and 1856 he visited Ceylon, Australia and New Zealand and various parts of the South Pacific (Huisman, 2000 & Papenfuss, 1976). His collection in Australia resulted in one of the most extensive collections of marine plants and it inspired others (Huisman, 2000). He published: Nereis Australis Or Algae of the Southern Ocean in 1847–1849 and in 1846–51 his Phycologia Britannica appeared. His Nereis Boreali-Americana was published in three parts (1852–1858) this was the first, and still is (1976) is the only marine algal flora of North America as it includes taxa from the Pacific coast (Papenfuss, 1976 p. 27). His five-volume Phycologia Australica was published in 1858 to 1863. These volumes remain to this day a most important reference to Australian algae (Huisman, 2000). His primary herbarium is in Trinity College, Dublin (TCD). However large collections of Harvey material are to be found in the Ulster Museum (BEL) (Morton, 1977; Morton, 1981); University of St Andrews (STA) and National Herbarium of Victoria (MEL), Melbourne, Australia (May, 1977).Many of the collectors of this period sent, and exchanged, specimens freely one to another, as a result Harvey's books show a remarkable knowledge of the distribution of algae elsewhere in the world. His Phycologia Britannica lists species recorded and collected from various parts of the British Isles. For example, he notes William Thompson (1805–1852), William McCalla (c.1814–1849), John Templeton (1766–1825) and D. Landsborough (1779–1854) who collected, as he did, from distinct sites in Ireland. The collections of these botanists, and many others, are represented separately by collections in the Ulster Museum (BEL).

Sir William Jackson Hooker (1785–1865) was a lifelong friend of Harvey (Papenfuss, 1976 p. 26), he was appointed Professor of Botany at Glasgow University in 1820 and became Director in Kew 1841–1865. Hooker recognized the talent in Harvey and lent him books, encouraged and invited him to write the section on algae in his British Flora. as well as the section on algae for The Botany of Captain Beechey's Voyage (Papenfuss, 1976). Margaret Gatty (1809–1873) (née Margaret Scott) (author of British Seaweeds, 1863), and others, corresponded with William Henry Harvey (Desmond, 1977 and Evans, 2003).

Late 19th Century

Much work was done in this period by many workers and the many specimens became very valuable. Harvey's specimens, are to be found in at least several herbaria as well as those of other phycologists whose names are to be found in historic publications. In the same period Friedrich Traugott Kützing (1807–1893) in Germany described more new genera than anyone either before or after (Chapman, 1968 p. 13). His publications span the period 1841 to 1869 and added materially to knowledge of algae of cold waters of the Arctic seas. Some of his specimens are stored in the Ulster Museum Herbarium (BEL) catalogued: F1171; F10281–F10318. In 1883 Frans Reinhold Kjellman, Professor of Botany at Uppsala University, published The Algae of the Arctic Sea. He divided the "Arctic Sea" into different regions which surround the North Pole (Kjellman, 1883). Further research work on the marine algae of the world included: Charles Lewis Anderson (1827–1910) who collaborated with William Gilson Farlow and with Professor Daniel Cady Eaton to produce on the first exsiccatae of North American Algae (Papenfuss, 1976). Edward Morell Holmes (1843–1930), was an expert on seaweeds, mosses, liverworts and lichens, specimens were sent to him from all over the British Isles, as well as from Norway, Sweden, Florida, Tasmania, France, Cape of Good Hope, Ceylon and Australia. He also exchanged specimens (Furley, 1989). and some are in the herbarium of the Ulster Museum (BEL). George Clifton (1823–1913) an Australian phycologist is mentioned in Harvey's Memoirs, as the Superintendent of the Water Police in Perth, West Australia sent algal specimens to Harvey (Blackler, H.1977). In these years there were many workers in this field: W.G. Farlow, mentioned above, who was appointed in 1879 Professor of Cryptogamic Botany at University of Harvard (U.S.A.) in 1879 and published, among other works, the Marine algae of New England and Adjacent Coasts.; in 1876 John Erhard Areschoug, a Swedish Professor of Botany at Upsalla University, reported on some brown algae collected in California by Gustavus A. Eisen (Papenfuss. 1976). George W.Traill (1836–1897) was a clerk in the Standard Life Company in Edinburgh where he worked long hours, yet he was one of the greatest authorities on Scottish algae. Despite bad health he was an indefatigable collector. In 1892 he gave his collection to the Herbarium of the Edinburgh Botanic Gardens (Furley, 1989).

Mikael Heggelund Foslie (M.Foslie) (1855–1905) published 69 papers between 1887–1909. During this time he increased the number of species and forms (of corallines) from 175 to 650 (Irvine and Chamberlain, 1994). After his death his collection of specimens was purchased by the Museum of the Royal Norwegian Society for Sciences and Letters (Thor et al., 2005) and there is a small collection of his in the Ulster Museum Herbarium: (Collection No. 42) entitled: Algae Norvegicae (Ulster Museum Herbarium catalogue (BEL): F10319–F10334). F.Heydrich also described 84 taxa and was a bitter foe of Foslie. This left a legacy of complicated and still unresolved problems.

It was in the 19th Century that the true nature of lichens, as organisms consisting of an alga and a fungus in specific association, was demonstrated by Schwendener in 1867. This removed a source of confusion in morphology and classification (Morton, 1981 p. 432). It was in this period (1859) that Charles Darwin (1809–1882) published his book on evolution:On the Origin of Species by Means of Natural Selection,....

20th Century

In 1895 Børgesen started his study of the Faeroe Islands and published his work in 1902. Later between 1920 and 1936 he published his research on the algae of the Canary Islands.

In 1935 and 1945 Felix Eugen Fritsch (1879–1954) published in two volumes his treatise: The Structure and Reproduction of the Algae. These two volumes detail virtually all that was then known about the morphology and reproduction of the algae. However knowledge of algae has so greatly increased since then it would be impossible for these to be brought up-to-date. Nevertheless, reference is often made to them. Other valuable works published in the 1950s include Cryptogamic Botany. written by Gilbert Morgan Smith (1885–1959), the algal volume (no.1) was published in 1955. In the following year (1956), Die Gattungen der Rhodophyceen. by Johan Harald Kylin (1879–1949) was published posthumously. Other phycologists who contributed massively to the knowledge of algae include: Elmer Yale Dawson (1918–1966) who published over 60 papers on the algae of the North American Pacific seas (Papenfuss, 1976).

DEVELOPMENT OF PUBLIC AWARENESS

The number of books published in the mid to late 19th century shows how interest in the natural world developed. Books on algae were written by: Isabella Gifford (1853) The Marine Botanist..., some of her specimens are in the Ulster Museum; D. Landsborough (c.1779–1854) A Popular History of British Seaweeds,... third edition published in 1857; Louisa Lane Clarke (c.1812–1883) The Common Seaweeds of the British Coast and Channel Islands;... in 1865; S.O.Gray (1828–1902) British Seaweeds:... published 1867 and W.H.Grattann British Marine Algae:...published about 1874. These books were for the common people.

In 1902 Edward Arthur Lionel Batters (1860–1907) published "A catalogue of the British Marine algae." (Batters, 1902). In this he detailed records of algae found on the shores of the British Isles with the localities. This was the start of a new approach, the bringing together of records, detailed keys, checklists and mapping schemes.

The process accelerated in the 20th century. Lilly Newton (née Batten) (1893–1981) Professor in Botany at the University College of Wales, Aberystwyth and Professor Emeritus in 1931 wrote: A Handbook of the British Seaweeds. This was the first, and for quite a time, the only book for identification of seaweeds in the British Isles using a botanical key. In 1962 Eifion Jones published: A key to the genera of the British seaweeds. This small booklet provided a valuable source in the period before the valuable series Seaweeds of the British Isles was produced by the British Museum (Natural History) or The Natural History Museum.

Research advanced so quickly that the need for an up-to-date checklist became apparent. Mary Parke (1902–1981), who was a founder member of the British Phycological Society, produced a preliminary checklist of British marine algae in 1953, corrections and additions of this were published in 1956, 1957 and 1959. In 1964 M.Parke and Peter Stanley Dixon (1929–1993) published a revised check-list, a second revision of this was produced in 1968 and a third revision in 1976. Distribution was added to the checklist in 1986 with G.R.South and I.Tittley's A Checklist and Distributional Index of the Benthic Marine Algae of the North Atlantic Ocean. In 2003 A Check-list and Atlas of the Seaweeds of Britain and Ireland was published by Gavin Hardy and Michael Guiry with a revised edition in 2006. This shows how rapidly knowledge of algae, at least in the British Isles, advanced. First efforts had been made by interested biologists and people capable of identifying the algae, this required books using the botanical names. Botanical keys to identify the plants then developed, followed by checklists. As more information was brought to light by interested workers, some volunteers, the checklists were improved and eventually a mapping scheme brought together all this information. The same pattern of knowledge developed with birds, mammals and flowering plants, though to a different time-scale and knowledge in other parts of the world has developed to this degree.

Numbers and Checklists

As records were collected the need to draw all the information together advanced. Checklists and annotated checklists were produced and updated so the actual numbers of different species became more precise. At first this was quite local. Threlkeld, in 1726, produced the first attempt at an enumeration of Irish Algae and in 1802 William Tighe published his "Marine plants observed at the County of Wexford," it included 58 marine and 2 freshwater species. In 1804 Wade published Plantae Rariores in Hibernia Inventae, in which 51 species of marine and 4 species of freshwater algae were enumerated. In the north of Ireland John Templeton and William Thompson were at work publishing on the algae of Ireland. In 1836 Mackay published his Flora Hibernica including 296 species. Adams, in his synopsis of 1908, listed a total of marine species reaching 843.

In more localised lists Adams (in 1907) listed the species of County Antrim noted that of the 747 species included in "Batter's List" he recorded 211 species from the Co. Antrim coast. In 1907 a list of marine aslgae from Lambay Island (County Dublin) was published by Batters. In 1960 A preliminary list of the marine algae of Galloway coast was published.

At the international level there are well over 3,000 species of alga in Australia.

Identification

As the study and identification of the different species became more extensive it became clear that identification was not at all easy. Harvey's 1846–51 Phycologia Britannica along with his other publications makes no effort to provide "keys" to help in the identification. In 1931 Newton's Handbook which gave the first key to assist in the identification of algae of the British Isles, in the same year Knight and Park gave a key in their "Manx Algae." Eifion Jones in 1962, wrote a key to the genera of British seaweeds. Others soon followed: Dickinson wrote one entitled British Seaweeds. and Adey and Adey (1973) gave keys to the identification of the Corallinaceae of the British Isles. Abott and Hollenberg, in 1976, published keys to the identification of algae of California.

EVOLUTION OF CLASSIFICATION IN THE ALGAE

Linnaeus's "sexual system" (Linnaeus, 1754) in which he grouped plants according to the number of stamens and carpels in their flowers, although wholly artificial was advantageous in that a newly discovered plant could be fitted in amongst those already known. He divided the plant kingdom into 25 classes, one of which was the Cryptogamia — plants with "concealed reproductive organs" (see above) (Smith, 1955). Linnaeus accepted 14 genera of algae of which only four, Conferva, Ulva, Fucus and Chara, contained organisms now regarded as algae (Dixon, 1973 p. 231). As a consequence of the great increase in the number of species the artificiality of the Linnaean system was appreciated so that during the 18th Century and early 19th Century considerable numbers of new genera were described. J.V.F.Lamouroux in 1813 was the first to separate the groups on the basis of colour, however this was not taken up by other botanists and it was Harvey who, in 1836, divided the algae into four major divisions solely on the basis of their pigmentation: Rhodospermae (red algae), Melanospermae (brown algae), Chlorospermae (green algae) and Diatomaceae (Dixon,1973 p. 232).

In 1883 and 1897 Schmitz separated the Rhodophyceae into two main groups. The first contained the Bangiales and the second the Nemoniales, Cryptonemiales, Gigartinales and Rhodymeniales (Newton, 1931). The Rhodophyta are now arranged in the Orders: Porphyridiales, Goniotrichales, Erythropeltidales, Bangiales, Acrochaetiales, Colaconematales, Palmariales, Ahnfeltiales, Nemaliales, Gelidiales, Gracilariales, Bonnemaisoniales, Cryptonemiales, Hildenbrandiales, Corallinales, Gigartinales, Plocamiales, Rhodymeniales and Ceramiales. The Chlorophyta are arranged in the Orders: Chlorococcales, Microsporales, Chaetophorales, Phaeophilales, Ulvales, Prasiolales, Acrosiphoniales, Cladiphorales, Bryopsidales, Chlorocystidales, Klebsormidiales and Ulotrichales. The Heterokontophyta: Sphacelariales, Dictyotales, Ectocarpales, Ralfsiales, Utleriales, Sporochniales, Tilopteridales, Desmarestiales, Laminariales and the Fucales (Hardy and Guiry, 2006).

Recently (1990s) The Kingdom: Protoctista has been recommended, however, this has not been accepted by many authors.

ALGAE

Algae is an informal term for a large, diverse group of photosynthetic organisms which are not necessarily closely related, and is thus polyphyletic. Included organisms range from unicellular genera, such as Chlorella and the diatoms, to multicellular forms, such as the giant kelp, a large brown alga which may grow up to 50 m in length. Most are aquatic and autotrophic and lack many of the distinct cell and tissue types, such as stomata, xylem, and phloem, which are found in land plants. The largest and most complex marine algae are called seaweeds, while the most complex freshwater forms are the Charophyta, a division of green algae which includes, for example, Spirogyra and the stoneworts.

No definition of algae is generally accepted. One definition is that algae "have chlorophyll as their primary photosynthetic pigment and lack a sterile covering of cells around their reproductive cells". Some authors exclude all prokaryotes thus do not consider cyanobacteria (blue-green algae) as algae.

Algae constitute a polyphyletic group since they do not include a common ancestor, and although their plastids seem to have a single origin, from cyanobacteria, they were acquired in different ways. Green algae are examples of algae that have primary chloroplasts derived from endosymbiotic cyanobacteria. Diatoms and brown algae are examples of algae with secondary chloroplasts derived from an endosymbiotic red alga.

Algae exhibit a wide range of reproductive strategies, from simple asexual cell division to complex forms of sexual reproduction.

Algae lack the various structures that characterize land plants, such as the phyllids (leaf-like structures) of bryophytes, rhizoids in nonvascular plants, and the roots, leaves, and other organs found in tracheophytes (vascular plants). Most are phototrophic, although some are mixotrophic, deriving energy both from photosynthesis and uptake of organic carbon either by osmotrophy, myzotrophy, or phagotrophy. Some unicellular species of green algae, many golden algae, euglenids, dinoflagellates, and other algae have become heterotrophs (also called colorless or apochlorotic algae), sometimes parasitic, relying entirely on external energy sources and have limited or no photosynthetic apparatus.

Some other heterotrophic organisms, such as the apicomplexans, are also derived from cells whose ancestors possessed plastids, but are not traditionally considered as algae. Algae have photosynthetic machinery ultimately derived from cyanobacteria that produce oxygen as a by-product of photosynthesis, unlike other photosynthetic bacteria such as purple and green sulfur bacteria. Fossilized filamentous algae from the Vindhya basin have been dated back to 1.6 to 1.7 billion years ago.

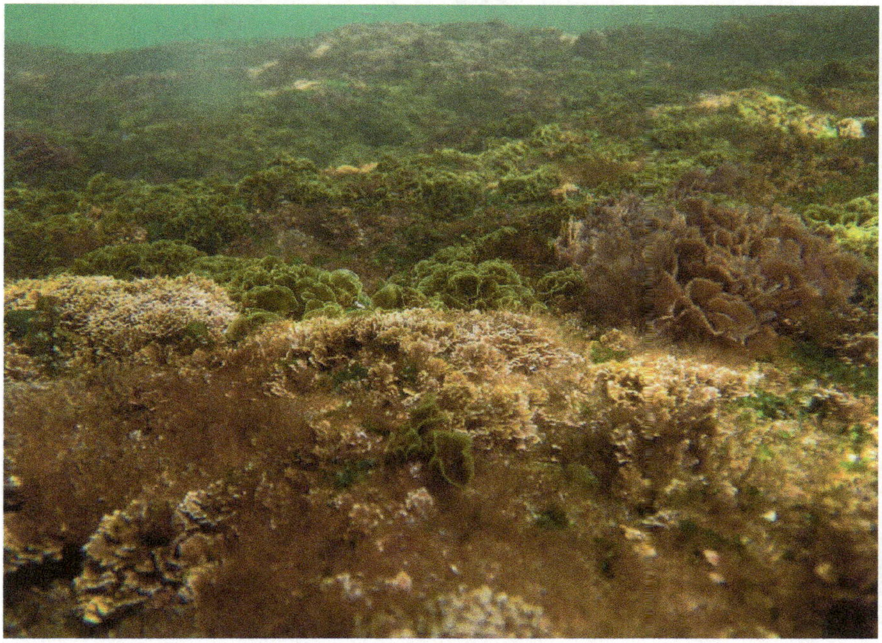

A variety of algae growing on the sea bed in shallow waters.

ETYMOLOGY AND STUDY

The singular alga is the Latin word for "seaweed" and retains that meaning in English. The etymology is obscure. Although some speculate that it is related to Latin algēre, "be cold", no reason is known to associate seaweed with temperature. A more likely source is alliga, "binding, entwining".

The Ancient Greek word for seaweed was fūkos or phykos, which could mean either the seaweed (probably red algae) or a red dye derived from it. The Latinization, fūcus, meant primarily the cosmetic rouge. The etymology is uncertain, but a strong candidate has long been some word related to the Biblical pūk, "paint" (if not that word itself), a cosmetic eye-shadow used by the ancient Egyptians and other inhabitants of the eastern Mediterranean. It could be any color: black, red, green, or blue.

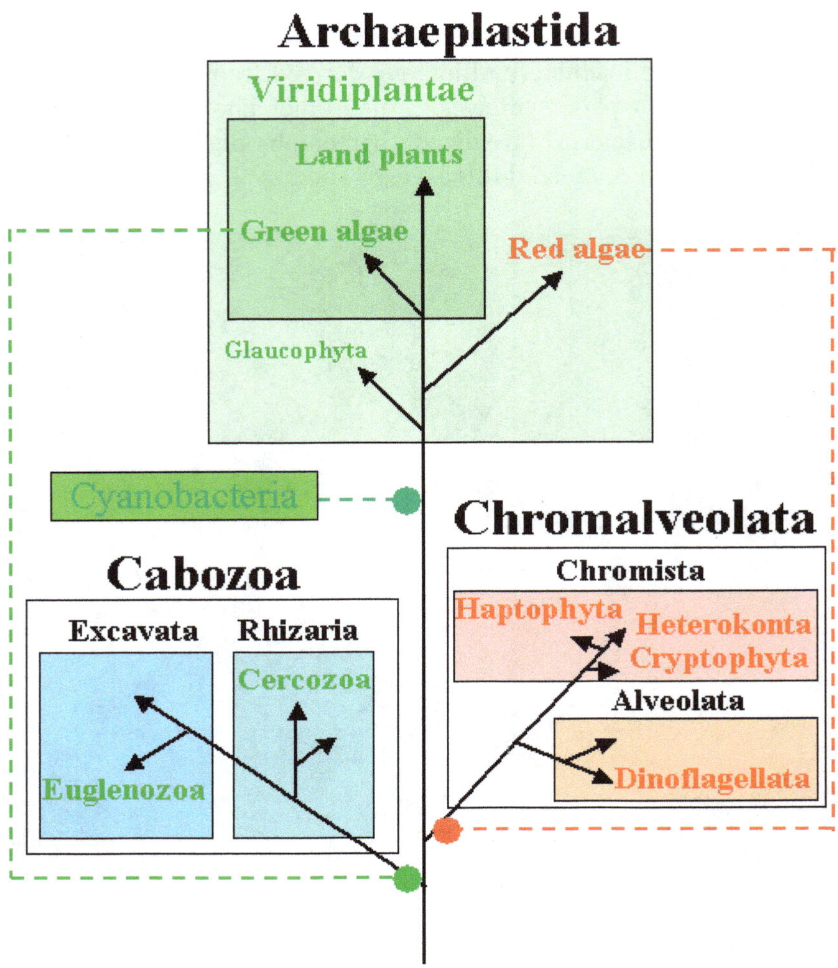

The lineage of algae according to Thomas Cavalier-Smith. The exact number and placement of endosymbiotic events is currently unknown, so this diagram can be taken only as a general guide. It represents the most parsimonious way of explaining the three types of endosymbiotic origins of plastids. These types include the endosymbiotic events of cyanobacteria, red algae and green algae, leading to the hypothesis of the supergroups Archaeplastida, Chromalveolata and Cabozoa respectively. Endosymbiotic events are noted with dotted lines.

Accordingly, the modern study of marine and freshwater algae is called either phycology or algology, depending on whether the Greek or Latin root is used. The name Fucus appears in a number of taxa.

CLASSIFICATION

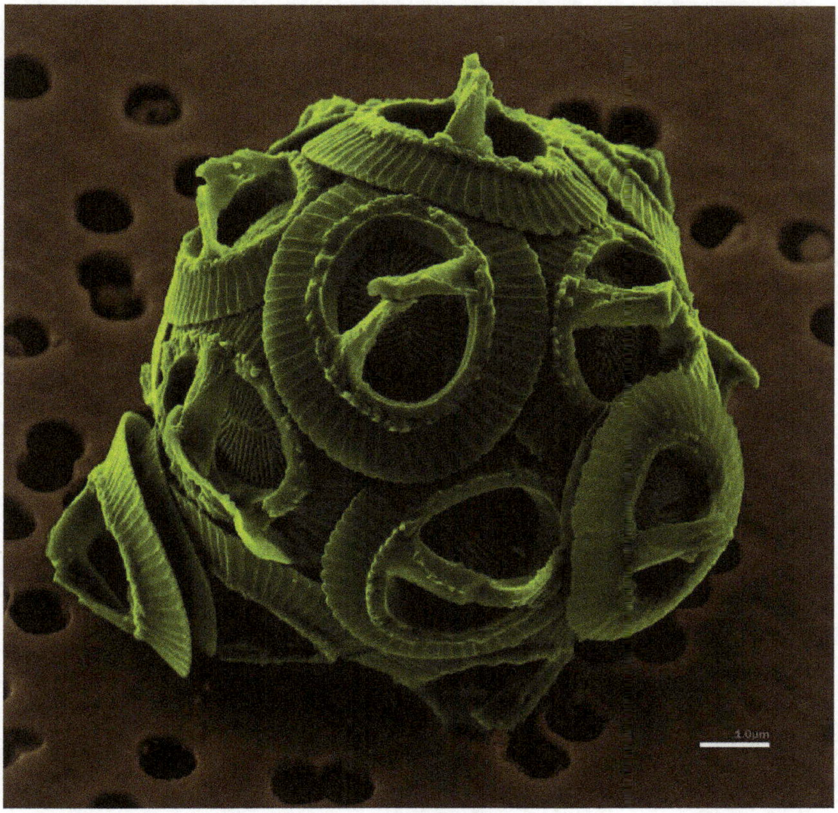

False-color scanning electron micrograph of the unicellular coccolithophore Gephyrocapsa oceanica.

Most algae contain chloroplasts that are similar in structure to cyanobacteria. Chloroplasts contain circular DNA like that in cyanobacteria and presumably represent reduced endosymbiotic cyanobacteria. However, the exact origin of the chloroplasts is different among separate lineages of algae, reflecting their acquisition during different endosymbiotic events. The table below describes the composition of the three major groups of algae. Their lineage relationships are shown in the figure in the upper right. Many of these groups contain some members that are no longer photosynthetic. Some retain plastids, but not chloroplasts, while others have lost plastids entirely.

Phylogeny based on plastid not nucleocytoplasmic genealogy:

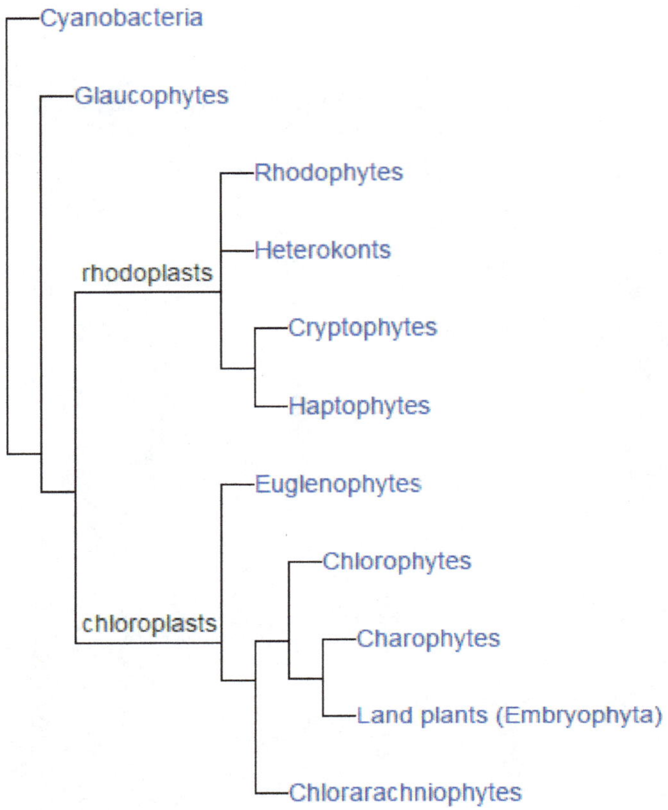

Supergroup affiliation	Members	Endosymbiont	Summary
Primoplantae/ Archaeplastida	• Chlorophyta • Rhodophyta • Glaucophyta	Cyanobacteria	These algae have 'primary' chloroplasts, i.e. the chloroplasts are surrounded by two membranes and probably developed through a single endosymbiotic event. The chloroplasts of red algae have chlorophylls a and c (often), and phycobilins, while those of green algae have chloroplasts with chlorophyll a and b without phycobilins. Land plants are pigmented similarly to green algae and probably developed from them, thus the Chlorophyta is a sister taxon to the plants; sometimes the Chlorophyta, the Charophyta, and land plants are grouped together as the Viridiplantae.

Excavata and Rhizaria	• Chlorarachniophytes • Euglenids	Green algae	These groups have green chloroplasts containing chlorophylls a and b. Their chloroplasts are surrounded by four and three membranes, respectively, and were probably retained from ingested green algae. **Chlorarachniophytes**, which belong to the phylum Cercozoa, contain a small nucleomorph, which is a relict of the algae's nucleus. **Euglenids**, which belong to the phylum Euglenozoa, live primarily in fresh water and have chloroplasts with only three membranes. The endosymbiotic green algae may have been acquired through myzocytosis rather than phagocytosis.
Chromista and Alveolata	• Heterokonts • Haptophyta • Cryptomonads • Dinoflagellates	Red algae	These groups have chloroplasts containing chlorophylls a and c, and phycobilins. The shape varies from plant to plant; they may be of discoid, plate-like, reticulate, cup-shaped, spiral, or ribbon shaped. They have one or more pyrenoids to preserve protein and starch. The latter chlorophyll type is not known from any prokaryotes or primary chloroplasts, but genetic similarities with red algae suggest a relationship there. In the first three of these groups (Chromista), the chloroplast has four membranes, retaining a nucleomorph in cryptomonads, and they likely share a common pigmented ancestor, although other evidence casts doubt on whether the heterokonts, Haptophyta, and cryptomonads are in fact more closely related to each other than to other groups. The typical dinoflagellate chloroplast has three membranes, but considerable diversity exists in chloroplasts within the group, and a number of endosymbiotic events apparently occurred. The Apicomplexa, a group of closely related parasites, also have plastids called apicoplasts, which are not photosynthetic, but appear to have a common origin with dinoflagellate chloroplasts.

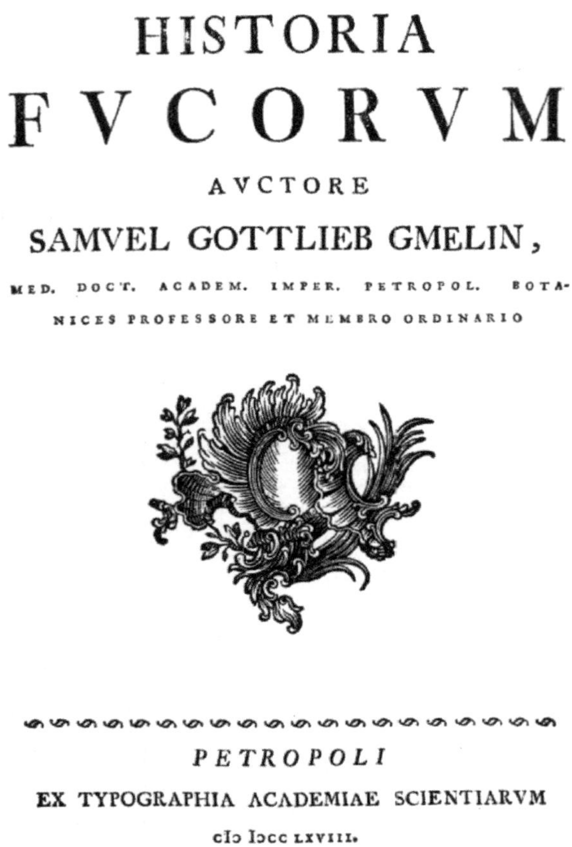

HISTORIA
FVCORVM
AVCTORE
SAMVEL GOTTLIEB GMELIN,
MED. DOCT. ACADEM. IMPER. PETROPOL. BOTANICES PROFESSORE ET MEMBRO ORDINARIO

PETROPOLI
EX TYPOGRAPHIA ACADEMIAE SCIENTIARVM
cIↃ IↃCC LXVIII.

Title page of Gmelin'sHistoria Fucorum, dated 1768.

Linnaeus, in Species Plantarum (1753), the starting point for modern botanical nomenclature, recognized 14 genera of algae, of which only four are currently considered among algae. In Systema Naturae, Linnaeus described the genera Volvox and Corallina, and a species of Acetabularia (as Madrepora), among the animals.

In 1768, Samuel Gottlieb Gmelin (1744–1774) published the Historia Fucorum, the first work dedicated to marine algae and the first book on marine biology to use the then new binomial nomenclature of Linnaeus. It included elaborate illustrations of seaweed and marine algae on folded leaves.

W.H.Harvey (1811—1866) and Lamouroux (1813) were the first to divide macroscopic algae into four divisions based on their pigmentation. This is the first use of a biochemical criterion in plant systematics. Harvey's four divisions are: red algae (Rhodospermae), brown algae (Melanospermae), green algae (Chlorospermae), and Diatomaceae.

At this time, microscopic algae were discovered and reported by a different group of workers (e.g., O. F. Müller and Ehrenberg) studying the Infusoria (microscopic organisms). Unlike macroalgae, which were clearly viewed as plants, microalgae were frequently considered animals because they are often motile. Even the nonmotile (coccoid) microalgae were sometimes merely seen as stages of the lifecycle of plants, macroalgae, or animals.

Although used as a taxonomic category in some pre-Darwinian classifications, e.g., Linnaeus (1753), de Jussieu (1789), Horaninow (1843), Agassiz (1859), Wilson & Cassin (1864), in further classifications, the "algae" are seen as an artificial, polyphyletic group.

Throughout the 20th century, most classifications treated the following groups as divisions or classes of algae: cyanophytes, rhodophytes, chrysophytes, xanthophytes, bacillariophytes, phaeophytes, pyrrhophytes (cryptophytes and dinophytes), euglenophytes, and chlorophytes. Later, many new groups were discovered (e.g., Bolidophyceae), and others were splintered from older groups: charophytes and glaucophytes (from chlorophytes), many heterokontophytes (e.g., synurophytes from chrysophytes, or eustigmatophytes from xanthophytes), haptophytes (from chrysophytes), and chlorarachniophytes (from xanthophytes).

With the abandonment of plant-animal dichotomous classification, most groups of algae (sometimes all) were included in Protista, later also abandoned in favour of Eukaryota. However, as a legacy of the older plant life scheme, some groups that were also treated as protozoans in the past still have duplicated classifications.

Some parasitic algae (e.g., the green algae Prototheca and Helicosporidium, parasites of metazoans, or Cephaleuros, parasites of plants) were originally classified as fungi, sporozoans, or protistans of incertae sedis, while others (e.g., the green algae Phyllosiphon and Rhodochytrium, parasites of plants, or the red algae Pterocladiophila and Gelidiocolax mammillatus, parasites of other red algae, or the dinoflagellates Oodinium, parasites of fish) had their relationship with algae conjectured early. In other cases, some groups were originally characterized as parasitic algae (e.g., Chlorochytrium), but later were seen as endophytic algae. Some filamentous bacteria (e.g., Beggiatoa) were originally seen as algae. Furthermore, groups like the apicomplexans are also parasites derived from ancestors that possessed plastids, but are not included in any group traditionally seen as algae.

RELATIONSHIP TO LAND PLANTS

The first land plants probably evolved from shallow freshwater charophyte algae much like Chara almost 500 million years ago. These probably had an isomorphic alternation of generations and were probably filamentous. Fossils of isolated land plant spores suggest land plants may have been around as long as 475 million years ago.

MORPHOLOGY

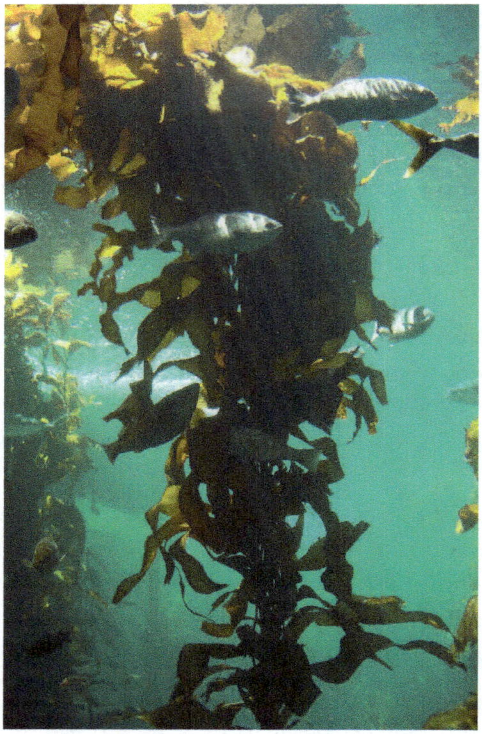

The kelp forest exhibit at the Monterey Bay Aquarium: A three-dimensional, multicellular thallus.

A range of algal morphologies is exhibited, and convergence of features in unrelated groups is common. The only groups to exhibit three-dimensional multicellular thalli are the reds and browns, and some chlorophytes. Apical growth is constrained to subsets of these groups: the florideophyte reds, various browns, and the charophytes. The form of charophytes is quite different from those of reds and browns, because they have distinct nodes, separated by internode 'stems'; whorls of branches reminiscent of the horsetails occur at the nodes. Conceptacles are another polyphyletic trait; they appear in the coralline algae and the Hildenbrandiales, as well as the browns.

Most of the simpler algae are unicellular flagellates or amoeboids, but colonial and nonmotile forms have developed independently among several of the groups. Some of the more common organizational levels, more than one of which may occur in the lifecycle of a species, are

- Colonial: small, regular groups of motile cells
- Capsoid: individual non-motile cells embedded in mucilage
- Coccoid: individual non-motile cells with cell walls
- Palmelloid: nonmotile cells embedded in mucilage

- Filamentous: a string of nonmotile cells connected together, sometimes branching
- Parenchymatous: cells forming a thallus with partial differentiation of tissues

In three lines, even higher levels of organization have been reached, with full tissue differentiation. These are the brown algae,—some of which may reach 50 m in length (kelps)—the red algae, and the green algae. The most complex forms are found among the green algae, in a lineage that eventually led to the higher land plants. The point where these nonalgal plants begin and algae stop is usually taken to be the presence of reproductive organs with protective cell layers, a characteristic not found in the other algal groups.

PHYSIOLOGY

Many algae, particularly members of the Characeae, have served as model experimental organisms to understand the mechanisms of the water permeability of membranes, osmoregulation, turgor regulation, salt tolerance, cytoplasmic streaming, and the generation of action potentials.

Phytohormones are found not only in higher plants, but in algae, too.

SYMBIOTIC ALGAE

Some species of algae form symbiotic relationships with other organisms. In these symbioses, the algae supply photosynthates (organic substances) to the host organism providing protection to the algal cells. The host organism derives some or all of its energy requirements from the algae. Examples are:

Lichens

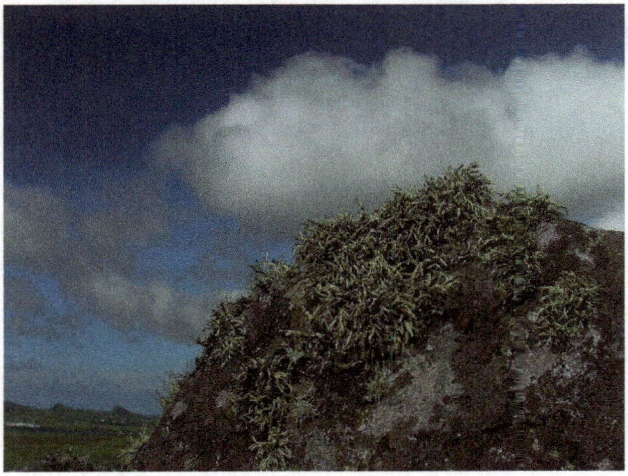

Rock lichens in Ireland.

Lichens are defined by the International Association for Lichenology to be "an association of a fungus and a photosynthetic symbiont resulting in a stable vegetative body having a specific structure." The fungi, or mycobionts, are mainly from the Ascomycota with a few from the Basidiomycota. They are not found alone in nature; but when they began to associate is not known. One mycobiont associates with the same phycobiont species, rarely two, from the green algae, except that alternatively, the mycobiont may associate with a species of cyanobacteria (hence "photobiont" is the more accurate term). A photobiont may be associated with many different mycobionts or may live independently; accordingly, lichens are named and classified as fungal species. The association is termed a morphogenesis because the lichen has a form and capabilities not possessed by the symbiont species alone (they can be experimentally isolated). The photobiont possibly triggers otherwise latent genes in the mycobiont.

Coral Reefs

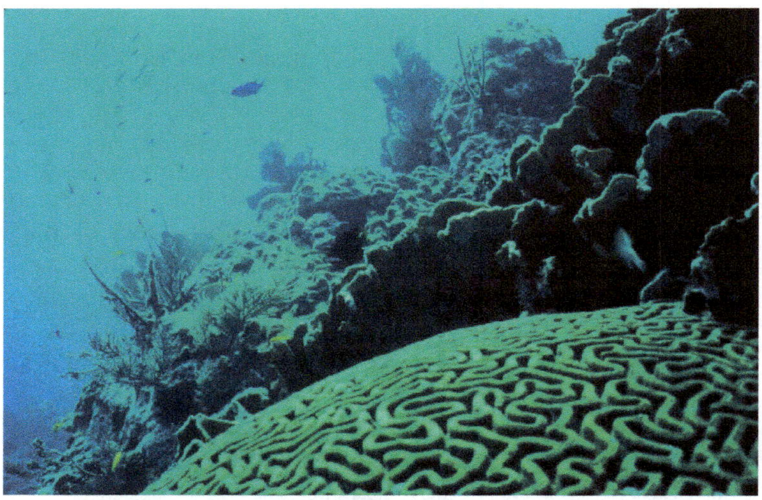

Floridian coral reef.

Coral reefs are accumulated from the calcareous exoskeletons of marine invertebrates of the order Scleractinia (stony corals). These animalsmetabolize sugar and oxygen to obtain energy for their cell-building processes, including secretion of the exoskeleton, with water and carbon dioxide as byproducts. Dinoflagellates (algal protists) are often endosymbionts in the cells of the coral-forming marine invertebrates, where they accelerate host-cell metabolism by generating immediately available sugar and oxygen through photosynthesis using incident light and the carbon dioxide produced by the host. Reef-building stony corals (hermatypic corals) require endosymbiotic algae from the genus Symbiodinium to be in a healthy condition. The loss of Symbiodinium from the host is known as coral bleaching, a condition which leads to the deterioration of a reef.

Sea Sponges

Green algae live close to the surface of some sponges, for example, breadcrumb sponge (Halichondria panicea). The alga is thus protected from predators; the sponge is provided with oxygen and sugars which can account for 50 to 80% of sponge growth in some species.

LIFECYCLE

Rhodophyta, Chlorophyta, and Heterokontophyta, the three main algal divisions, have lifecycles which show considerable variation and complexity. In general, an asexual phase exists where the seaweed's cells are diploid, a sexual phase where the cells are haploid, followed by fusion of the male and female gametes. Asexual reproduction permits efficient population increases, but less variation is possible. Commonly, in sexual reproduction of unicellular and colonial algae, two specialized, sexually compatible, haploid gametes make physical contact and fuse to form a zygote. To ensure a successful mating, the development and release of gametes is highly synchronized and regulated; pheromones may play a key role in these processes. Sexual reproduction allows for more variation and provides the benefit of efficient recombinational repair of DNA damages during meiosis, a key stage of the sexual cycle.However, sexual reproduction is more costly than asexual reproduction. Meiosis has been shown to occur in many different species of algae.

Numbers

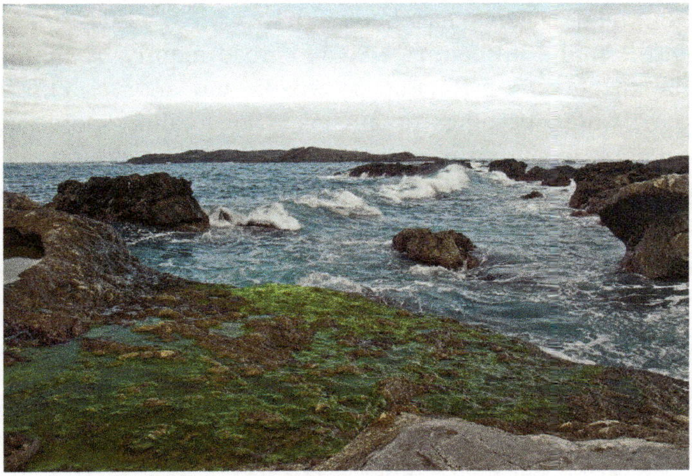

Algae on coastal rocks at Shihtiping in Taiwan

The Algal Collection of the US National Herbarium (located in the National Museum of Natural History) consists of approximately 320,500 dried specimens, which, although not exhaustive (no exhaustive collection exists), gives an idea of the order of magnitude of the number of algal species (that number remains unknown). Estimates vary widely. For example, according to one standard textbook, in the British Isles the UK Biodiversity Steering Group Report estimated there to be 20,000 algal species in the UK. Another checklist reports only about 5,000 species. Regarding the difference of about 15,000 species, the text concludes: "It will require many detailed field surveys before it is possible to provide a reliable estimate of the total number of species ..."

Regional and group estimates have been made, as well:

- 5,000–5,500 species of red algae worldwide
- "some 1,300 in Australian Seas"
- 400 seaweed species for the western coastline of South Africa, and 212 species from the coast of KwaZulu-Natal. Some of these are duplicates, as the range extends across both coasts, and the total recorded is probably about 500 species. Most of these are listed in List of seaweeds of South Africa. These exclude phytoplankton and crustose corallines.
- 669 marine species from California (US)
- 642 in the check-list of Britain and Ireland

and so on, but lacking any scientific basis or reliable sources, these numbers have no more credibility than the British ones mentioned above. Most estimates also omit microscopic algae, such as phytoplankton.

The most recent estimate suggests 72,500 algal species worldwide.

DISTRIBUTION

The distribution of algal species has been fairly well studied since the founding of phytogeography in the mid-19th century. Algae spread mainly by the dispersal of spores analogously to the dispersal of Plantae by seeds and spores. This dispersal can be accomplished by air, water, or other organisms. Due to this, spores can be found in a variety of environments: fresh and marine waters, air, soil, and in or on other organisms. Whether a spore is to grow into an organism depends on the combination of the species and the environmental conditions where the spore lands.

The spores of freshwater algae are dispersed mainly by running water and wind, as well as by living carriers. However, not all bodies of water can carry all species of algae, as the chemical composition of certain water bodies limits the algae that can survive within them. Marine spores are often spread by ocean currents. Ocean water presents many vastly different habitats based on temperature and nutrient availability, resulting in phytogeographic zones, regions, and provinces.

To some degree, the distribution of algae is subject to floristic discontinuities caused by geographical features, such as Antarctica, long distances of ocean or general land masses. It is, therefore, possible to identify species occurring by locality, such as "Pacific algae" or "North Sea algae". When they occur out of their localities, hypothesizing a transport mechanism is usually possible, such as the hulls of ships. For example, Ulva reticulata and U. fasciata travelled from the mainland to Hawaii in this manner.

Mapping is possible for select species only: "there are many valid examples of confined distribution patterns." For example, Clathromorphum is an arctic genus and is not mapped far south of there. However, scientists regard the overall data as insufficient due to the "difficulties of undertaking such studies."

Ecology

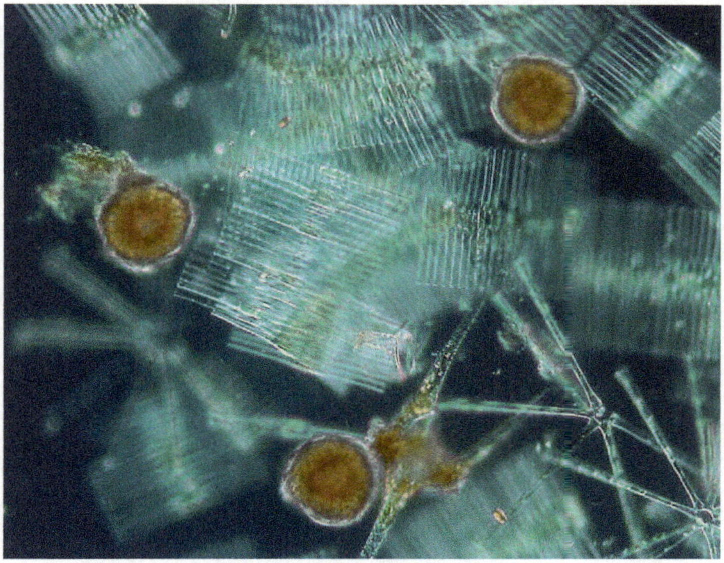

Phytoplankton, Lake Chuzenji

Algae are prominent in bodies of water, common in terrestrial environments, and are found in unusual environments, such as on snow and ice. Seaweeds grow mostly in shallow marine waters, under 100 m (330 ft) deep; however, some such as Navicula pennata have been recorded to a depth of 360 m (1,180 ft).

The various sorts of algae play significant roles in aquatic ecology. Microscopic forms that live suspended in the water column (phytoplankton) provide the food base for most marine food chains. In very high densities (algal blooms), these algae may discolor the water and outcompete, poison, or asphyxiate other life forms.

Algae can be used as indicator organisms to monitor pollution in various aquatic systems. In many cases, algal metabolism is sensitive to various pollutants. Due to this, the species composition of algal populations may shift in the presence of chemical pollutants. To detect these changes, algae can be sampled from the environment and maintained in laboratories with relative ease.

On the basis of their habitat, algae can be categorized as: aquatic (planktonic, benthic, marine, freshwater, lentic, lotic), terrestrial, aerial (subareial), lithophytic, halophytic (or euryhaline), psammon, thermophilic, cryophilic, epibiont (epiphytic, epizoic), endosymbiont (endophytic, endozoic), parasitic, calcifilic or lichenic (phycobiont).

Cultural Associations

In classical Chinese, the word 藻 is used both for "algae" and (in the modest tradition of the imperial scholars) for "literary talent". The third island in Kunming Lake beside the Summer Palace in Beijing is known as the Zaojian Tang Dao, which thus simultaneously means "Island of the Algae-Viewing Hall" and "Island of the Hall for Reflecting on Literary Talent".

Uses

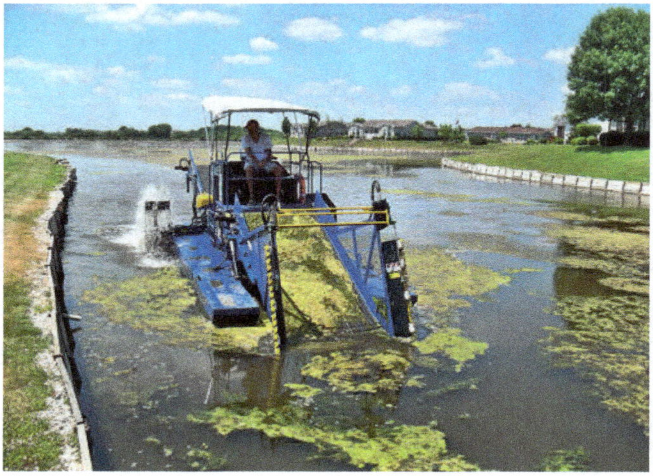

Harvesting algae

Agar

Agar, a gelatinous substance derived from red algae, has a number of commercial uses. It is a good medium on which to grow bacteria and fungi, as most microorganisms cannot digest agar.

Alginates

Alginic acid, or alginate, is extracted from brown algae. Its uses range from gelling agents in food, to medical dressings. Alginic acid also has been used in the field of biotechnology as a biocompatible medium for cell encapsulation and cell immobilization. Molecular cuisine is also a user of the substance for its gelling properties, by which it becomes a delivery vehicle for flavours.

Between 100,000 and 170,000 wet tons of Macrocystis are harvested annually in New Mexico for alginate extraction and abalone feed.

Energy Source

To be competitive and independent from fluctuating support from (local) policy on the long run, biofuels should equal or beat the cost level of fossil fuels. Here, algae-based fuels hold great promise, directly related to the potential to produce more biomass per unit area in a year than any other form of biomass. The break-even point for algae-based biofuels is estimated to occur by 2025.

Fertilizer

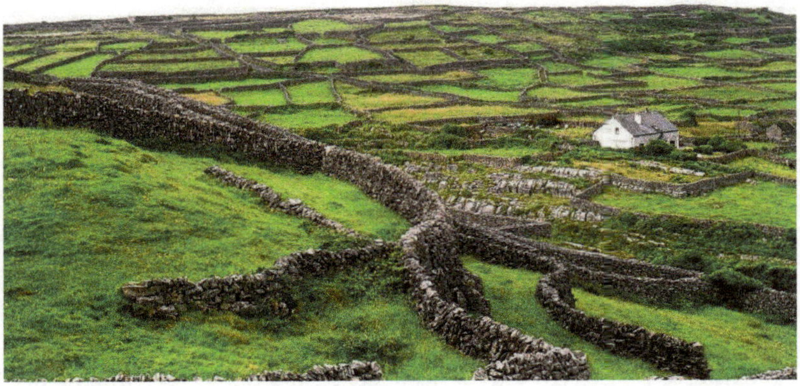

Seaweed-fertilized gardens on Inisheer

For centuries, seaweed has been used as a fertilizer; George Owen of Henllys writing in the 16th century referring to drift weed in South Wales:

This kind of ore they often gather and lay on great heapes, where it heteth and rotteth, and will have a strong and loathsome smell; when being so rotten they cast on the land, as they do their muck, and thereof springeth good corn, especially barley ... After spring-tydes or great rigs of the sea, they fetch it in sacks on horse backes, and carie the same three, four, or five miles, and cast it on the lande, which doth very much better the ground for corn and grass.

Today, algae are used by humans in many ways; for example, as fertilizers, soil conditioners, and livestock feed. Aquatic and microscopic species are cultured in clear tanks or ponds and are either harvested or used to treat effluents pumped through the ponds. Algaculture on a large scale is an important type of aquaculture in some places. Maerl is commonly used as a soil conditioner.

Nutrition

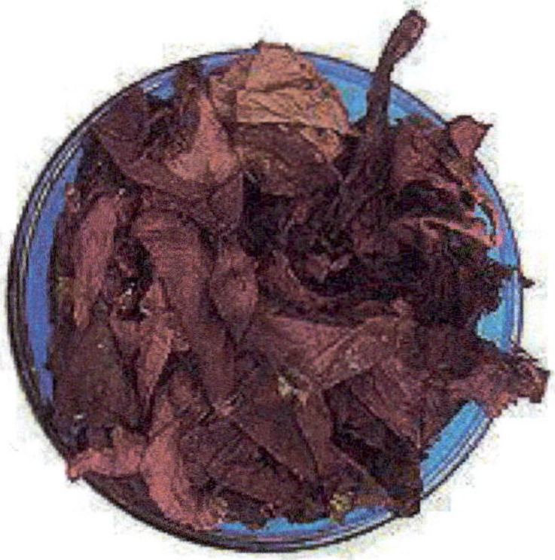

Dulse, a type of food

Naturally growing seaweeds are an important source of food, especially in Asia. They provide many vitamins including: A, B_1, B_2, B_6, niacin, and C, and are rich in iodine, potassium, iron, magnesium, and calcium. In addition, commercially cultivated microalgae, including both algae and cyanobacteria, are marketed as nutritional supplements, such as spirulina, Chlorella and the vitamin-C supplement from Dunaliella, high in beta-carotene.

Algae are national foods of many nations: China consumes more than 70 species, including fat choy, a cyanobacterium considered a vegetable; Japan, over 20 species; Ireland, dulse; Chile, cochayuyo. Laver is used to make "laver bread" in Wales, where it is known as bara lawr; in Korea, gim; in Japan, nori and aonori. It is also used along the west coast of North America from California to British Columbia, in Hawaii and by the Māori of New Zealand. Sea lettuce and badderlocks are salad ingredients in Scotland, Ireland, Greenland, and Iceland.

The oils from some algae have high levels of unsaturated fatty acids. For example, Parietochloris incisa is very high in arachidonic acid, where it reaches up to 47% of the triglyceride pool. Some varieties of algae favored by vegetarianism and veganism contain the long-chain, essential omega-3 fatty acids, docosahexaenoic acid (DHA) and eicosapentaenoic acid (EPA). Fish oil contains the omega-3 fatty acids, but the original source is algae (microalgae in particular), which are eaten by marine life such as copepods and are passed up the food chain. Algae have emerged in recent years as a popular source of omega-3 fatty acids for vegetarians who cannot get long-chain EPA and DHA from other vegetarian sources such as flaxseed oil, which only contains the short-chain alpha-linolenic acid (ALA).

Pollution Control

- Sewage can be treated with algae, reducing the use of large amounts of toxic chemicals that would otherwise be needed.

- Algae can be used to capture fertilizers in runoff from farms. When subsequently harvested, the enriched algae can be used as fertilizer.
- Aquaria and ponds can be filtered using algae, which absorb nutrients from the water in a device called an algae scrubber, also known as an algae turf scrubber.

Agricultural Research Service scientists found that 60–90% of nitrogen runoff and 70–100% of phosphorus runoff can be captured from manure effluents using a horizontal algae scrubber, also called an algal turf scrubber (ATS). Scientists developed the ATS, which consists of shallow, 100-foot raceways of nylon netting where algae colonies can form, and studied its efficacy for three years. They found that algae can readily be used to reduce the nutrient runoff from agricultural fields and increase the quality of water flowing into rivers, streams, and oceans. Researchers collected and dried the nutrient-rich algae from the ATS and studied its potential as an organic fertilizer. They found that cucumber and corn seedlings grew just as well using ATS organic fertilizer as they did with commercial fertilizers. Algae scrubbers, using bubbling upflow or vertical waterfall versions, are now also being used to filter aquaria and ponds.

Bioremediation

The alga Stichococcus bacillaris has been seen to colonize silicone resins used at archaeological sites; biodegrading the synthetic substance.

Pigments

The natural pigments (carotenoids and chlorophylls) produced by algae can be used as alternatives to chemical dyes and coloring agents. The presence of some individual algal pigments, together with specific pigment concentration ratios, are taxon-specific: analysis of their concentrations with various analytical methods, particularly high-performance liquid chromatography, can therefore offer deep insight into the taxonomic composition and relative abundance of natural alga populations in sea water samples.

Stabilizing Substances

Carrageenan, from the red alga Chondrus crispus, is used as a stabilizer in milk products.

REFERENCES

1. N. J. Butterfield (2000). "Bangiomorpha pubescens n. gen., n. sp.: implications for the evolution of sex, multicellularity, and the Mesoproterozoic/Neoproterozoic radiation of eukaryotes". Paleobiology. 26 (3): 386–404. doi:10.1666/0094-8373(2000)026<0386:BPNGNS>2.0.CO;2. ISSN 0094-8373.
2. Patrick J. Keeling (2004). "Diversity and evolutionary history of plastids and their hosts". American Journal of Botany. 91 (10): 1481–1493. doi:10.3732/ajb.91.10.1481Freely accessible. PMID 21652304.
3. Laura Wegener Parfrey, Erika Barbero, Elyse Lasser, Micah Dunthorn, Debashish Bhattacharya, David J Patterson, and Laura A Katz (December 2006). "Evaluating

Support for the Current Classification of Eukaryotic Diversity". PLoS Genet. 2 (12): e220. doi:10.1371/journal.pgen.0020220. PMC 1713255Freely accessible. PMID 17194223.

4. Lee, R. E. (2008). Phycology. Cambridge University Press.
5. Nabors, Murray W. (2004). Introduction to Botany. San Francisco, CA: Pearson Education, Inc. ISBN 978-0-8053-4416-5.
6. Allaby, M., ed. (1992). "Algae". The Concise Dictionary of Botany. Oxford: Oxford University Press.
7. J.D. Palmer, D.E. Soltis, M.W. Chase (2004). "The plant tree of life: an overview and some points of view". Am. J. Bot. 91 (10): 1437–1445. doi:10.3732/ajb.91.10.1437Freely accessible. PMID 21652302.
8. Smithsonian National Museum of Natural History; Department of Botany. http://botany.si.edu/projects/algae/introduction.htm
9. Pringsheim, E.G. 1963. Farblose Algen. Ein beitrag zur Evolutionsforschung. Gustav Fischer Verlag, Stuttgart. 471 pp., species:Algae#Pringsheim .281963.29.
10. Tartar, A., Boucias, D. G., Becnel, J. J., and Adams, B. J. (2003). "Comparison of plastid 16S rRNA (rrn 16) genes from Helicosporidium spp.: evidence supporting the reclassification of Helicosporidia as green algae (Chlorophyta)". International Journal of Systematic and Evolutionary Microbiology. 53 (Pt 6): 1719–1723. doi:10.1099/ijs.0.02559-0Freely accessible. PMID 14657099.
11. Figueroa-Martinez, F.; Nedelcu, A. M.; Smith, D. R.; Reyes-Prieto, A. (2015). "When the lights go out: the evolutionary fate of free-living colorless green algae". New Phytologist. 206 (3): 972–982. doi:10.1111/nph.13279.
12. Bengtson, S; Belivanova, V; Rasmussen, B; Whitehouse, M (2009). "The controversial "Cambrian" fossils of the Vindhyan are real but more than a billion years older". Proceedings of the National Academy of Sciences of the United States of America. 106 (19): 7729–34. Bibcode:2009PNAS..106.7729B. doi:10.1073/pnas.0812460106. PMC 2683128Freely accessible. PMID 19416859.
13. "alga, algae". Webster's Third New International Dictionary of the English Language Unabridged with Seven Language Dictionary. 1. Encyclopædia Britannica, Inc. 1986.
14. Partridge, Eric (1983). "algae". Origins.
15. Lewis, Charlton T.; Charles Short (1879). alga. Oxford: Clarendon Press. ISBN 978-0-19-864201-5.
16. Thomas Kelly Cheyne; John Sutherland Black (1902). Encyclopædia biblica: a critical dictionary of the literary, political and religious history, the archæology, geography, and natural history of the Bible. Macmillan Company. p. 3525.
17. Bhattacharya, D.; Medlin, L. (1998). "Algal Phylogeny and the Origin of Land Plants" (PDF). Plant Physiology. 116 (1): 9–15. doi:10.1104/pp.116.1.9.
18. Losos, Jonathan B.; Mason, Kenneth A.; Singer, Susan R. (2007). Biology (8 ed.). McGraw-Hill. ISBN 978-0-07-304110-0.
19. Archibald JM; Keeling PJ (November 2002). "Recycled plastids: a 'green

movement' in eukaryotic evolution". Trends in Genetics. 18 (11): 577–584. doi:10.1016/S0168-9525(02)02777-4. PMID 12414188.

20. Janson, Sven; Graneli, Edna (September 2003). "Genetic analysis of the psbA gene from single cells indicates a cryptomonad origin of the plastid in Dinophysis (Dinophyceae)". Phycologia. Allen Press Publishing Services. 42 (5): 473–477. doi:10.2216/i0031-8884-42-5-473.1. ISSN 0031-8884.
21. Burki F, Shalchian-Tabrizi K, Minge M, Skjæveland Å, Nikolaev SI et al. (2007). Butler, Geraldine, ed. Phylogenomics Reshuffles the Eukaryotic Supergroups. PLOS ONE. 2 (8): e790. Bibcode:2007PLoSO...2..790B. doi:10.1371/journal.pone.0000790. PMC 1949142Freely accessible. PMID 17726520.
22. Linnæus, C. (1753). Species Plantarum, vol. 2, p. 1131, .
23. Sharma, O. P. (1986). Textbook of Algae. McGraw Hill. p. 22, .
24. Gmelin S G (1768) Historia Fucorum Ex typographia Academiae scientiarum, St. Petersburg.
25. Silva PC, Basson PW and Moe RL (1996) Catalogue of the Benthic Marine Algae of the Indian Ocean page 2, University of California Press. ISBN 978-0-520-91581-7.
26. Medlin, L. K., W. H. C. F. Kooistra, D. Potter, G. W. Saunders, and R. A. Anderson (1997). Phylogenetic relationships of the golden algae (haptophytes, heterokont chromophytes) and their plastids. Plant Systematics and Evolution, p. 188.
27. Dixon, P S (1973). Biology of the Rhodophyta. Edinburgh: Oliver & Boyd. p. 232. ISBN 978-0-05-002485-0.
28. Harvey, D. (1836). Flora hibernica.
29. Medlin et al. (1997), p. 188.
30. Braun, A. Algarum unicellularium genera nova et minus cognita, praemissis observationibus de algis unicellularibus in genere (New and less known genera of unicellular algae, preceded by observations respecting unicellular algae in general). Lipsiae, Apud W. Engelmann, 1855. Translation at: Lankester, E. & Busk, G. (eds.). Quarterly Journal of Microscopical Science, 1857, vol. 5, (17), 13-16; (18), 90-96; (19), 143-149.
31. Siebold, C. Th. v. Ueber einzellige Pflanzen und Thiere (On unicellular plants and animals). In: Siebold, C. Th. v. & Kölliker, A. (1849). Zeitschrift für wissenschaftliche Zoologie, Bd. 1, p. 270. Translation at: Lankester, E. & Busk, G. (eds.). Quarterly Journal of Microscopical Science, 1853, vol. 1, (2), 111-121; (3), 195-206.
32. Williams, B. A.; Keeling, P. J. (2003). Cryptic organelles in parasitic protists and fungi. In Littlewood, D. T. J. The Evolution of Parasitism. London: Elsevier Academic Press. p. 46. ISBN 0-12-031754-0.
33. Round (1981). pp. 398–400, .
34. Ivan Noble (18 September 2003). When plants conquered land. BBC.
35. Wellman, C.H.; Osterloff, P.L.; Mohiuddin, U. (2003). Fragments of the earliest

land plants. Nature. 425 (6955): 282–285. Bibcode:2003Natur.425..282W. doi:10.1038/nature01884. PMID 13679913.

36. Xiao, S.; Knoll, A.H.; Yuan, X.; Pueschel, C.M. (2004). Phosphatized multicellular algae in the Neoproterozoic Doushantuo Formation, China, and the early evolution of florideophyte red algae. American Journal of Botany. 91 (2): 214–227. doi:10.3732/ajb.91.2.214Freely accessible. PMID 21653378.
37. Waggoner, Ben (1994–2008). Introduction to the Phaeophyta: Kelps and brown Algae. University of California Museum of Palaeontology (UCMP). Archived from the original on 21 December 2008. Retrieved 19 December 2008.
38. Thomas, D N (2002). Seaweeds. London: The Natural History Museum. ISBN 978-0-565-09175-0.
39. Waggoner, Ben (1994–2008). Introduction to the Rhodophyta, The red algae. University of California Museum of Palaeontology (UCMP). Archived from the original on 18 December 2008. Retrieved 19 December 2008.
40. Introduction to the Green Algae. berkeley.edu.
41. Tazawa, Masashi (2010). Sixty Years Research with Characean Cells: Fascinating Material for Plant Cell Biology. Progress in Botany. Progress in Botany. Springer. 72: 5–34. doi:10.1007/978-3-642-13145-5_1. ISBN 978-3-642-13145-5. Retrieved 7 October 2012.
42. Tarakhovskaya, E. R.; Maslov, Yu. I.; Shishova, M. F. (April 2007). Phytohormones in algae. Russian Journal of Plant Physiology. 54 (2): 163–170. doi:10.1134/s1021443707020021.
43. Brodo, Irwin M; Sharnoff, Sylvia Duran; Sharnoff, Stephen; Laurie-Bourque, Susan (2001). Lichens of North America. New Haven: Yale University Press. p. 8. ISBN 978-0-300-08249-4.
44. Pearson, Lorentz C (1995). The Diversity and Evolution of Plants. CRC Press. p. 221. ISBN 978-0-8493-2483-3.
45. Brodo et al. (2001), page 6: A species of lichen collected anywhere in its range has the same lichen-forming fungus and, generally, the same photobiont. (A particular photobiont, though, may associate with scores of different lichen fungi).
46. Brodo et al. (2001), page 8.
47. Taylor, Dennis L (1983). The coral-algal symbiosis. In Goff, Lynda J. Algal Symbiosis: A Continuum of Interaction Strategies. CUP Archive. pp. 19–20. ISBN 978-0-521-25541-7.
48. http://uwsp.edu/cnr/UWEXlakes/laketides/vol26-4/vol26-4.pdf
49. Frenkel J, Vyverman W, Pohnert G (2014). Pheromone signaling during sexual reproduction in algae. Plant J. 79 (4): 632–44. doi:10.1111/tpj.12496. PMID 24597605.
50. Harris Bernstein, Carol Bernstein and Richard E. Michod (2011). Meiosis as an Evolutionary Adaptation for DNA Repair. Chapter 19 pages 357–382 in DNA Repair (Inna Kruman editor). InTech Open Publisher. DOI: 10.5772/25117 ISBN 978-953-307-697-3 http://www.intechopen.com/books/dna-repair/meiosis-as-an-

evolutionary-adaptation-for-dna-repair

51. Otto SP (2009). The evolutionary enigma of sex. Am. Nat. 174 Suppl 1: S1–S14. doi:10.1086/599084. PMID 19441962.
52. Heywood P, Magee PT (1976). Meiosis in protists. Some structural and physiological aspects of meiosis in algae, fungi, and protozoa. Bacteriol Rev. 40 (1): 190–240. PMC 413949Freely accessible. PMID 773364.
53. Algae Herbarium. National Museum of Natural History, Department of Botany. 2008. Archived from the original on 1 December 2008. Retrieved 19 December 2008.
54. John (2002), page 1.
55. Huisman (2000), page 25.
56. Stegenga (1997).
57. Clerck, Olivier (2005). Guide to the seaweeds of KwaZulu-Natal. ISBN 978-90-72619-64-8.
58. Abbott and Hollenberg (1976), page 2.
59. Hardy and Guiry (2006).
60. Guiry, M. D. (2012). How Many Species of Algae Are There?. Journal of Phycology. 48 (5): 1057–1063. doi:10.1111/j.1529-8817.2012.01222.x. PMID 27011267.
61. Round, FE (1981). Chapter 8, Dispersal, continuity and phytogeography. The ecology of algae. pp. 357–361. Retrieved 6 February 2015.
62. Wan Maznah Wan Omar (Dec 2010). Perspectives on the Use of Algae as Biological Indicators for Monitoring and Protecting Aquatic Environments, with Special Reference to Malaysian Freshwater Ecosystems. Trop Life Sci Res. 21 (2): 51–67. PMC 3819078Freely accessible. PMID 24575199.
63. Necchi Jr., O. (ed.) (2016). River Algae. Springer, .
64. Johansen, J. R. 2012. Diatoms of aerial habitats. In: Smol, J. P. & Stoermer, E. F. (Eds.). The Diatoms: Applications for the Environmental and Earth Sciences, 2nd ed. Cambridge University Press. Cambridge, UK. pp. 465–472, .
65. Sharma, O. P. (1986). pp. 2–6, .
66. Lewis, J G; Stanley, N F; Guist, G G (1988). 9 Commercial production of algal hydrocolloides. In Lembi, C.A.; Waaland, J.R. Algae and Human Affairs. Cambridge: Cambridge University Press. ISBN 978-0-521-32115-0.
67. Macrocystis C. Agardh 1820: 46. AlgaeBase. Retrieved 28 December 2008.
68. Secondary Products of Brown Algae. Algae Research. Smithsonian National Museum of Natural History. Retrieved 29 December 2008.
69. Chisti, Y (May–Jun 2007). Biodiesel from microalgae.. Biotechnology advances. 25 (3): 294–306. doi:10.1016/j.biotechadv.2007.02.001. PMID 17350212.
70. Yang, ZK; Niu, YF; Ma, YH; Xue, J; Zhang, MH; Yang, WD; Liu, JS; Lu, SH; Guan, Y; Li, HY (4 May 2013). Molecular and cellular mechanisms of neutral

lipid accumulation in diatom following nitrogen deprivation.. Biotechnology for biofuels. 6 (1): 67. doi:10.1186/1754-6834-6-67. PMC 3662598Freely accessible. PMID 23642220.

71. An Outlook on Microalgal Biofuels René H. Wijffels and Maria J. Barbosa Science 13 August 2010: 329 (5993), 796–799. [DOI:10.1126/science.1189003]
72. Read, Clare Sewell (1849). On the Farming of South Wales: Prize Report. Journal of the Royal Agricultural Society of England. London: John Murray. 10: 142–143. Downloadable Google Books.
73. McHugh, Dennis J. (2003). 9, Other Uses of Seaweeds. A Guide to the Seaweed Industry: FAO Fisheries Technical Paper 441. Rome: Fisheries and Aquaculture Department, Food and Agriculture Organization (FAO) of the United Nations. ISBN 978-92-5-104958-7.
74. Simoons, Frederick J (1991). 6, Seaweeds and Other Algae. Food in China: A Cultural and Historical Inquiry. CRC Press. pp. 179–190. ISBN 978-0-936923-29-1.
75. Morton, Steve L. Modern Uses of Cultivated Algae. Ethnobotanical Leaflets. Southern Illinois University Carbondale. Archived from the original on 23 December 2008. Retrieved 26 December 2008.
76. Mondragón, Jennifer; Mondragón, Jeff (2003). Seaweeds of the Pacific Coast. Monterey, California: Sea Challengers Publications. ISBN 978-0-930118-29-7.
77. Durvillaea antarctica (Chamisso) Hariot. AlgaeBase.
78. Bigogno, C; I Khozin-Goldberg; S Boussiba; A Vonshak; Z Cohen (2002). Lipid and fatty acid composition of the green oleaginous alga Parietochloris incisa, the richest plant source of arachidonic acid. Phytochemistry. 60 (5): 497–503. doi:10.1016/S0031-9422(02)00100-0. PMID 12052516.
79. Allison Aubrey (1 November 2007). Morning Edition: Getting Brain Food Straight from the Source. National Public Radio.
80. Morrissey, J., M.S. Jones and V. Harriott (1988). ReefBase :: Main Publications : Nutrient cycling in the Great Barrier Reef Aquarium - Proceedings of the 6th International Coral Reef Symposium, Australia. reefbase.org.
81. Patent US4333263 - Algal turf scrubber. google.com.
82. Hydromentia Water Treatment Technologies
83. ALGAL RESPONSE TO NUTRIENT ENRICHMENT IN FORESTED OLIGOTROPHIC STREAM - Veraart - 2008 - Journal of Phycology - Wiley Online Library. wiley.com.
84. Algae: A Mean, Green Cleaning Machine. USDA Agricultural Research Service. 7 May 2010.
85. Cappitelli, Francesca; Sorlini, Claudia (2008). Microorganisms Attack Synthetic Polymers in Items Representing Our Cultural Heritage. Applied and Environmental Microbiology. 74 (3): 564–569. doi:10.1128/AEM.01768-07. PMC 2227722Freely accessible. PMID 18065627.
86. Arad, Shoshana; Spharim, Ishai (1998). Production of Valuable Products

from Microalgae: An Emerging Agroindustry. In Altman, Arie. Agricultural Biotechnology. Books in Soils, Plants, and the Environment. 61. CRC Press. p. 638. ISBN 978-0-8247-9439-2.

87. C. Rathbun; A. Doyle; T. Waterhouse (June 1994). Measurement of Algal Chlorophylls and Carotenoids by HPLC (PDF). Joint Global Ocean Flux Study protocols. Global Ocean Data Analysis Project. 13: 91–96.

88. M. Latasa; R. Bidigare (1998). A comparison of phytoplankton populations of the Arabian Sea during the Spring Intermonsoon and Southwest Monsoon of 1995 as described by HPLC-analyzed pigments. Deep-Sea Research Part II. Pergamon Press. 45 (10-11): 2133–2170. Bibcode:1998DSRII..45.2133L. doi:10.1016/S0967-0645(98)00066-6.

CHAPTER 9

Microbial Ecology

Chapter Contents

- **Introduction**
- **History**
- **Symbiosis**
- **Roles**
- **Microbial Resource Management**

Microbial ecology is the study of the interactions of microorganisms with their environment, each other, and plant and animal species. It includes the study of symbioses, biogeochemical cycles and the interaction of microbes with anthropogenic effects such as pollution and climate change.

The study of microbial ecology can help us improve our lives via the use of microbes in environmental restoration, food production, bioengineering of useful products such as antibiotics, food supplements, and chemicals. The study of these bizarre and diverse creatures that are everywhere yet nowhere to be seen is fascinating and a pursuit that appeals to the curiosity and playfulness in us.

Most types of microbes remain unknown. It is estimated that we know fewer than 1% of the microbial species on Earth. Yet microbes surround us everywhere -- air, water, soil. An average gram of soil contains one billion (1,000,000,000) microbes representing probably several thousand species.

INTRODUCTION

Microbial ecology (or environmental microbiology) is the ecology of microorganisms: their relationship with one another and with their environment. It concerns the three major domains of life—Eukaryota, Archaea, and Bacteria—as well as viruses.

Microorganisms, by their omnipresence, impact the entire biosphere. Microbial life plays a primary role in regulating biogeochemical systems in virtually all of our planet's environments, including some of the most extreme, from frozen environments and acidic lakes, to hydrothermal vents at the bottom of deepest oceans, and some of the most familiar, such as the human small intestine. As a consequence of the quantitative magnitude of microbial life (Whitman and coworkers calculated 5.0×10^{30} cells, eight orders of magnitude greater than the number of stars in the observable universe) microbes, by virtue of their biomass alone, constitute a significant carbon sink. Aside from carbon fixation, microorganisms' key collective metabolic processes (including nitrogen fixation, methane metabolism, and sulfur metabolism) control global biogeochemical cycling. The immensity of microorganisms' production is such that, even in the total absence of eukaryotic life, these processes would likely continue unchanged.

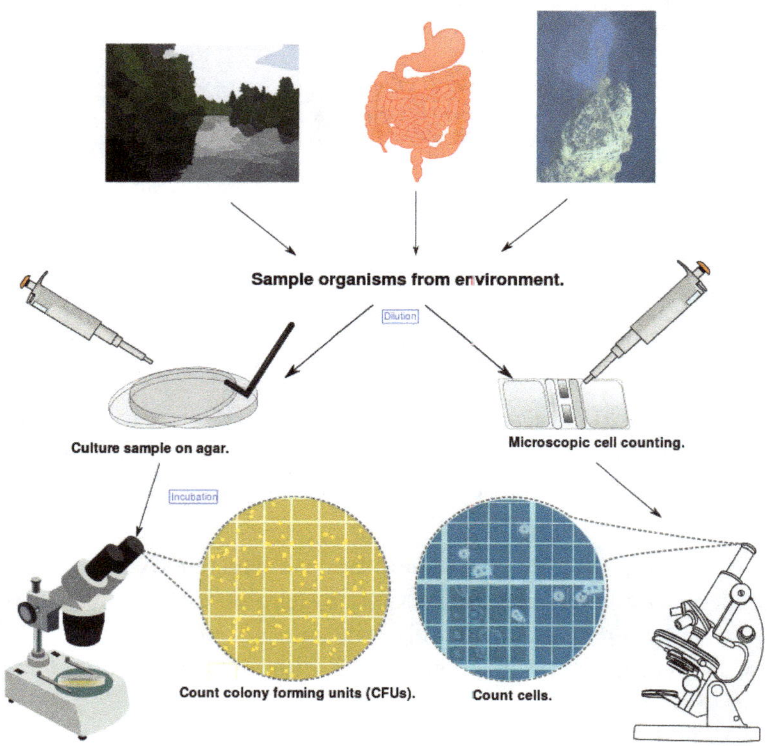

The great plate count anomaly. Counts of cells obtained via cultivation are orders of magnitude lower than those directly observed under the microscope. This is because microbiologists are able to cultivate only a minority of naturally occurring microbes using current laboratory techniques, depending on the environment.

HISTORY

While microbes have been studied since the seventeenth-century, this research was from a primarily physiological perspective rather than an ecological one. Martinus Beijerinck invented the enrichment culture, a fundamental method of studying microbes from the environment. He is often incorrectly credited with framing the microbial biogeographic idea that "everything is everywhere, but, the environment selects", which was stated by Lourens Baas Becking. Sergei Winogradsky was one of the first researchers to attempt to understand microorganisms outside of the medical context—making him among the first students of microbial ecology and environmental microbiology—discovering chemosynthesis, and developing the Winogradsky column in the process.

Beijerinck and Windogradsky, however, were focused on the physiology of microorganisms, not the microbial habitat or their ecological interactions. Modern microbial ecology was launched by Robert Hungate and coworkers, who investigated the rumen ecosystem. The study of the rumen required Hungate to develop techniques for culturing anaerobic microbes, and he also pioneered a quantitative approach to the study of microbes and their ecological activities that differentiated the relative contributions of species and catabolic pathways.

SYMBIOSIS

Microbes, especially bacteria, often engage in symbiotic relationships (either positive or negative) with other organisms, and these relationships affect the ecosystem. One example of these fundamental symbioses are chloroplasts, which allow eukaryotes to conduct photosynthesis. Chloroplasts are considered to be endosymbiotic cyanobacteria, a group of bacteria that are thought to be the origins of aerobic photosynthesis. Some theories state that this invention coincides with a major shift in the early earth's atmosphere, from a reducing atmosphere to an oxygen-rich atmosphere. Some theories go as far as saying that this shift in the balance of gases might have triggered a global ice-age known as the Snowball Earth.

ROLES

Microorganisms are the backbone of all ecosystems, but even more so in the zones where photosynthesis is unable to take place because of the absence of light. In such zones, chemosynthetic microbes provide energy and carbon to the other organisms.

Other microbes are decomposers, with the ability to recycle nutrients from other organisms' waste products. These microbes play a vital role in biogeochemical cycles. The nitrogen cycle, the phosphorus cycle, the sulphur cycle and the carbon cycle all depend on microorganisms in one way or another. For example, the nitrogen gas which makes up 78% of the earth's atmosphere is unavailable to most organisms, until it is converted to a biologically available form by the microbial process of nitrogen fixation.

Due to the high level of horizontal gene transfer among microbial communities, microbial ecology is also of importance to studies of evolution.

MICROBIAL RESOURCE MANAGEMENT

Biotechnology may be used alongside microbial ecology to address a number of environmental and economic challenges. For example, molecular techniques such as community fingerprinting can be used to track changes in microbial communities over time or assess their biodiversity. Managing the carbon cycle to sequester carbon dioxide and prevent excess methanogenesis is important in mitigating global warming, and the prospects of bioenergy are being expanded by the development of microbial fuel cells. Microbial resource management advocates a more progressive attitude towards disease, whereby biological control agents are favored over attempts at eradication. Fluxes in microbial communities has to be better characterized for this field's potential to be realized. In addition, there are also clinical implications, as marine microbial symbioses are a valuable source of existing and novel antimicrobial agents, and thus offer another line of inquiry in the evolutionary arms race of antibiotic resistance, a pressing concern for researchers.

In Built Environment and Human Interaction

Microbes exist in all areas, including homes, offices, commercial centers, and hospitals. In 2016, the journal *Microbiome* published a collection of various works studying the microbial ecology of the built environment.

A 2006 study of pathogenic bacteria in hospitals found that their ability to survive varied by the type, with some surviving for only a few days while others survived for months.

The lifespan of microbes in the home varies similarly. Generally bacteria and viruses require a wet environment with a humidity of over 10 percent. *E. coli* can survive for a few hours to a day. Bacteria which form spores can survive longer, with *Staphylococcus aureus* surviving potentially for weeks or, in the case of *Bacillus anthracis*, years.

In the home, pets can be carriers of bacteria; for example, reptiles in particular are commonly carriers of salmonella.

S. aureus is particularly common, and asymptomatically colonizes about 30% of the human population; attempts to decolonize carriers have met with limited success and generally involve mupirocin nasally and chlorhexidine washing, potentially along with vancomycin and cotrimoxazole to address intestinal and urinary tract infections.

Antimicrobials

Some metals, particularly copper and silver, are relatively microbial. Using antimicrobial copper-alloy touch surfaces is a technique which has began to be used in the 21st century to prevent transmission of bacteria. Silver, particularly in nanoparticle form, has also began to be incorporated into building surfaces and fabrics, although concerns have been raised about the potential unhealthy side-effects of the tiny particles on the body.

REFERENCES

1. Hugenholtz, P. (2002). "Exploring prokaryotic diversity in the genomic era". Genome Biology. 3 (2): reviews0003.reviews0001–reviews0003.reviews0001. doi:10.1186/gb-2002-3-2-reviews0003. PMC 139013Freely accessible. PMID 11864374.
2. Barton, Larry L.; Northup, Diana E. (9 September 2011). Microbial Ecology. Wiley-Blackwell. Oxford: John Wiley & Sons. p. 22. ISBN 978-1-118-01582-7. Retrieved 25 May 2013.
3. Bowler, Chris; Karl, David M.; Colwell, Rita R. (2009). "Microbial oceanography in a sea of opportunity". Nature. 459 (7244): 180–4. Bibcode:2009Natur.459..180B. doi:10.1038/nature08056. PMID 19444203.
4. Konopka, Allan (2009). "What is microbial community ecology?". The ISME Journal. 3 (11): 1223–30. doi:10.1038/ismej.2009.88. PMID 19657372.
5. Whitman, W. B.; Coleman, DC; Wiebe, WJ (1998). "Prokaryotes: The unseen majority". Proceedings of the National Academy of Sciences. 95 (12): 6578–83. Bibcode:1998PNAS...95.6578W. doi:10.1073/pnas.95.12.6578. JSTOR 44981. PMC 33863Freely accessible. PMID 9618454.
6. "number of stars in the observable universe - Wolfram|Alpha". Retrieved 2011-11-22.
7. Reddy, K. Ramesh; DeLaune, Ronald D. (15 July 2004). Biogeochemistry of Wetlands: Science and Applications. Boca Raton: Taylor & Francis. p. 116. ISBN 978-0-203-49145-4. Retrieved 25 May 2013
8. Delong, Edward F. (2009). "The microbial ocean from genomes to biomes". Nature. 459 (7244): 200–6. Bibcode:2009Natur.459..200D. doi:10.1038/nature08059. PMID 19444206.
9. Lupp, Claudia (2009). "Microbial oceanography" Nature. 459 (7244): 179. Bibcode:2009Natur.459..179L. doi:10.1038/459179a. PMID 19444202.
10. Konopka, A. (2009). "Ecology, Microbial in Encyclopedia of Microbiology": 91–106. doi:10.1016/B978-012373944-5.00002-X. ISBN 978-0-12-373944-5.
11. De Wit, Rutger; Bouvier, Thierry (2006). "'Everything is everywhere, but, the environment selects'; what did Baas Becking and Beijerinck really say?". Environmental Microbiology. 8 (4): 755–8. doi:10.1111/j.1462-2920.2006.01017.x. PMID 16584487.
12. Madigan, Michael T. (2012). Brock biology of microorganisms (13th ed.). San Francisco: Benjamin Cummings. ISBN 9780321649638.
13. Fenchel, Tom; Blackburn, Henry; King, Gary M (24 July 2012). Bacterial Biogeochemistry: The Ecophysiology of Mineral Cycling (3 ed.). Boston, Mass.: Academic Press/Elsevier. p. 3. ISBN 978-0-12-415974-7. Retrieved 25 May 2013.
14. McDaniel, L. D.; Young, E.; Delaney, J.; Ruhnau, F.; Ritchie, K. B.; Paul, J. H. (2010). "High Frequency of Horizontal Gene Transfer in the Oceans". Science. 330 (6000): 50. Bibcode:2010Sci...330...50M. doi:10.1126/science.1192243.

PMID 20929803.

15. Smets, Barth F.; Barkay, Tamar (2005). "Horizontal gene transfer: Perspectives at a crossroads of scientific disciplines". Nature Reviews Microbiology. 3 (9): 675–8. doi:10.1038/nrmicro1253. PMID 16145755.
16. Verstraete, Willy (2007). "Microbial ecology and environmental biotechnology". The ISME Journal. 1 (1): 4–8. doi:10.1038/ismej.2007.7. PMID 18043608.
17. Ott, J. (2005). "Marine Microbial Thiotrophic Ectosymbioses". Oceanography and Marine Biology: An Annual Review. 42: 95–118. ISBN 9780203507810.
18. "Microbiology of the Built Environment". www.biomedcentral.com. Retrieved 2016-09-18.
19. Kramer, Axel; Schwebke, Ingeborg; Kampf, Günter (2006-08-16). "How long do nosocomial pathogens persist on inanimate surfaces? A systematic review". BMC Infectious Diseases. 6 (1): 1–8. doi:10.1186/1471-2334-6-130. PMC 1564025Freely accessible. PMID 16914034.
20. "How long do microbes like bacteria and viruses live on surfaces in the home at normal room temperatures?". Retrieved 2016-09-18.
21. "Raw Diets Linked To Salmonella". Retrieved 2016-09-18.
22. Tong SY; Davis JS; Eichenberger E; Holland TL; Fowler VG (July 2015). "Staphylococcus aureus infections: epidemiology, pathophysiology, clinical manifestations, and management". Clinical Microbiology Reviews. 28 (3): 603–661. doi:10.1128/CMR.00134-14. PMC 4451395Freely accessible. PMID 26016486.
23. "Many factors involved in decolonization of S. aureus". www.healio.com. Retrieved 2016-09-18.
24. Buehlmann, M.; Frei, R.; Fenner, L.; Dangel, M.; Fluckiger, U.; Widmer, A. F. (2008-06-01). "Highly effective regimen for decolonization of methicillin-resistant Staphylococcus aureus carriers". Infection Control and Hospital Epidemiology. 29 (6): 510–516. doi:10.1086/588201. ISSN 0899-823X. PMID 18510460.
25. "The bacteria-fighting super element making a return to hospitals: Copper". Washington Post. Retrieved 2016-09-18.
26. "Silver nanoparticles kill germs, raise health concerns". Retrieved 2016-09-18.

CHAPTER 10

Microbial Genetics

Chapter Contents

- **Introduction**
- **Microorganisms Whose Study is Encompassed by Microbial Genetics**
- **Applications of Microbial Genetics**

Microorganisms include prokaryotes like bacteria, unicellular or mycelial eukaryotes e.g., yeasts and other fungi, and viruses, notably bacterial viruses (bacteriophages). Microbial genetics is concerned with the transmission of hereditary characters in microorganisms. Microbial genetics has played a unique role in developing the fields of molecular and cell biology and also has found applications in medicine, agriculture, and the food and pharmaceutical industries.

Hereditary processes in microorganisms are analogous to those in multicellular organisms. In both prokaryotic and eukaryotic microbes, the genetic material is DNA; the only known exceptions to this rule are the RNA viruses. Mutations, heritable changes in the DNA, occur spontaneously and the rate of mutation can be increased by mutagenic agents. In practice, the susceptibility of bacteria to mutagenic agents has been used to identify potentially hazardous chemicals in the environment. For example, the Ames test was developed to evaluate the mutagenicity of a chemical in the following way. Plates containing a medium lacking in, for example, the nutrient histidine are inolculated with a histidine requiring strain of the bacterium Salmonella typhimurium. Thus, only cells that revert back to the wild type can grow on the medium. If plates are exposed to a mutagenic agent, the increase in the number of mutants compared with unexposed plates can be observed and a large number of revertants would indicate a strong mutagenic agent. For such studies, microorganisms offer the advantage that they have short mean generation times, are easily cultured in a small space under controlled conditions and have a relatively uncomplicated structure.

INTRODUCTION

Microbial genetics is a subject area within microbiology and genetic engineering. It studies the genetics of very small (micro) organisms; bacteria, archaea, viruses and some protozoa and fungi. This involves the study of the genotype of microbial species and also the expression system in the form of phenotypes.

Since the discovery of microorganisms by two Fellows of The Royal Society, Robert Hooke and Antoni van Leeuwenhoek during the period 1665-1885 they have been used to study many processes and have had applications in various areas of study in genetics. For example: Microorganisms' rapid growth rates and short generation times are used by scientists to study evolution. Microbial genetics also has applications in being able to study processes and pathways that are similar to those found in humans such as drug metabolism.

MICROORGANISMS WHOSE STUDY IS ENCOMPASSED BY MICROBIAL GENETICS

Bacteria

Bacteria have been on this planet for approximately 3.5 billion years, and are classified by their shape. Bacterial genetics studies the mechanisms of their heritable information, their chromosomes, plasmids, transposons, and phages.

Gene transfer systems that have been extensively studied in bacteria include genetic transformation, conjugation and transduction. Natural transformation is a bacterial adaptation for DNA transfer between two cells through the intervening medium. The uptake of donor DNA and its recombinational incorporation into the recipient chromosome depends on the expression of numerous bacterial genes whose products direct this process. In general, transformation is a complex, energy-requiring developmental process that appears to be an adaptation for repairing DNA damage.

Bacterial conjugation is the transfer of genetic material between bacterial cells by direct cell-to-cell contact or by a bridge-like connection between two cells. Bacterial conjugation has been extensively studied in *Escherichia coli*, but also occurs in other bacteria such as *Mycobacterium smegmatis*. Conjugation requires stable and extended contact between a donor and a recipient strain, is DNase resistant, and the transferred DNA is incorporated into the recipient chromosome by homologous recombination. *E. coli* conjugation is mediated by expression of plasmid genes, whereas mycobacterial conjugation is mediated by genes on the bacterial chromosome.

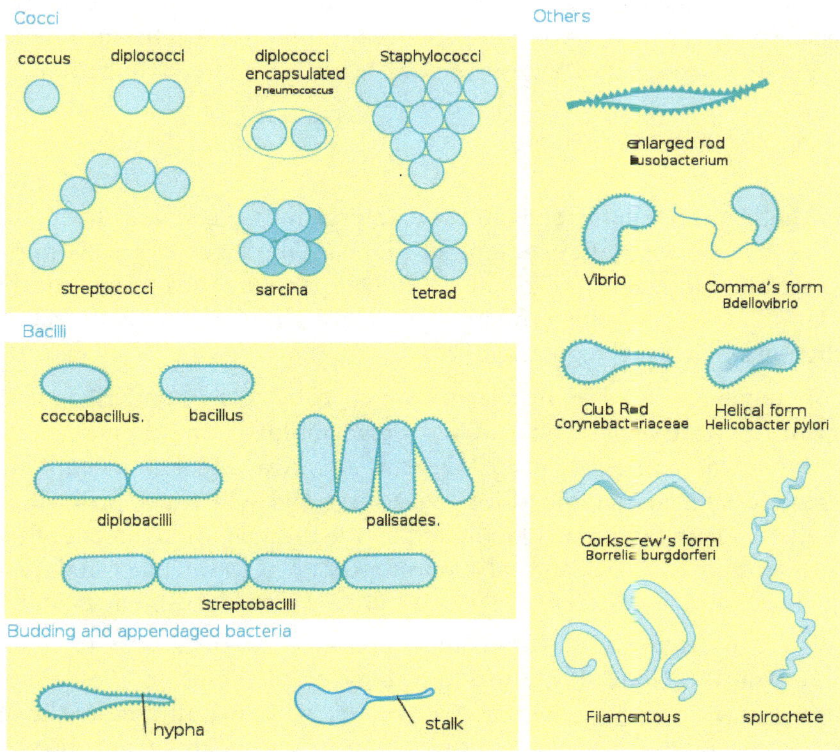

Bacteria are classified by their shape.

Transduction is the process by which foreign DNA is introduced into a cell by a virus or viral vector. Transduction is a common tool used by molecular biologists to stably introduce a foreign gene into a host cell's genome.

Archaea

Archaea is a domain of organisms that are prokaryotic, single-celled, and are thought to have developed 4 billion years ago. They share a common ancestor with bacteria, but are more closely related to eukaryotes in comparison to bacteria. Some Archaea are able to survive extreme environments, which leads to many applications in the field of genetics. One of such applications is the use of archaeal enzymes, which would be better able to survive harsh conditions *in vitro*.

Gene transfer and genetic exchange have been studied in the halophilic archaeon *Halobacterium volcanii* and the hyperthermophilic archaeons *Sulfolobus solfataricus* and *Sulfolobus acidocaldarius*. *H. volcani* forms cytoplasmic bridges between cells that appear to be used for transfer of DNA from one cell to another in either direction. When *S. solfataricus* and *S. acidocaldarius* are exposed to DNA damaging agents, species-specific cellular aggregation is induced. Cellular aggregation mediates chromosomal marker exchange and genetic recombination with high frequency. Cellular aggregation is thought to enhance species specific DNA transfer between *Sulfolobus* cells in order to provide increased repair of damaged DNA by means of homologous recombination.

Fungi

Fungi can be both multicellular and unicellular organisms, and are distinguished from other microbes by the way they obtain nutrients. Fungi secrete enzymes into their surroundings, to break down organic matter. Fungal genetics uses yeast, and filamentous fungi as model organisms for eukaryotic genetic research, including cell cycle regulation, chromatin structure and gene regulation.

Studies of the fungus *Neurospora crassa* have contributed substantially to understanding how genes work. *N. crassa* is a type of red bread mold of the phylum *Ascomycota*. It is used as a model organism because it is easy to grow and has a haploid life cycle that makes genetic analysis simple since recessive traits will show up in the offspring. Analysis of genetic recombination is facilitated by the ordered arrangement of the products of meiosis in ascospores. In its natural environment, *N. crassa* lives mainly in tropical and sub-tropical regions. It often can be found growing on dead plant matter after fires.

Neurospora was used by Edward Tatum and George Beadle in their experiments for which they won the Nobel Prize in Physiology or Medicine in 1958. The results of these experiments led directly to the one gene-one enzyme hypothesis that specific genes code for specific proteins. This concept proved to be the opening gun in what became molecular genetics and all the developments that have followed from that.

Saccharomyces cerevisiae is a yeast of the phylum *Ascomycota*. During vegetative growth that ordinarily occurs when nutrients are abundant, *S. cerevisiae* reproduces by mitosis as diploid cells. However, when starved, these cells undergo meiosis to form haploid spores. Mating occurs when haploid cells of opposite mating types MATa and MATα come into contact. Ruderfer et al. pointed out that, in nature, such contacts are frequent between closely related yeast cells for two reasons. The first is that cells of opposite mating type are present together in the same acus, the sac that contains the cells directly produced by a single meiosis, and these cells can mate with each other. The second reason is that haploid cells of one mating type, upon cell division, often produce cells of the opposite mating type. An analysis of the ancestry of natural *S. cerevisiae* strains concluded that outcrossing occurs very infrequently (only about once every 50,000 cell divisions). The relative rarity in nature of meiotic events that result from outcrossing suggests that the possible long-term benefits of outcrossing (e.g. generation of diversity) are unlikely to be sufficient for generally maintaining sex from one generation to the next. Rather, a short term benefit, such as meiotic recombinational repair of DNA damages caused by stressful conditions (such as starvation) may be the key to the maintenance of sex in *S. cerevisiae*.

Candida albicans is a diploid fungus that grows both as a yeast and as a filament. *C. albicans* is the most common fungal pathogen in humans. It causes both debilitating mucosal infections and potentially life-threatening systemic infections. *C. albicans* has maintained an elaborate, but largely hidden, mating apparatus. Johnson suggested that mating strategies may allow *C. albicans* to survive in the hostile environment of a mammalian host.

Among the 250 known species of aspergilli, about 33% have an identified sexual state. Among those *Aspergillus* species that exhibit a sexual cycle the overwhelming majority in nature are homothallic (self-fertilizing). Selfing in the homothallic fungus *Aspergillus nidulans* involves activation of the same mating pathways characteristic of sex in outcrossing species, i.e. self-fertilization does not bypass required pathways for outcrossing sex but instead requires activation of these pathways within a single individual. Fusion of haploid nuclei occurs within reproductive structures termed *cleistothecia*, in which the diploid zygote undergoes meiotic divisions to yield haploid ascospores.

Protozoa

Protozoa are unicellular organisms, which have nuclei, and ultramicroscopic cellular bodies within their cytoplasm. One particular aspect of protozoa that are of interest to human geneticists are their flagella, which are very similar to human sperm flagella.

Studies of *Paramecia* have contributed to our understanding of the function of meiosis. Like all ciliates, *Paramecia* have a polyploid macronucleus, and one or more diploid micronuclei. The macronucleus controls non-reproductive cell functions, expressing the genes needed for daily functioning. The micronucleus is the generative, or germline nucleus, containing the genetic material that is passed along from one generation to the next.

In the asexual fission phase of growth, during which cell divisions occur by mitosis rather than meiosis, clonal aging occurs leading to a gradual loss of vitality. In some species, such as the well studied *Paramecium tetraurelia*, the asexual line of clonally aging paramecia loses vitality and expires after about 200 fissions if the cells fail to undergo meiosis followed by either autogamy (self-fertilizaion) or conjugation (outcrossing). DNA damage increases dramatically during successive clonal cell divisions and is a likely cause of clonal aging in *P. tetraurelia*.

When clonally aged *P. tetraurelia* are stimulated to undergo meiosis in association with either autogamy or conjugation, the progeny are rejuvenated and are able to have many more mitotic binary fission divisions. During either of these processes the micronuclei of the cell(s) undergo meiosis, the old macronucleus disintegrates and a new macronucleus is formed by replication of the micronuclear DNA that had recently undergone meiosis. There is apparently little, if any, DNA damage in the new macronucleus, suggesting that rejuvenation is associated with the repair of these damages in the micronucleus during meiosis.

Viruses

Viruses are capsid-encoding organisms composed of proteins and nucleic acids that can self-assemble after replication in a host cell using the host's replication machinery. There is a disagreement in science about whether viruses are living due to their lack of ribosomes. Comprehending the viral genome is important not only for studies in genetics but also for understanding their pathogenic properties.

Many types of virus are capable of genetic recombination. When two or more individual viruses of the same type infect a cell, their genomes may recombine with each other to produce recombinant virus progeny. Both DNA and RNA viruses can undergo recombination. When two or more viruses, each containing lethal genomic damage infect the same host cell, the virus genomes often can pair with each other and undergo homologous recombinational repair to produce viable progeny. This process is known as multiplicity reactivation. Enzymes employed in multiplicity reactivation are functionally homologous to enzymes employed in bacterial and eukaryotic recombinational repair. Multiplicity reactivation has been found to occur with pathogenic viruses including influenza virus, HIV-1, adenovirus simian virus 40, vaccinia virus, reovirus, poliovirus and herpes simplex virus as well as numerous bacteriophages.

APPLICATIONS OF MICROBIAL GENETICS

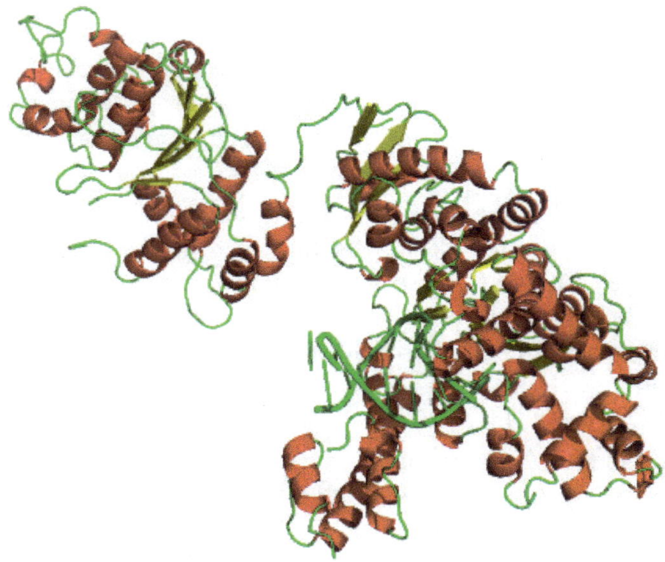

Taq polymerase which is used in Polymerase Chain Reaction(PCR).

Microbes are ideally suited for biochemical and genetics studies and have made huge contributions to these fields of science such as the demonstration that DNA is the genetic material, that the gene has a simple linear structure, that the genetic code is a triplet code, and that gene expression is regulated by specific genetic processes. Jacques Monod and François Jacob used *Escherichia coli*, a type of bacteria, in order to develop the operon model of gene expression, which lay down the basis of gene expression and regulation. Furthermore the hereditary processes of single-celled eukaryotic microorganisms are similar to those in multi-cellular organisms allowing researchers to gather information on this process as well. Another bacterium which has greatly contributed to the field of genetics is *Thermus aquaticus*, which is a bacterium that tolerates high temperatures. From this microbe scientists isolated the enzyme Taq polymerase, which is now used in the powerful experimental technique, Polymerase chain reaction(PCR). Additionally the development of recombinant DNA technology through the use of bacteria has led to the birth of modern genetic engineering and biotechnology.

Using microbes, protocols were developed to insert genes into bacterial plasmids, taking advantage of their fast reproduction, to make biofactories for the gene of interest. Such genetically engineered bacteria can produce pharmaceuticals such as insulin, human growth hormone, interferons and blood clotting factors. Microbes synthesize a variety of enzymes for industrial applications, such as fermented foods, laboratory test reagents, dairy products (such as renin), and even in clothing (such as *Trichoderma* fungus whose enzyme is used to give jeans a stone washed appearance).

REFERENCES

1. "Microbial genetics". Nature. Nature Publishing Group, A division of Macmillan Publishers Limmited. Retrieved 2015-09-24.
2. Gest, Hau (22 May 2004). "The discovery of microorganisms by Robert Hooke and Antoni van Leeuwenhoek, Fellows of The Royal Society". The Royal Society. 58: 137–201. doi:10.1098/rsnr.2004.0055. PMID 15209075. Retrieved 2015-09-25.
3. Mortlock, Robert (2013). Microorganisms As Model Systems for Studying Evolution. Springer Verlag. p. 2. ISBN 978-1-4684-4846-7.
4. Murphy, Cormac D. (2 September 2014). "Drug metabolism in microorganisms". Biotechnology Letters. 37 (1): 19–28. doi:10.1007/s10529-014-1653-8.
5. Weeks, Benjamin S. (2012). Alcamo's microbes and society (3rd ed.). Sudbury, MA: Jones & Bartlett Learning. ISBN 978-0-7637-9064-6.
6. "Bacterial genetics". Nature. Macmillan Publishers Limmited. Retrieved 8 November 2015.
7. Chen I, Dubnau D (2004). "DNA uptake during bacterial transformation". Nat. Rev. Microbiol. 2 (3): 241–9. doi:10.1038/nrmicro844. PMID 15083159.
8. Johnsborg O, Eldholm V, Håvarstein LS (2007). "Natural genetic transformation: prevalence, mechanisms and function". Res. Microbiol. 158 (10): 767–78. doi:10.1016/j.resmic.2007.09.004. PMID 17997281.
9. Michod RE, Bernstein H, Nedelcu AM (2008). "Adaptive value of sex in microbial pathogens". Infect. Genet. Evol. 8 (3): 267–85. doi:10.1016/j.meegid.2008.01.002. PMID 18295550.
10. Gray TA, Krywy JA, Harold J, Palumbo MJ, Derbyshire KM (2013). "Distributive conjugal transfer in mycobacteria generates progeny with meiotic-like genome-wide mosaicism, allowing mapping of a mating identity locus". PLoS Biol. 11 (7): e1001602. doi:10.1371/journal.pbio.1001602. PMC 3706393Freely accessible. PMID 23874149.

11. "Archaea". Microbe WORLD. Microbe WORLD. Retrieved 8 November 2015.
12. Chambers, Cecilia R.; Patrick, Wayne M. (2015). "Archaeal Nucleic Acid Ligases and Their Potential in Biotechnology". Archaea. 2015: 1–10. doi:10.1155/2015/170571.
13. Rosenshine I, Tchelet R, Mevarech M (1989). "The mechanism of DNA transfer in the mating system of an archaebacterium". Science. 245 (4924): 1387–9. doi:10.1126/science.2818746. PMID 2818746.
14. Fröls S, Ajon M, Wagner M, Teichmann D, Zolghadr B, Folea M, Boekema EJ, Driessen AJ, Schleper C, Albers SV (2008). "UV-inducible cellular aggregation of the hyperthermophilic archaeon Sulfolobus solfataricus is mediated by pili formation". Mol. Microbiol. 70 (4): 938–52. doi:10.1111/j.1365-2958.2008.06459.x. PMID 18990182.
15. Fröls S, White MF, Schleper C (2009). "Reactions to UV damage in the model archaeon Sulfolobus solfataricus". Biochem. Soc. Trans. 37 (Pt 1): 36–41. doi:10.1042/BST0370036. PMID 19143598.
16. Ajon M, Fröls S, van Wolferen M, Stoecker K, Teichmann D, Driessen AJ, Grogan DW, Albers SV, Schleper C (2011). "UV-inducible DNA exchange in hyperthermophilic archaea mediated by type IV pili". Mol. Microbiol. 82 (4): 807–17. doi:10.1111/j.1365-2958.2011.07861.x. PMID 21999488.
17. "Fungal Genetics". Nature.com. Macmillan Publishers Limited. Retrieved 9 November 2015.
18. Beadle GW, Tatum EL (1941). "Genetic Control of Biochemical Reactions in Neurospora". Proc. Natl. Acad. Sci. U.S.A. 27 (11): 499–506. doi:10.1073/pnas.27.11.499. PMC 1078370Freely accessible. PMID 16588492.
19. Horowitz NH, Berg P, Singer M, Lederberg J, Susman M, Doebley J, Crow JF (2004). "A centennial: George W. Beadle, 1903-1989". Genetics. 166 (1): 1–10. doi:10.1534/genetics.166.1.1. PMC 1470705Freely accessible. PMID 15020400.
20. Herskowitz I (1988). "Life cycle of the budding yeast Saccharomyces cerevisiae". Microbiol. Rev. 52 (4): 536–53. PMC 373162Freely accessible. PMID 3070323.
21. Ruderfer DM, Pratt SC, Seidel HS, Kruglyak L (2006). "Population genomic analysis of outcrossing and recombination in yeast". Nat. Genet. 38 (9): 1077–81. doi:10.1038/ng1859. PMID 16892060.
22. Birdsell JA, Wills C (2003). The evolutionary origin and maintenance of sexual recombination: A review of contemporary models. Evolutionary Biology Series >> Evolutionary Biology, Vol. 33 pp. 27-137. MacIntyre, Ross J.; Clegg, Michael, T (Eds.), Springer. Hardcover ISBN 978-0306472619, ISBN 0306472619 Softcover ISBN 978-1-4419-3385-0.
23. Elvira Hörandl (2013). Meiosis and the Paradox of Sex in Nature, Meiosis, ISBN 978-953-51-1197-9, InTech, DOI: 10.5772/56542. Available from: http://www.intechopen.com/books/meiosis/meiosis-and-the-paradox-of-sex-in-nature
24. Bernstein H and Bernstein C (2013). Evolutionary Origin and Adaptive Function of Meiosis. In Meiosis: Bernstein C and Bernstein H, editors. ISBN 978-953-51-

1197-9, InTech, http://www.intechopen.com/books/meiosis/evolutionary-origin-and-adaptive-function-of-meiosis

25. Johnson A (2003). "The biology of mating in Candida albicans". Nat. Rev. Microbiol. 1 (2): 106–16. doi:10.1038/nrmicro752. PMID 15035040.
26. Dyer PS, O'Gorman CM (2012). "Sexual development and cryptic sexuality in fungi: insights from Aspergillus species". FEMS Microbiol. Rev. 36 (1): 165–92. doi:10.1111/j.1574-6976.2011.00308.x. PMID 22091779.
27. Paoletti M, Seymour FA, Alcocer MJ, Kaur N, Calvo AM, Archer DB, Dyer PS (2007). "Mating type and the genetic basis of self-fertility in the model fungus Aspergillus nidulans". Curr. Biol. 17 (16): 1384–9. doi:10.1016/j.cub.2007.07.012. PMID 17669651.
28. Prescott DM (1994). "The DNA of ciliated protozoa". Microbiol. Rev. 58 (2): 233–67. PMC 372963Freely accessible. PMID 8078435.
29. Smith-Sonneborn J (1979). "DNA repair and longevity assurance in Paramecium tetraurelia". Science. 203 (4385): 1115–7. doi:10.1126/science.424739. PMID 424739.
30. Holmes GE, Holmes NR (1986). "Accumulation of DNA damages in aging Paramecium tetraurelia". Mol. Gen. Genet. 204 (1): 108–14. doi:10.1007/bf00330196. PMID 3091993.
31. Gilley D, Blackburn EH (1994). "Lack of telomere shortening during senescence in Paramecium". Proc. Natl. Acad. Sci. U.S.A. 91 (5): 1955–8. doi:10.1073/pnas.91.5.1955. PMC 43283Freely accessible. PMID 8127914.
32. Raoult, Didier; Forterre, Patrick (3 March 2008). "Redefining viruses: lessons from Mimivirus". Nature Reviews Microbiology. 6 (4): 315–319. doi:10.1038/nrmicro1858.
33. Seto, Donald (30 November 2010). "Viral Genomics and Bioinformatics". Viruses. 2 (12): 2587–2593. doi:10.3390/v2122587.
34. Bernstein C (1981). "Deoxyribonucleic acid repair in bacteriophage". Microbiol. Rev. 45 (1): 72–98. PMC 281499Freely accessible PMID 6261109.
35. Chen D, Bernstein C (1987). "Recombinational repair of hydrogen peroxide-induced damages in DNA of phage T4". Mutat. Res. 184 (2): 87–98. doi:10.1016/0167-8817(87)90064-2. PMID 3627145.
36. Michod RE, Bernstein H, Nedelcu AM (May 2008). "Adaptive value of sex in microbial pathogens". Infection, Genetics and Evolution. 8 (3): 267–85. doi:10.1016/j.meegid.2008.01.002. PMID 18295550.http://www.hummingbirds.arizona.edu/Faculty/Michod/Downloads/IGE%20review%20sex.pdf
37. Avery OT, MacLeod CM, McCarty M (1979). "Studies on the chemical nature of the substance inducing transformation of pneumococcal types. Inductions of transformation by a desoxyribonucleic acid fraction isolated from pneumococcus type III". J. Exp. Med. 149 (2): 297–326. doi:10.1084/jem.149.2.297. PMC 2184805Freely accessible. PMID 33226.

38. HERSHEY AD, CHASE M (1952). "Independent functions of viral protein and nucleic acid in growth of bacteriophage". J. Gen. Physiol. 36 (1): 39–56. doi:10.1085/jgp.36.1.39. PMC 2147348Freely accessible. PMID 12981234.

39. Benzer S (1959). "ON THE TOPOLOGY OF THE GENETIC FINE STRUCTURE". Proc. Natl. Acad. Sci. U.S.A. 45 (11): 1607–20. PMC 222769Freely accessible. PMID 16590553.

40. CRICK FH, BARNETT L, BRENNER S, WATTS-TOBIN RJ (1961). "General nature of the genetic code for proteins". Nature. 192: 1227–32. doi:10.1038/1921227a0. PMID 13882203.

41. JACOB F, MONOD J (1961). "Genetic regulatory mechanisms in the synthesis of proteins". J. Mol. Biol. 3: 318–56. doi:10.1016/S0022-2836(61)80072-7. PMID 13718526.

42. "Microbial Genetics". World Of Micorbiology and Immunology. 2003. Retrieved 9 November 2015.

43. Bainbridge, B.W. (1987). Genetics of microbes (2nd ed.). Glasgow: Blackie. ISBN 0-412-01281-2.

44. Terpe, Kay (1 November 2013). "Overview of thermostable DNA polymerases for classical PCR applications: from molecular and biochemical fundamentals to commercial systems". Applied Microbiology and Biotechnology. 97 (24): 10243–10254. doi:10.1007/s00253-013-5290-2.

CHAPTER 11

Immunology

Chapter Contents

- Introduction
- Classical Immunology
- Clinical Immunology
- Developmental Immunology
- Immunotherapy
- Diagnostic Immunology
- Cancer Immunology
- Reproductive Immunology
- Theoretical Immunology

The science of Immunology encompasses the study of the development, anatomy functions and malfunctions of the immune system, all of which are of fundamental importance to the understanding of human disease. The immune system is made up of many types of molecules and cells that are distributed in every tissue of the body, as well as specialized lymphoid organs, which act in a coordinated manner to prevent or eliminate microbial infections, to suppress the growth of tumors, and to initiate repair of damaged tissues. The immune system normally recognizes and responds to foreign molecules or damaged self, but not healthy host cells and tissues. The innate immune system maintains barriers to microbial invasion and provides critical biochemical and cellular first responders to infections that are absolutely essential for survival in a world teeming with microbes. Innate immune recognition initiates stereotypical inflammatory or anti-viral responses to a limited number of molecular patterns that are shared by different pathogens or expressed by injured or infected host cells. The more highly evolved adaptive immune system relies on collections of millions of clones of B and T lymphocytes to provide protection for the host, each clone capable of recognizing a distinct molecule. Furthermore, B and T lymphocytes are capable of differentiating into several different types of effector cells that perform distinct functions, and into long-lived memory cells that prevent or minimize repeat infections by a microbe.

INTRODUCTION

Immunology is a branch of biology that covers the study of immune systems in all organisms. It was the Russian biologist Ilya Ilyich Mechnikov who boosted studies on immunology, and received the Nobel Prize in 1908 for his work. He jabbed the thorn of a rose on a starfish and noted that, 24 hours later, cells were surrounding the tip. It was an active response of the body, trying to maintain its integrity. It was Mechnikov who first observed the phenomenon of phagocytosis, in which the body defends itself against a foreign body, and coined the term. It charts, measures, and contextualizes the: physiological functioning of the immune system in states of both health and diseases; malfunctions of the immune system in immunological disorders (such as autoimmune diseases, hypersensitivities, immune deficiency, and transplant rejection); the physical, chemical and physiological characteristics of the components of the immune system *in vitro*, *in situ*, and *in vivo*. Immunology has applications in numerous disciplines of medicine, particularly in the fields of organ transplantation, oncology, virology, bacteriology, parasitology, psychiatry, and dermatology.

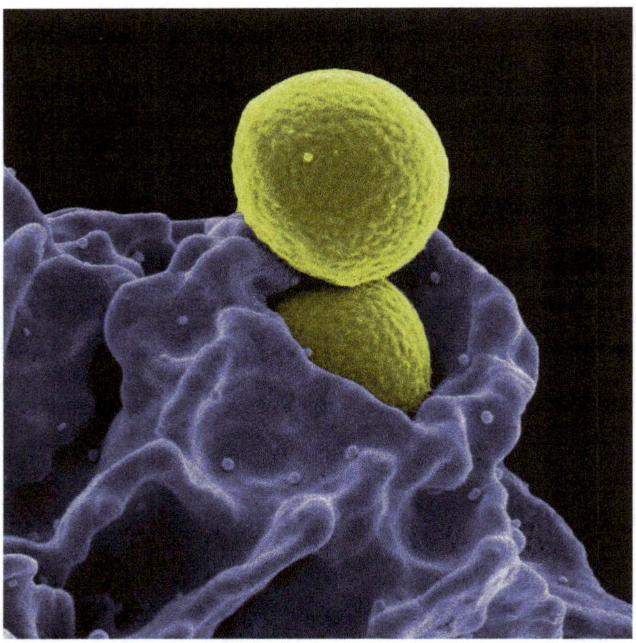

A bacterium (MRSA, yellow) being ingested by an immune cell (Neutrophil, purple).

Prior to the designation of immunity from the etymological root *immunis*, which is Latin for "exempt"; early physicians characterized organs that would later be proven as essential components of the immune system. The important lymphoid organs of the immune system are the thymus and bone marrow, and chief lymphatic tissues such as spleen, tonsils, lymph vessels, lymph nodes, adenoids, and liver. When health conditions worsen to emergency status, portions of immune system organs including the thymus, spleen, bone marrow, lymph nodes and other lymphatic tissues can be surgically excised for examination while patients are still alive.

Many components of the immune system are typically cellular in nature and not associated with any specific organ; but rather are embedded or circulating in various tissues located throughout the body.

CLASSICAL IMMUNOLOGY

Classical immunology ties in with the fields of epidemiology and medicine. It studies the relationship between the body systems, pathogens, and immunity. The earliest written mention of immunity can be traced back to the plague of Athens in 430 BCE. Thucydides noted that people who had recovered from a previous bout of the disease could nurse the sick without contracting the illness a second time. Many other ancient societies have references to this phenomenon, but it was not until the 19th and 20th centuries before the concept developed into scientific theory.

The study of the molecular and cellular components that comprise the immune system, including their function and interaction, is the central science of immunology. The immune system has been divided into a more primitive innate immune system and, in vertebrates, an acquired or adaptive immune system. The latter is further divided into humoral (or antibody) and cell-mediated components.

The humoral (antibody) response is defined as the interaction between antibodies and antigens. Antibodies are specific proteins released from a certain class of immune cells known as B lymphocytes, while antigens are defined as anything that elicits the generation of antibodies ("anti"body "gen"erators). Immunology rests on an understanding of the properties of these two biological entities and the cellular response to both.

Immunological research continues to become more specialized, pursuing non-classical models of immunity and functions of cells, organs and systems not previously associated with the immune system (Yemeserach 2010).

CLINICAL IMMUNOLOGY

Clinical immunology is the study of diseases caused by disorders of the immune system (failure, aberrant action, and malignant growth of the cellular elements of the system). It also involves diseases of other systems, where immune reactions play a part in the pathology and clinical features.

The diseases caused by disorders of the immune system fall into two broad categories:

- immunodeficiency, in which parts of the immune system fail to provide an adequate response (examples include chronic granulomatous disease and primary immune diseases);

- autoimmunity, in which the immune system attacks its own host's body (examples include systemic lupus erythematosus, rheumatoid arthritis, Hashimoto's disease and myasthenia gravis).

Other immune system disorders include various hypersensitivities (such as in asthma and other allergies) that respond inappropriately to otherwise harmless compounds.

The most well-known disease that affects the immune system itself is AIDS, an immunodeficiency characterized by the suppression of CD4+ ("helper") T cells, dendritic cells and macrophages by the Human Immunodeficiency Virus (HIV).

Clinical immunologists also study ways to prevent the immune system's attempts to destroy allografts (transplant rejection).

DEVELOPMENTAL IMMUNOLOGY

The body's capability to react to antigen depends on a person's age, antigen type, maternal factors and the area where the antigen is presented. Neonates are said to be in a state of physiological immunodeficiency, because both their innate and adaptive immunological responses are greatly suppressed. Once born, a child's immune system responds favorably to protein antigens while not as well to glycoproteins and polysaccharides. In fact, many of the infections acquired by neonates are caused by low virulence organisms like *Staphylococcus* and *Pseudomonas*. In neonates, opsonic activity and the ability to activate the complement cascade is very limited. For example, the mean level of C3 in a newborn is approximately 65% of that found in the adult. Phagocytic activity is also greatly impaired in newborns. This is due to lower opsonic activity, as well as diminished up-regulation of integrin and selectin receptors, which limit the ability of neutrophils to interact with adhesion molecules in the endothelium. Their monocytes are slow and have a reduced ATP production, which also limits the newborn's phagocytic activity. Although, the number of total lymphocytes is significantly higher than in adults, the cellular and humoral immunity is also impaired. Antigen-presenting cells in newborns have a reduced capability to activate T cells. Also, T cells of a newborn proliferate poorly and produce very small amounts of cytokines like IL-2, IL-4, IL-5, IL-12, and IFN-g which limits their capacity to activate the humoral response as well as the phagocitic activity of macrophage. B cells develop early during gestation but are not fully active.

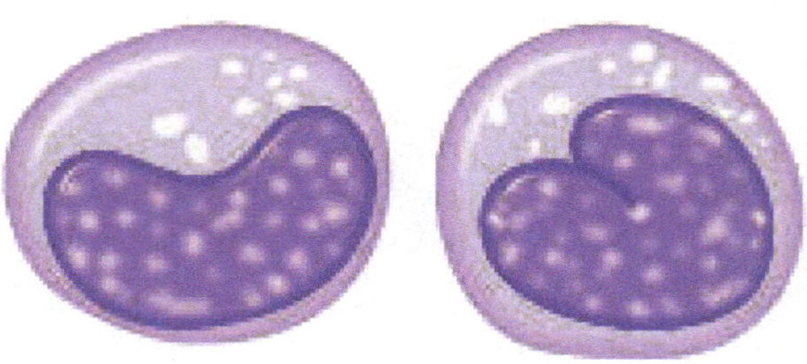

Artist's impression of monocytes.

Maternal factors also play a role in the body's immune response. At birth, most of the immunoglobulin present is maternal IgG. Because IgM, IgD, IgE and IgA don't cross the placenta, they are almost undetectable at birth. Some IgA is provided by breast milk. These passively-acquired antibodies can protect the newborn for up to 18 months, but their response is usually short-lived and of low affinity. These antibodies can also produce a negative response. If a child is exposed to the antibody for a particular antigen before being exposed to the antigen itself then the child will produce a dampened response. Passively acquired maternal antibodies can suppress the antibody response to active immunization. Similarly the response of T-cells to vaccination differs in children compared to adults, and vaccines that induce Th1 responses in adults do not readily elicit these same responses in neonates. Between six and nine months after birth, a child's immune system begins to respond more strongly to glycoproteins, but there is usually no marked improvement in their response to polysaccharides until they are at least one year old. This can be the reason for distinct time frames found in vaccination schedules.

During adolescence, the human body undergoes various physical, physiological and immunological changes triggered and mediated by hormones, of which the most significant in females is 17-β-oestradiol (an oestrogen) and, in males, is testosterone. Oestradiol usually begins to act around the age of 10 and testosterone some months later. There is evidence that these steroids not only act directly on the primary and secondary sexual characteristics but also have an effect on the development and regulation of the immune system, including an increased risk in developing pubescent and post-pubescent autoimmunity. There is also some evidence that cell surface receptors on B cells and macrophages may detect sex hormones in the system.

The female sex hormone 17-β-oestradiol has been shown to regulate the level of immunological response, while some male androgens such as testosterone seem to suppress the stress response to infection. Other androgens, however, such as DHEA, increase immune response. As in females, the male sex hormones seem to have more control of the immune system during puberty and post-puberty than during the rest of a male's adult life.

Physical changes during puberty such as thymic involution also affect immunological response.

IMMUNOTHERAPY

Immunotherapy is the "treatment of disease by inducing, enhancing, or suppressing an immune response". Immunotherapies designed to elicit or amplify an immune response are classified as activation immunotherapies, while immunotherapies that reduce or suppress are classified as suppression immunotherapies.

Immunomodulatory regimens often have fewer side effects than existing drugs, including less potential for creating resistance when treating microbial disease.

Cell-based immunotherapies are effective for some cancers. Immune effector cells such as lymphocytes, macrophages, dendritic cells, natural killer cells (NK Cell), cytotoxic T lymphocytes (CTL), etc., work together to defend the body against cancer by targeting abnormal antigens expressed on the surface of tumor cells.

Therapies such as granulocyte colony-stimulating factor (G-CSF), interferons, imiquimod and cellular membrane fractions from bacteria are licensed for medical use. Others including IL-2, IL-7, IL-12, various chemokines, synthetic cytosine phosphate-guanosine (CpG) oligodeoxynucleotides and glucans are involved in clinical and preclinical studies.

Immunomodulators

Immunomodulators are the active agents of immunotherapy. They are a diverse array of recombinant, synthetic and natural preparations.

Class	Example agents
Interleukins	IL-2, IL-7, IL-12
Cytokines	Interferons, G-CSF, Imiquimod
Chemokines	CCL3, CCL26, CXCL7
Immunomodulatory imide drugs (IMiDs)	thalidomide and its analogues (lenalidomide, pomalidomide, and apremilast)
Other	cytosine phosphate-guanosine, oligodeoxynucleotides, glucans

Activation Immunotherapies

Cancer

Cancer immunotherapy attempts to stimulate the immune system to destroy tumors. A variety of strategies are in use or are undergoing research and testing. Randomized controlled studies in different cancers resulting in significant increase in survival and disease free period have been reported and its efficacy is enhanced by 20–30% when cell-based immunotherapy is combined with conventional treatment methods.

The extraction of G-CSF lymphocytes from the blood and expanding in vitro against a tumour antigen before reinjecting the cells with appropriate stimulatory cytokines. The cells then destroy the tumor cells that express the antigen.

BCG immunotherapy for early stage (non-invasive) bladder cancer instills attenuated live bacteria into the bladder and is effective in preventing recurrence in up to two thirds of cases.

Topical immunotherapy utilizes an immune enhancement cream (imiquimod) which produces interferon, causing the recipient's killer T cells to destroy warts, actinic keratoses, basal cell cancer, vaginal intraepithelial neoplasia, squamous cell cancer, cutaneous lymphoma, and superficial malignant melanoma.

Injection immunotherapy ("intralesional" or "intratumoral") uses mumps, candida, the HPV vaccine or trichophytin antigen injections to treat warts (HPV induced tumors).

Adoptive cell transfer has been tested on lung and other cancers.

Dendritic Cell-Based Pump-Priming

Dendritic cells can be stimulated to activate a cytotoxic response towards an antigen. Dendritic cells, a type of antigen presenting cell, are harvested from the person needing the immunotherapy. These cells are then either pulsed with an antigen or tumor lysate or transfected with a viral vector, causing them to display the antigen. Upon transfusion into the person, these activated cells present the antigen to the effector lymphocytes (CD4+ helper T cells, cytotoxic CD8+ T cells and B cells). This initiates a cytotoxic response against tumor cells expressing the antigen (against which the adaptive response has now been primed). The cancer vaccine Sipuleucel-T is one example of this approach.

T-Cell Adoptive Transfer

Adoptive cell transfer *in vitro* cultivates autologous, extracted T cells for later transfusion. The T cells may already target tumor cells. Alternatively, they may be genetically engineered to do so. These T cells, referred to as tumor-infiltrating lymphocytes (TIL), are multiplied using high concentrations of Interleukin-2, anti-CD3 and allo-reactive feeder cells. These T cells are then transferred back into the person along with administration of IL-2 to further boost their anti-cancer activity.

Before reinfusion, lymphodepletion of the recipient is required to eliminate regulatory T cells as well as unmodified, endogenous lymphocytes that compete with the transferred cells for homeostatic cytokines. Lymphodepletion can be achieved by total body irradiation. Transferred cells multiplied *in vivo* and persisted in peripheral blood in many people, sometimes representing levels of 75% of all $CD8^+$ T cells at 6–12 months after infusion. As of 2012, clinical trials for metastatic melanoma were ongoing at multiple sites.

Immune Enhancement Therapy

Autologous immune enhancement therapy use a person's own peripheral blood-derived natural killer cells, cytotoxic T lymphocytes and other relevant immune cells are expanded *in vitro* and then reinfused. The therapy has been tested against Hepatitis C, Chronic fatigue syndrome and HHV6 infection.

Genetically Engineered T Cells

Genetically engineered T cells are created by harvesting T cells and then infecting the T cells with a retrovirus that contains a copy of a T cell receptor (TCR) gene that is specialised to recognise tumour antigens. The virus integrates the receptor into the T cells' genome. The cells are expanded non-specifically and/or stimulated. The cells are then reinfused and produce an immune response against the tumour cells. The technique has been tested on refractory stage IV metastatic melanomas and advanced skin cancer

Immune Recovery

Another potential use of immunotherapy is to restore the immune system of people with immune deficiencies. Cytokines, Interleukin-7 and Interleukin-2 have been tested in clinical trials.

Vaccination

Antimicrobial immunotherapy, which includes vaccination, involves activating the immune system to respond to an infectious agent.

Suppression Immunotherapies

Immune suppression dampens an abnormal immune response in autoimmune diseases or reduces a normal immune response to prevent rejection of transplanted organs or cells.

Immunosuppressive Drugs

Immunosuppressive drugs help manage organ transplantation and autoimmune disease. Immune responses depend on lymphocyte proliferation. Cytostatic drugs are immunosuppressive. Glucocorticoids are somewhat more specific inhibitors of lymphocyte activation, whereas inhibitors of immunophilins more specifically target T lymphocyte activation. Immunosuppressive antibodies target steps in the immune response. Other drugs modulate immune responses.

Immune Tolerance

The body naturally does not launch an immune system attack on its own tissues. Immune tolerance therapies seek to reset the immune system so that the body stops mistakenly attacking its own organs or cells in autoimmune disease or accepts foreign tissue in organ transplantation. Creating immunity reduces or eliminates the need for lifelong immunosuppression and attendant side effects. It has been tested on transplantations, and type 1 diabetes or other autoimmune disorders.

Allergies

Immunotherapy is used to treat allergies. While allergy treatments (such as antihistamines or corticosteroids) treat allergic symptoms, immunotherapy can reduce sensitivity to allergens, lessening its severity.

Immunotherapy may produce long-term benefits. Immunotherapy is partly effective in some people and ineffective in others, but it offers allergy sufferers a chance to reduce or stop their symptoms.

The therapy is indicated for people who are extremely allergic or who cannot avoid specific allergens. Immunotherapy is generally not indicated for food or medicinal allergies. This therapy is particularly useful for people with allergic rhinitis or asthma.

The first dose contain tiny amounts of the allergen or antigen. Dosages increase over time, as the person becomes desensitized. This technique has been tested on infants to prevent peanut allergies.

Helminthic Therapies

Whipworm ova (*Trichuris suis*) and Hookworm (*Necator americanus*) have been tested for immunological diseases and allergies. Helminthic therapy has been investigated as a treatment for relapsing remitting multiple sclerosis Crohn's, allergies and asthma. The mechanism of how the helminths modulate the immune response, is unknown. Hypothesized mechanisms include re-polarisation of the Th1 / Th2 response and modulation of dendritic cell function. The helminths down regulate the pro-inflammatory Th1 cytokines, Interleukin-12 (IL-12), Interferon-Gamma (IFN-γ) and Tumour Necrosis Factor-Alpha (TNF-ά), while promoting the production of regulatory Th2 cytokines such as IL-10, IL-4, IL-5 and IL-13.

Co-evolution with helminths has shaped some of the genes associated with Interleukin expression and immunological disorders, such Crohn's, ulcerative colitis and Celiac disease. Helminth's relationship to humans as hosts should be classified as mutualistic or symbiotic.

DIAGNOSTIC IMMUNOLOGY

The specificity of the bond between antibody and antigen has made the antibody an excellent tool for the detection of substances by a variety of diagnostic techniques. Antibodies specific for a desired antigen can be conjugated with an isotopic (radio) or fluorescent label or with a color-forming enzyme in order to detect it. However, the similarity between some antigens can lead to false positives and other errors in such tests by antibodies cross-reacting with antigens that aren't exact matches.

CANCER IMMUNOLOGY

Cancer immunology is a branch of immunology that studies interactions between the immune system and cancer cells (also called tumors or malignancies). It is a field of research that aims to discover cancer immunotherapies to treat and retard progression of the disease. The immune response, including the recognition of cancer-specific antigens, forms the basis of targeted therapy (such as vaccines and antibody therapies) and tumor marker-based diagnostic tests. For instance tumour infiltrating lymphocytes are significant in human colorectal cancer. The host was given a better chance at survival if the cancer tissue showed infiltration of inflammatory cells, in particular those prompting lymphocytic reactions. The results yielded suggest some extent of anti-tumour immunity is present in colorectal cancers in humans.

Cancer immunosurveillance and immunoediting is based on (i) protection against development of spontaneous and chemically induced tumors in animal systems and (ii) identification of targets for immune recognition of human cancer.

Immunosurveillance

Cancer immunosurveillance is a theory formulated in 1957 by Burnet and Thomas, who proposed that lymphocytes act as sentinels in recognizing and eliminating continuously arising, nascent transformed cells. Cancer immunosurveillance appears to be an important host protection process that decreases cancer rates through inhibition of carcinogenesis and maintaining of regular cellular homeostasis. It has also been suggested that immunosurveillance primarily functions as a component of a more general process of cancer immunoediting.

Immunoediting

Immunoediting is a process by which a person is protected from cancer growth and the development of tumour immunogenicity by their immune system. It has three main phases: elimination, equilibrium and escape.

Elimination

The elimination phase consists of the following four phases:

The first phase of elimination involves the initiation of an antitumor immune response. Cells of the innate immune system recognize the presence of a growing tumor which has undergone stromal remodeling, causing local tissue damage. This is followed by the induction of inflammatory signals which is essential for recruiting cells of the innate immune system (e.g. natural killer cells, natural killer T cells, macrophages and dendritic cells) to the tumor site. During this phase, the infiltrating lymphocytes such as the natural killer cells and natural killer T cells are stimulated to produce IFN-gamma.

In the second phase of elimination, newly synthesized IFN-gamma induces tumor death (to a limited amount) as well as promoting the production of chemokines CXCL10, CXCL9 and CXCL11. These chemokines play an important role in promoting tumor death by blocking the formation of new blood vessels. Tumor cell debris produced as a result of tumor death is then ingested by dendritic cells, followed by the migration of these dendritic cells to the draining lymph nodes. The recruitment of more immune cells also occurs and is mediated by the chemokines produced during the inflammatory process.

In the third phase, natural killer cells and macrophages transactivate one another via the reciprocal production of IFN-gamma and IL-12. This again promotes more tumor killing by these cells via apoptosis and the production of reactive oxygen and nitrogen intermediates. In the draining lymph nodes, tumor-specific dendritic cells trigger the differentiation of Th1 cells which in turn facilitates the development of cytotoxic $CD8^+$ T cells also known as *killer T-cells*.

In the final phase of elimination, tumor-specific $CD4^+$ and $CD8^+$ T cells home to the tumor site and the cytotoxic T lymphocytes then destroy the antigen-bearing tumor cells which remain at the site.

Equilibrium and Escape

Tumor cell variants which have survived the elimination phase enter the equilibrium phase. In this phase, lymphocytes and IFN-gamma exert a selection pressure on tumor cells which are genetically unstable and rapidly mutating. Tumor cell variants which have acquired resistance to elimination then enter the escape phase.

In the escape phase, tumor cells continue to grow and expand in an uncontrolled manner and may eventually lead to malignancies. In the study of cancer immunoediting, knockout mice have been used for experimentation since human testing is not possible. Tumor infiltration by lymphocytes is seen as a reflection of a tumor-related immune response.

Cancer Immunology and Chemotherapy

Obeid et al. investigated how inducing immunogenic cancer cell death ought to become a priority of cancer chemotherapy. He reasoned, the immune system would be able to play a factor via a 'bystander effect' in eradicating chemotherapy-resistant cancer cells. However, extensive research is still needed on how the immune response is triggered against dying tumour cells.

Professionals in the field have hypothesized that 'apoptotic cell death is poorly immunogenic whereas necrotic cell death is truly immunogenic'. This is perhaps because cancer cells being eradicated via a necrotic cell death pathway induce an immune response by triggering dendritic cells to mature, due to inflammatory response stimulation. On the other hand, apoptosis is connected to slight alterations within the plasma membrane causing the dying cells to be attractive to phagocytic cells. However, numerous animal studies have shown the superiority of vaccination with apoptotic cells, compared to necrotic cells, in eliciting anti-tumor immune responses.

Thus Obeid *et al.* propose that the way in which cancer cells die during chemotherapy is vital. Anthracyclins produce a beneficial immunogenic environment. The researchers report that when killing cancer cells with this agent uptake and presentation by antigen presenting dendritic cells is encouraged, thus allowing a T-cell response which can shrink tumours. Therefore activating tumour-killing T-cells is crucial for immunotherapy success.

However, advanced cancer patients with immunosuppression have left researchers in a dilemma as to how to activate their T-cells. The way the host dendritic cells react and uptake tumour antigens to present to $CD4^+$ and $CD8^+$ T-cells is the key to success of the treatment.

The Role of Viruses in Cancer Development

Various strains of human papillomavirus (HPV) have been found to play an important role in the development of cervical cancer. The HPV oncogenes E6 and E7 that these viruses possess have been shown to immortalise some human cells and thus promote cancer development. Although these strains of HPV have not been found in all cervical cancers, they have been found to be the cause in roughly 70% of cases. The study of these viruses and their role in the development of various cancers is still continuing, however a vaccine has been developed that can prevent infection of certain HPV strains, and thus prevent those HPV strains from causing cervical cancer, and possibly other cancers as well.

A virus that has been shown to cause breast cancer in mice is mouse mammary tumor virus. It is from discoveries such as this and the role of HPV in cervical cancer development that research is currently being undertaken to discover whether or not *human mammary tumour virus* is a cause of breast cancer in humans.

REPRODUCTIVE IMMUNOLOGY

Reproductive immunology refers to a field of medicine that studies interactions (or the absence of them) between the immune system and components related to the reproductive system, such as maternal immune tolerance towards the fetus, or immunological interactions across the blood-testis barrier. The concept has been used by fertility clinics to explain the fertility problems, recurrent miscarriages and pregnancy complications observed when this state of immunological tolerance is not successfully achieved. Immunological therapy is the new up and coming method for treating many cases of previously "unexplained infertility" or recurrent miscarriage.

Between Mother and Fetus

The fact that the embryo's tissue is half foreign and unlike mismatched organ transplant, it is not normally rejected, suggests that the immunological system of the mother plays an important role in pregnancy. The placenta also plays an important part in protecting the embryo for the immune attack from the mother's system. Studies also propose that proteins in semen may help woman's immune system prepare for conception and pregnancy. For example, there is substantial evidence for exposure to partner's semen as prevention for pre-eclampsia, largely due to the absorption of several immune modulating factors present in seminal fluid, such as transforming growth factor beta (TGFβ).

Sperm Cells within a Male

The presence of anti-sperm antibodies in infertile men was first reported in 1954 by Rumke and Wilson. It has been noticed that the number of cases of sperm autoimmunity is higher in the infertile population leading to the idea that autoimmunity could be a cause of infertility.Anti sperm antigen has been described as three immunoglobulin isotopes (IgG, IgA, IgM) each of which targets different part of the spermatozoa. If more than 10% of the sperm are bound to anti-sperm antibodies (ASA), then infertility is suspected. The blood-testis barrier separates the immune system and the developing spermatozoa. The tight junction between the Sertoli cells form the blood-testis barrier but it is usually breached by physiological leakage. Not all sperms are protected by the barrier because spermatogonia and early spermatocytes are located below the junction. They are protected by other means like immunologic tolerance and immunomodulation.

Infertility after anti-sperm antibody binding can be caused by autoagglutination, sperm cytotoxicity, blockage of sperm-ovum interaction, and inadequate motility. Each presents itself depending on the binding site of ASA.

Immunocontraceptive Vaccine

Experiments are undergoing to test the effectiveness of an immunocontraceptive vaccine that inhibits the fusing of spermatozoa to the zona pellucida. This vaccine is currently being tested in animals and hopefully will be an effective contraceptive for humans. Normally, spermatozoa fuse with the zona pellucida surrounding the mature oocyte; the resulting acrosome reaction breaks down the egg's tough coating so that the sperm can fertilize the oovum. The mechanism of the vaccine is injection with cloned ZP cDNA, therefore this vaccine is a DNA based vaccine. This results in the production of antibodies against the ZP, which stop the sperm from binding to the zona pellucida and ultimately from fertilizing the oovum.

Another vaccine in investigation is one against HCG. This immunization would produce antibodies against hCG and TT. Antibodies against hCG would prevent the maintenance of the uterus for a viable pregnancy therefore preventing contraception. Another vaccine that is utilized is the peptide β-hCG that is more specific to hCG and a more rapid and effective response occurs in the absence of LH, FSH, and TSH.

THEORETICAL IMMUNOLOGY

Immunology is strongly experimental in everyday practice but is also characterized by an ongoing theoretical attitude. Many theories have been suggested in immunology from the end of the nineteenth century up to the present time. The end of the 19th century and the beginning of the 20th century saw a battle between "cellular" and "humoral" theories of immunity. According to the cellular theory of immunity, represented in particular by Elie Metchnikoff, it was cells – more precisely, phagocytes – that were responsible for immune responses. In contrast, the humoral theory of immunity, held by Robert Koch and Emil von Behring, among others, stated that the active immune agents were soluble components (molecules) found in the organism's "humors" rather than its cells.

In the mid-1950s, Frank Burnet, inspired by a suggestion made by Niels Jerne, formulated the clonal selection theory (CST) of immunity. On the basis of CST, Burnet developed a theory of how an immune response is triggered according to the self/nonself distinction: "self" constituents (constituents of the body) do not trigger destructive immune responses, while "nonself" entities (e.g., pathogens, an allograft) trigger a destructive immune response. The theory was later modified to reflect new discoveries regarding histocompatibility or the complex "two-signal" activation of T cells. The self/nonself theory of immunity and the self/nonself vocabulary have been criticized, but remain very influential.

More recently, several theoretical frameworks have been suggested in immunology, including "autopoietic" views, "cognitive immune" views, the "danger model" (or "danger theory"), and the "discontinuity" theory. The danger model, suggested by Polly Matzinger and colleagues, has been very influential, arousing many comments and discussions.

Immunologist

Immunologist	
Occupation	
Occupation type	Profession / Specialty
Activity sectors	• Medicine • Physiology • Science • Laboratorial
Description	
Education required	• MD • PhD • DO
Related jobs	• Physician • Research scientist

According to the American Academy of Allergy, Asthma, and Immunology (AAAAI), "an immunologist is a research scientist who investigates the immune system of vertebrates (including the human immune system). Immunologists include research scientists (PhDs) who work in laboratories. Immunologists also include physicians who, for example, treat patients with immune system disorders. Some immunologists are physician-scientists who combine laboratory research with patient care."

Career in Immunology

Bioscience is the overall major in which undergraduate students who are interested in general well-being take in college. Immunology is a branch of bioscience for undergraduate programs but the major gets specified as students move on for graduate program in immunology. The aim of immunology is to study the health of humans and animals through effective yet consistent research, (AAAAI, 2013). The most important thing about being immunologists is the research because it is the biggest portion of their jobs.

Most graduate immunology schools follow the AAI courses immunology which are offered throughout numerous schools in the United States. For example, in New York State, there are several universities that offer the AAI courses immunology: Albany Medical College, Cornell University, Icahn School of Medicine at Mount Sinai, New York University Langone Medical Center, University at Albany (SUNY), University at Buffalo (SUNY), University of Rochester Medical Center and Upstate Medical University (SUNY). The AAI immunology courses include an Introductory Course and an Advance Course. The Introductory Course is a course that gives students an overview of the basics of immunology.

In addition, this Introductory Course gives students more information to complement general biology or science training. It also has two different parts: Part I is an introduction to the basic principles of immunology and Part II is a clinically-oriented lecture series. On the other hand, the Advanced Course is another course for those who are willing to expand or update their understanding of immunology. It is advised for students who want to attend the Advanced Course to have a background of the principles of immunology. Most schools require students to take electives in other to complete their degrees. A Master's degree requires two years of study following the attainment of a bachelor's degree. For a doctoral programme it is required to take two additional years of study.

The expectation of occupational growth in immunology is an increase of 36 percent from 2010 to 2020. The median annual wage was $76,700 in May 2010. However, the lowest 10 percent of immunologists earned less than $41,550, and the top 10 percent earned more than $142,800, (Bureau of Labor Statistics, 2013). The practice of immunology itself is not specified by the U.S. Department of Labor but it belongs to the practice of life science in general.

REFERENCES

1. Goldsby RA; Kindt TK; Osborne BA & Kuby J (2003). Immunology (5th ed.). San Francisco: W.H. Freeman. ISBN 0-7167-4947-5.
2. Jaspan HB; Lawn SD; Safrit JT; Bekker LG (February 2006). "The maturing immune system: implications for development and testing HIV-1 vaccines for children and adolescents". AIDS. 20 (4): 483–94. doi:10.1097/01.aids.0000210602.40267.60. PMID 16470112.
3. Glezen WP (December 2001). "Maternal vaccines". Prim. Care. 28 (4): 791–806, vi–vii. doi:10.1016/S0095-4543(05)70041-5. PMID 11739030.
4. Holt PG; Macaubas C; Cooper D; Nelson DJ; et al. (1997). "Th-1/Th-2 switch regulation in immune responses to inhaled antigens. Role of dendritic cells in the aetiology of allergic respiratory disease". Adv. Exp. Med. Biol. Advances in Experimental Medicine and Biology. 417: 301–6. doi:10.1007/978-1-4757-9966-8_49. ISBN 978-1-4757-9968-2. PMID 9286377.
5. Sizonenko PC; Paunier L (November 1975). "Hormonal changes in puberty III: Correlation of plasma dehydroepiandrosterone, testosterone, FSH, and LH with stages of puberty and bone age in normal boys and girls and in patients with Addison's disease or hypogonadism or with premature or late adrenarche". J. Clin. Endocrinol. Metab. 41 (5): 894–904. doi:10 1210/jcem-41-5-894. PMID 127002.
6. Verthelyi D (June 2001). "Sex hormones as immunomodulators in health and disease". Int. Immunopharmacol. 1 (6): 983–93. doi:10.1016/S1567-5769(01)00044-3. PMID 11407317.
7. Stimson WH (September 1988). "Oestrogen and human T lymphocytes: presence of specific receptors in the T-suppressor/cytotoxic subset". Scand. J. Immunol. 28 (3): 345–50. doi:10.1111/j.1365-3083.1988.tb01459.x. PMID 2973658.
8. Benten WP; Stephan C; Wunderlich F (June 2002). 'B cells express intracellular

but not surface receptors for testosterone and estradiol". Steroids. 67 (7): 647–54. doi:10.1016/S0039-128X(02)00013-2. PMID 11996938.

9. Beagley KW; Gockel CM (August 2003). "Regulation of innate and adaptive immunity by the female sex hormones oestradiol and progesterone". FEMS Immunol. Med. Microbiol. 38 (1): 13–22. doi:10.1016/S0928-8244(03)00202-5. PMID 12900050.
10. Kanda N; Tamaki K (February 1999). "Estrogen enhances immunoglobulin production by human PBMCs". J. Allergy Clin. Immunol. 103 (2 Pt 1): 282–8. doi:10.1016/S0091-6749(99)70503-8. PMID 9949320.
11. McFarland RD; Douek DC; Koup RA; Picker LJ (April 2000). "Identification of a human recent thymic emigrant phenotype". Proc. Natl. Acad. Sci. U.S.A. 97 (8): 4215–20. doi:10.1073/pnas.070061597. PMC 18202Freely accessible. PMID 10737767.
12. Miller JJ; Valdes R (February 1991). "Approaches to minimizing interference by cross-reacting molecules in immunoassays". Clin. Chem. 37 (2): 144–53. PMID 1993317.
13. Silverstein A (1989). A History of Immunology. New York: Academic Press.
14. Tauber AI & Chernyak L (1991). Metchnikoff and the Origins of Immunology. New York: Oxford University Press.
15. Tauber AI (1994). The Immune Self: Theory or Metaphor?. Cambridge: Cambridge University Press.
16. Jerne NK (1955). "The natural selection theory of antibody formation". Proceedings of the National Academy of Sciences USA. 41: 849–57. doi:10.1073/pnas.41.11.849. PMC 534292Freely accessible. PMID 16589759.
17. Burnet FM (1959). The Clonal Selection Theory of Acquired Immunity. Cambridge: Cambridge University Press.
18. Burnet FM (1969). Cellular Immunology: Self and Notself. Cambridge: Cambridge University Press.
19. Bretscher P; Cohn M (1970). "A theory of self-nonself discrimination". Science. 169 (3950): 1042–49. doi:10.1126/science.169.3950.1042.
20. Matzinger P (2002). "The danger model: A renewed sense of self". Science. 296 (5566): 301–5. doi:10.1126/science.1071059. PMID 11951032.
21. Pradeu (2012). The Limits of the Self: Immunology and Biological Identity. New York: Oxford University Press.
22. Langman RE; Cohn M (2000). "A minimal model for the self-nonself discrimination: a return to the basics". Seminars in Immunology. 12: 189–195. doi:10.1006/smim.2000.0231. PMID 10910739.
23. Clark WR (2008). In Defense of Self: How the Immune System Really Works. New York: Oxford University Press.
24. Coutinho A; et al. (1984). "From an antigen-centered, clonal perspective of immune responses to an organism-centered network perspective of autonomous reactivity of self-referential immune systems". Immunological Reviews. 79:

151–168. doi:10.1111/j.1600-065x.1984.tb00492.x.

25. Irun C (2000). Tending Adam's garden: Evolving the cognitive immune self. San Diego: Academic Press.

26. Pradeu T; Carosella ED (2006). "On the definition of a criterion of immunogenicity". Proc Natl Acad Sci U S A. 103 (47): 17858–17861. doi:10.1073/pnas.0608683103. PMID 17101995.

27. Pradeu T; Jaeger S; Vivier E (2013). "The speed of change: towards a discontinuity theory of immunity?". Nature Reviews Immunology. 13 (10): 764–769. doi:10.1038/nri3521. PMID 23995627.

28. Janeway CA Jr.; Goodnow CC; Medzhitov R (1996). "Immunological tolerance: Danger – pathogen on the premises!". Current Biology. 6 (5): 519–522. doi:10.1016/S0960-9822(02)00531-6. PMID 8805259.

29. Vance RE (2000). "Cutting edge commentary: a Copernican revolution? Doubts about the danger theory". Journal of Immunology. 165 (4): 1725–1728. doi:10.4049/jimmunol.165.4.1725.

30. Matzinger P (2012). "The evolution of the danger theory. Interview by Lauren Constable". Expert Rev Clin Immunol. 8 (4): 311–317. doi:10.1586/eci.12.21. PMID 22607177.

31. Pradeu T; Cooper EL (2012). "The danger theory: 20 years later". Frontiers in Immunology. 3: 287. doi:10.3389/fimmu.2012.00287. PMC 3443751Freely accessible. PMID 23060876.

32. "Office of Science Education – LifeWorks – Immunologist". Retrieved 2009-09-10.

33. http://www.aaaai.org/about-the-aaaai/allergist---immunologists--specialized-skills.aspx.

34. North Carolina Association for Biomedical Research, 2013.

35. American Association of Immunology, n.d.

36. http://www.aai.org/Careers/Graduate_Programs.html.

37. The American Association of Immunologists, n.d.

38. Stanford School of Medicine.

39. http://www.bls.gov/bls/confidentiality.htm Bureau of Labor Statistics, 2013, May 02.

40. http://www.bls.gov/bls/confidentiality.htm Bureau of Labor Statistics, 2013.

41. "immunotherapies definition". Dictionary.com. Retrieved 2009-06-02.

42. Masihi KN (July 2001). "Fighting infection using immunomodulatory agents". Expert Opin Biol Ther. 1 (4): 641–53. doi:10.1517/14712598.1.4.641. PMID 11727500.

43. Fujita K, Ikarashi H, Takakuwa K, Kodama S, Tokunaga A, Takahashi T, Tanaka K (May 1995). "Prolonged disease-free period in patients with advanced epithelial ovarian cancer after adoptive transfer of tumor-infiltrating lymphocytes". Clin.

Cancer Res. 1 (5): 501–7. PMID 9816009.

44. Kimura H, Yamaguchi Y (July 1997). "A phase III randomized study of interleukin-2 lymphokine-activated killer cell immunotherapy combined with chemotherapy or radiotherapy after curative or noncurative resection of primary lung carcinoma". Cancer. 80 (1): 42–9. doi:10.1002/(SICI)1097-0142(19970701)80:1<42::AID-CNCR6>3.0.CO;2-H. PMID 9210707.

45. Takayama T, Sekine T, Makuuchi M, Yamasaki S, Kosuge T, Yamamoto J, Shimada K, Sakamoto M, Hirohashi S, Ohashi Y, Kakizoe T (September 2000). "Adoptive immunotherapy to lower postsurgical recurrence rates of hepatocellular carcinoma: a randomised trial". Lancet. 356 (9232): 802–7. doi:10.1016/S0140-6736(00)02654-4. PMID 11022927.

46. Kono K, Takahashi A, Ichihara F, Amemiya H, Iizuka H, Fujii H, Sekikawa T, Matsumoto Y (June 2002). "Prognostic significance of adoptive immunotherapy with tumor-associated lymphocytes in patients with advanced gastric cancer: a randomized trial". Clin. Cancer Res. 8 (6): 1767–71. PMID 12060615.

47. Li K, Li CK, Chuen CK, Tsang KS, Fok TF, James AE, Lee SM, Shing MM, Chik KW, Yuen PM (February 2005). "Preclinical ex vivo expansion of G-CSF-mobilized peripheral blood stem cells: effects of serum-free media, cytokine combinations and chemotherapy". Eur. J. Haematol. 74 (2): 128–35. doi:10.1111/j.1600-0609.2004.00343.x. PMID 15654904.

48. Järvinen R, Kaasinen E, Sankila A, Rintala E (August 2009). "Long-term efficacy of maintenance bacillus Calmette-Guérin versus maintenance mitomycin C instillation therapy in frequently recurrent TaT1 tumours without carcinoma in situ: a subgroup analysis of the prospective, randomised FinnBladder I study with a 20-year follow-up". Eur. Urol. 56 (2): 260–5. doi:10.1016/j.eururo.2009.04.009. PMID 19395154.

49. van Seters M, van Beurden M, ten Kate FJ, Beckmann I, Ewing PC, Eijkemans MJ, Kagie MJ, Meijer CJ, Aaronson NK, Kleinjan A, Heijmans-Antonissen C, Zijlstra FJ, Burger MP, Helmerhorst TJ (April 2008). "Treatment of vulvar intraepithelial neoplasia with topical imiquimod". N. Engl. J. Med. 358 (14): 1465–73. doi:10.1056/NEJMoa072685. PMID 18385498.

50. Buck HW, Guth KJ (October 2003). "Treatment of vaginal intraepithelial neoplasia (primarily low grade) with imiquimod 5% cream". J Low Genit Tract Dis. 7 (4): 290–3. doi:10.1097/00128360-200310000-00011. PMID 17051086.

51. Davidson HC, Leibowitz MS, Lopez-Albaitero A, Ferris RL (September 2009). "Immunotherapy for head and neck cancer". Oral Oncol. 45 (9): 747–51. doi:10.1016/j.oraloncology.2009.02.009. PMID 19442565.

52. Dani T, Knobler R (2009). "Extracorporeal photoimmunotherapy-photopheresis". Front. Biosci. 14 (14): 4769–77. doi:10.2741/3566. PMID 19273388.

53. Eggermont AM, Schadendorf D (June 2009). "Melanoma and immunotherapy". Hematol. Oncol. Clin. North Am. 23 (3): 547–64, ix–x. doi:10.1016/j.hoc.2009.03.009. PMID 19464602.

54. Chuang CM, Monie A, Wu A, Hung CF (2009). "Combination of apigenin treatment with therapeutic HPV DNA vaccination generates enhanced therapeutic anti tumor effects". J. Biomed. Sci. 16 (1): 49. doi:10.1186/1423-0127-16-49. PMC 2705346Freely accessible. PMID 19473507.

55. Pawlita M, Gissmann L (April 2009). "[Recurrent respiratory papillomatosis: indication for HPV vaccination?]". Dtsch. Med. Wochenschr. (in German). 134 Suppl 2: S100–2. doi:10.1055/s-0029-1220219. PMID 19353471.

56. Kang N, Zhou J, Zhang T, Wang L, Lu F, Cui Y, Cui L, He W (August 2009). "Adoptive immunotherapy of lung cancer with immobilized anti-TCRgammadelta antibody-expanded human gammadelta T-cells in peripheral blood". Cancer Biol. Ther. 8 (16): 1540–9. doi:10.4161/cbt.8.16.8950. PMID 19471115.

57. Gao, Daiqing; Li, Changyou; Xie, Xihe; Zhao, Peng; Wei, Xiaofang; Sun, Weihong; Liu, Hsin-Chen; Alexandrou, Aris T.; Jones, Jennifer (2014-01-01). "Autologous tumor lysate-pulsed dendritic cell immunotherapy with cytokine-induced killer cells improves survival in gastric and colorectal cancer patients". PloS One. 9 (4): e93886. doi:10.1371/journal.pone.0093886. ISSN 1932-6203. PMC 3974849Freely accessible. PMID 24699863.

58. Overes IM, Fredrix H, Kester MG, Falkenburg JH, van der Voort R, de Witte TM, Dolstra H (2009). "Efficient activation of LRH-1-specific CD8+ T-cell responses from transplanted leukemia patients by stimulation with P2X5 mRNA-electroporated dendritic cells". J. Immunother. 32 (6): 539–51. doi:10.1097/CJI.0b013e3181987c22. PMID 19483655.

59. Di Lorenzo G, Buonerba C, Kantoff PW (September 2011). "Immunotherapy for the treatment of prostate cancer". Nature Reviews Clinical Oncology. 8 (9): 551–61. doi:10.1038/nrclinonc.2011.72. PMID 21606971.

60. Rosenberg SA, Restifo NP, Yang JC, Morgan RA, Dudley ME (April 2008). "Adoptive cell transfer: a clinical path to effective cancer immunotherapy". Nature Reviews Cancer. 8 (4): 299–308. doi:10.1038/nrc2355. PMC 2553205Freely accessible. PMID 18354418.

61. Antony PA, Piccirillo CA, Akpinarli A, Finkelstein SE, Speiss PJ, Surman DR, Palmer DC, Chan CC, Klebanoff CA, Overwijk WW, Rosenberg SA, Restifo NP (March 2005). "CD8+ T cell immunity against a tumor/self-antigen is augmented by CD4+ T helper cells and hindered by naturally occurring T regulatory cells". Journal of Immunology. 174 (5): 2591–601. doi:10.4049/jimmunol.174.5.2591. PMC 1403291Freely accessible. PMID 15728465.

62. Gattinoni L, Finkelstein SE, Klebanoff CA, Antony PA, Palmer DC, Spiess PJ, Hwang LN, Yu Z, Wrzesinski C, Heimann DM, Surh CD, Rosenberg SA, Restifo NP (October 2005). "Removal of homeostatic cytokine sinks by lymphodepletion enhances the efficacy of adoptively transferred tumor-specific CD8+ T cells". J. Exp. Med. 202 (7): 907–12. doi:10.1084/jem.20050732. PMC 1397916Freely accessible. PMID 16203864.

63. Dummer W, Niethammer AG, Baccala R, Lawson BR, Wagner N, Reisfeld RA, Theofilopoulos AN (July 2002). "T cell homeostatic proliferation elicits effective antitumor autoimmunity". J. Clin. Invest. 110 (2): 185–92. doi:10.1172/

JCI15175. PMC 151053Freely accessible. PMID 12122110.

64. Dudley ME, Yang JC, Sherry R, Hughes MS, Royal R, Kammula U, Robbins PF, Huang J, Citrin DE, Leitman SF, Wunderlich J, Restifo NP, Thomasian A, Downey SG, Smith FO, Klapper J, Morton K, Laurencot C, White DE, Rosenberg SA (November 2008). "Adoptive cell therapy for patients with metastatic melanoma: evaluation of intensive myeloablative chemoradiation preparative regimens". J. Clin. Oncol. 26 (32): 5233–9. doi:10.1200/JCO.2008.16.5449. PMC 2652090Freely accessible. PMID 18809613.
65. Dudley ME, Wunderlich JR, Robbins PF, Yang JC, Hwu P, Schwartzentruber DJ, Topalian SL, Sherry R, Restifo NP, Hubicki AM, Robinson MR, Raffeld M, Duray P, Seipp CA, Rogers-Freezer L, Morton KE, Mavroukakis SA, White DE, Rosenberg SA (October 2002). "Cancer regression and autoimmunity in patients after clonal repopulation with antitumor lymphocytes". Science. 298 (5594): 850–4. doi:10.1126/science.1076514. PMC 1764179Freely accessible. PMID 12242449.
66. Pilon-Thomas S, Kuhn L, Ellwanger S, Janssen W, Royster E, Marzban S, Kudchadkar R, Zager J, Gibney G, Sondak VK, Weber J, Mulé JJ, Sarnaik AA (October 2012). "Efficacy of adoptive cell transfer of tumor-infiltrating lymphocytes after lymphopenia induction for metastatic melanoma". J. Immunother. 35 (8): 615–20. doi:10.1097/CJI.0b013e31826e8f5f. PMID 22996367.
67. Manjunath SR, Ramanan G, Dedeepiya VD, Terunuma H, Deng X, Baskar S, Senthilkumar R, Thamaraikannan P, Srinivasan T, Preethy S, Abraham SJ (January 2012). "Autologous immune enhancement therapy in recurrent ovarian cancer with metastases: a case report". Case Rep Oncol. 5 (1): 114–8. doi:10.1159/000337319. PMC 3364094Freely accessible. PMID 22666198.
68. Li Y, Zhang T, Ho C, Orange JS, Douglas SD, Ho WZ (December 2004). "Natural killer cells inhibit hepatitis C virus expression". J. Leukoc. Biol. 76 (6): 1171–9. doi:10.1189/jlb.0604372. PMID 15339939.
69. Doskali M, Tanaka Y, Ohira M, Ishiyama K, Tashiro H, Chayama K, Ohdan H (March 2011). "Possibility of adoptive immunotherapy with peripheral blood-derived CD3⁻CD56+ and CD3+CD56+ cells for inducing antihepatocellular carcinoma and antihepatitis C virus activity". J. Immunother. 34 (2): 129–38. doi:10.1097/CJI.0b013e3182048c4e. PMID 21304407.
70. Terunuma H, Deng X, Dewan Z, Fujimoto S, Yamamoto N (2008). "Potential role of NK cells in the induction of immune responses: implications for NK cell-based immunotherapy for cancers and viral infections". Int. Rev. Immunol. 27 (3): 93–110. doi:10.1080/08830180801911743. PMID 18437601.
71. See DM, Tilles JG (1996). "alpha-Interferon treatment of patients with chronic fatigue syndrome". Immunol. Invest. 25 (1–2): 153–64. doi:10.3109/08820139609059298. PMID 8675231.
72. Ojo-Amaize EA, Conley EJ, Peter JB (January 1994). "Decreased natural killer cell activity is associated with severity of chronic fatigue immune dysfunction syndrome". Clin. Infect. Dis. 18 Suppl 1: S157–9. doi:10.1093/clinids/18.

Supplement_1.S157. PMID 8148445.

73. Kida K, Isozumi R, Ito M (December 2000). "Killing of human Herpes virus 6-infected cells by lymphocytes cultured with interleukin-2 or -12". Pediatr Int. 42 (6): 631–6. doi:10.1046/j.1442-200x.2000.01315.x. PMID 11192519.

74. Morgan RA, Dudley ME, Wunderlich JR, Hughes MS, Yang JC, Sherry RM, Royal RE, Topalian SL, Kammula US, Restifo NP, Zheng Z, Nahvi A, de Vries CR, Rogers-Freezer LJ, Mavroukakis SA, Rosenberg SA (October 2006). "Cancer regression in patients after transfer of genetically engineered lymphocytes". Science. 314 (5796): 126–9. doi:10.1126/science.1129003. PMC 2267026Freely accessible. PMID 16946036.

75. Hunder NN, Wallen H, Cao J, Hendricks DW, Reilly JZ, Rodmyre R, Jungbluth A, Gnjatic S, Thompson JA, Yee C (June 2008). "Treatment of metastatic melanoma with autologous CD4+ T cells against NY-ESO-1". N. Engl. J. Med. 358 (25): 2698–703. doi:10.1056/NEJMoa0800251. PMC 3277288Freely accessible. PMID 18565862.

76. "2008 Symposium Program & Speakers". Cancer Research Institute.

77. http://www.telegraph.co.uk/earth/main.jhtml?xml=/earth/2008/06/18/scicanc118.xml

78. Rotrosen D, Matthews JB, Bluestone JA (July 2002). "The immune tolerance network: a new paradigm for developing tolerance-inducing therapies". The Journal of Allergy and Clinical Immunology. 110 (1): 17–23. doi:10.1067/mai.2002.124258. PMID 12110811.

79. Durham SR, Walker SM, Varga EM, Jacobson MR, O'Brien F, Noble W, Till SJ, Hamid QA, Nouri-Aria KT (August 1999). "Long-term clinical efficacy of grass-pollen immunotherapy". N. Engl. J. Med. 341 (7): 468–75. doi:10.1056/NEJM199908123410702. PMID 10441602.

80. "Clinical Trials Search Results - Stanford University School of Medicine". med.stanford.edu. Retrieved 2016-04-03.

81. Correale J, Farez M (February 2007). "Association between parasite infection and immune responses in multiple sclerosis". Annals of Neurology. 61 (2): 97–108. doi:10.1002/ana.21067. PMID 17230481.

82. Croese J, O'neil J, Masson J, Cooke S, Melrose W, Pritchard D, Speare R (January 2006). "A proof of concept study establishing Necator americanus in Crohn's patients and reservoir donors". Gut. 55 (1): 136–7. doi:10.1136/gut.2005.079129. PMC 1856386Freely accessible. PMID 16344586.

83. Reddy A, Fried B (January 2009). "An update on the use of helminths to treat Crohn's and other autoimmunune diseases". Parasitol. Res. 104 (2): 217–21. doi:10.1007/s00436-008-1297-5. PMID 19050918.

84. Laclotte C, Oussalah A, Rey P, Bensenane M, Pluvinage N, Chevaux JB, Trouilloud I, Serre AA, Boucekkine T, Bigard MA, Peyrin-Biroulet L (December 2008). "[Helminths and inflammatory bowel diseases]". Gastroenterol. Clin. Biol. (in French). 32 (12): 1064–74. doi:10.1016/j.gcb.2008.04.030. PMID 18619749.

85. Zaccone P, Fehervari Z, Phillips JM, Dunne DW, Cooke A (October 2006). "Parasitic worms and inflammatory diseases". Parasite Immunol. 28 (10): 515–23. doi:10.1111/j.1365-3024.2006.00879.x. PMC 1618732Freely accessible. PMID 16965287.

86. Brooker S, Bethony J, Hotez PJ (2004). "Human Hookworm Infection in the 21st Century". Advances in Parasitology. 58: 197–288. doi:10.1016/S0065-308X(04)58004-1. ISBN 9780120317585. PMC 2268732Freely accessible. PMID 15603764.

87. Fujiwara RT, Cançado GG, Freitas PA, Santiago HC, Massara CL, Dos Santos Carvalho O, Corrêa-Oliveira R, Geiger SM, Bethony J (2009). Yazdanbakhsh M, ed. "Necator americanus infection: a possible cause of altered dendritic cell differentiation and eosinophil profile in chronically infected individuals". PLoS Negl Trop Dis. 3 (3): e399. doi:10.1371/journal.pntd.0000399. PMC 2654967Freely accessible. PMID 19308259.

88. Carvalho L, Sun J, Kane C, Marshall F, Krawczyk C, Pearce EJ (January 2009). "Review series on helminths, immune modulation and the hygiene hypothesis: mechanisms underlying helminth modulation of dendritic cell function". Immunology. 126 (1): 28–34. doi:10.1111/j.1365-2567.2008.03008.x. PMC 2632707Freely accessible. PMID 19120496.

89. Fumagalli M, Pozzoli U, Cagliani R, Comi GP, Riva S, Clerici M, Bresolin N, Sironi M (June 2009). "Parasites represent a major selective force for interleukin genes and shape the genetic predisposition to autoimmune conditions". J. Exp. Med. 206 (6): 1395–408. doi:10.1084/jem.20082779. PMC 2715056Freely accessible. PMID 19468064.

90. Vinzenz K, Schönthal E, Zekert F, Wunderer S (Oct 1987). "Diagnosis of head and neck carcinomas by means of immunological tumour markers (Beta-2-microglobulin, immunoglobulin E, ferritin, N-acetyl-neuraminic acid, phosphohexose-isomerase)". Journal of Cranio-Maxillo-Facial Surgery. 15 (5): 270–7. doi:10.1016/s1010-5182(87)80066-5. PMID 3316283.

91. Méhes G, Luegmayr A, Hattinger CM, Lörch T, Ambros IM, Gadner H, Ambros PF (Jan 2001). "Automatic detection and genetic profiling of disseminated neuroblastoma cells". Medical and Pediatric Oncology. 36 (1): 205–9. doi:10.1002/1096-911X(20010101)36:1<205::AID-MPO1050>3.0.CO;2-G. PMID 11464886{{inconsistent citations}}

92. Dunn GP, Dunn IF, Curry WT (2007). "Focus on TILs: Prognostic significance of tumor infiltrating lymphocytes in human glioma". Cancer Immunity. 7: 12. PMC 2935751Freely accessible. PMID 17691714.

93. Dunn GP, Bruce AT, Ikeda H, Old LJ, Schreiber RD (Nov 2002). "Cancer immunoediting: from immunosurveillance to tumor escape". Nature Immunology. 3 (11): 991–8. doi:10.1038/ni1102-991. PMID 12407406.

94. Burnet M (Apr 1957). "Cancer; a biological approach. I. The processes of control". British Medical Journal. 1 (5022): 779–86. doi:10.1136/bmj.1.3356.779. JSTOR 25382096. PMC 1973174Freely accessible. PMID 13404306.

95. Kim R, Emi M, Tanabe K (May 2007). "Cancer immunoediting from immune surveillance to immune escape". Immunology. 121 (1): 1–14. doi:10.1111/j.1365-2567.2007.02587.x. PMC 2265921Freely accessible. PMID 17386080.

96. Dunn GP, Old LJ, Schreiber RD (2004). "The three Es of cancer immunoediting". Annual Review of Immunology. 22: 329–60. doi:10.1146/annurev.immunol.22.012703.104803. PMID 15032581.

97. Odunsi K, Old LJ (2007). "Tumor infiltrating lymphocytes: indicators of tumor-related immune responses". Cancer Immunity. 7: 3. PMC 2935754Freely accessible. PMID 17311362.

98. Obeid M, Tesniere A, Ghiringhelli F, Fimia GM, Apetoh L, Perfettini JL, Castedo M, Mignot G, Panaretakis T, Casares N, Métivier D, Larochette N, van Endert P, Ciccosanti F, Piacentini M, Zitvogel L, Kroemer G (Jan 2007). "Calreticulin exposure dictates the immunogenicity of cancer cell death". Nature Medicine. 13 (1): 54–61. doi:10.1038/nm1523. PMID 17187072.

99. Steinman RM, Mellman I (Jul 2004). "Immunotherapy: bewitched, bothered, and bewildered no more". Science. 305 (5681): 197–200. doi:10.1126/science.1099688. PMID 15247468.

100. Lake RA, van der Most RG (Jun 2006). "A better way for a cancer cell to die". The New England Journal of Medicine. 354 (23): 2503–4. doi:10.1056/NEJMcibr061443. PMID 16760453.

101. Zitvogel L, Tesniere A, Kroemer G (Oct 2006). "Cancer despite immunosurveillance: immunoselection and immunosubversion". Nature Reviews. Immunology. 6 (10): 715–27. doi:10.1038/nri1936. PMID 16977338.

102. Zitvogel L, Casares N, Péquignot MO, Chaput N, Albert ML, Kroemer G (2004). "Immune response against dying tumor cells". Advances in Immunology. Advances in Immunology. 84: 131–79. doi:10.1016/S0065-2776(04)84004-5. ISBN 978-0-12-022484-5. PMID 15246252.

103. Bellamy CO, Malcomson RD, Harrison DJ, Wyllie AH (Feb 1995). "Cell death in health and disease: the biology and regulation of apoptosis". Seminars in Cancer Biology. 6 (1): 3–16. doi:10.1006/scbi.1995.0002. PMID 7548839.

104. Thompson CB (Mar 1995). "Apoptosis in the pathogenesis and treatment of disease". Science. 267 (5203): 1456–62. doi:10.1126/science.7878464. PMID 7878464.

105. Igney FH, Krammer PH (Apr 2002). "Death and anti-death: tumour resistance to apoptosis". Nature Reviews. Cancer. 2 (4): 277–88. doi:10.1038/nrc776. PMID 12001989.

106. Steinman RM, Turley S, Mellman I, Inaba K (Feb 2000). "The induction of tolerance by dendritic cells that have captured apoptotic cells". The Journal of Experimental Medicine. 191 (3): 411–6. doi:10.1084/jem.191.3.411. PMC 2195815Freely accessible. PMID 10662786.

107. Liu K, Iyoda T, Saternus M, Kimura Y, Inaba K, Steinman RM (Oct 2002). "Immune tolerance after delivery of dying cells to dendritic cells in situ". The Journal of Experimental Medicine. 196 (8): 1091–7. doi:10.1084/jem.20021215.

PMC 2194037Freely accessible. PMID 12391020.

108. Kroemer G, El-Deiry WS, Golstein P, Peter ME, Vaux D, Vandenabeele P, Zhivotovsky B, Blagosklonny MV, Malorni W, Knight RA, Piacentini M, Nagata S, Melino G (Nov 2005). "Classification of cell death: recommendations of the Nomenclature Committee on Cell Death". Cell Death and Differentiation. 12 Suppl 2: 1463–7. doi:10.1038/sj.cdd.4401724. PMID 16247491.

109. Buckwalter MR, Srivastava PK (2013). "Mechanism of dichotomy between CD8+ responses elicited by apoptotic and necrotic cells". Cancer Immunity. 13: 2. PMC 3559190Freely accessible. PMID 23390373.

110. Gamrekelashvili J, Ormandy LA, Heimesaat MM, Kirschning CJ, Manns MP, Korangy F, Greten TF (Oct 2012). "Primary sterile necrotic cells fail to cross-prime CD8(+) T cells". Oncoimmunology. 1 (7): 1017–1026. doi:10.4161/onci.21098. PMC 3494616Freely accessible. PMID 23170250.

111. Janssen E, Tabeta K, Barnes MJ, Rutschmann S, McBride S, Bahjat KS, Schoenberger SP, Theofilopoulos AN, Beutler B, Hoebe K (Jun 2006). "Efficient T cell activation via a Toll-Interleukin 1 Receptor-independent pathway". Immunity. 24 (6): 787–99. doi:10.1016/j.immuni.2006.03.024. PMID 16782034.

112. Ronchetti A, Rovere P, Iezzi G, Galati G, Heltai S, Protti MP, Garancini MP, Manfredi AA, Rugarli C, Bellone M (Jul 1999). "Immunogenicity of apoptotic cells in vivo: role of antigen load, antigen-presenting cells, and cytokines". Journal of Immunology. 163 (1): 130–6. PMID 10384108.

113. Scheffer SR, Nave H, Korangy F, Schlote K, Pabst R, Jaffee EM, Manns MP, Greten TF (Jan 2003). "Apoptotic, but not necrotic, tumor cell vaccines induce a potent immune response in vivo". International Journal of Cancer. 103 (2): 205–11. doi:10.1002/ijc.10777. PMID 12455034.

114. Storkus WJ, Falo LD (Jan 2007). "A 'good death' for tumor immunology". Nature Medicine. 13 (1): 28–30. doi:10.1038/nm0107-28. PMID 17206130.

115. Dunn GP, Koebel CM, Schreiber RD (Nov 2006). "Interferons, immunity and cancer immunoediting". Nature Reviews. Immunology. 6 (11): 836–48. doi:10.1038/nri1961. PMID 17063185.

116. zur Hausen H (May 2000). "Papillomaviruses causing cancer: evasion from host-cell control in early events in carcinogenesis". Journal of the National Cancer Institute. 92 (9): 690–8. doi:10.1093/jnci/92.9.690. PMID 10793105.

117. Brittner, J.J. (1943). "Possible relationship of the oestrogenic hormones, genetic susceptibility and milk influence in the production of mammary cancer in mice". Cancer Research. 2: 710–721.

118. Callahan R, Smith GH (Feb 2000). "MMTV-induced mammary tumorigenesis: gene discovery, progression to malignancy and cellular pathways". Oncogene. 19 (8): 992–1001. doi:10.1038/sj.onc.1203276. PMID 10713682.

119. Lawson JS, Tran DD, Carpenter E, Ford CE, Rawlinson WD, Whitaker NJ, Delprado W (Dec 2006). "Presence of mouse mammary tumour-like virus gene sequences may be associated with morphology of specific human breast cancer".

Journal of Clinical Pathology. 59 (12): 1287–92. doi:10.1136/jcp.2005.035907. PMC 1860546Freely accessible. PMID 16698952.

Index

A

B

C

D

E

F

H

I

M

N

P

R

S

T

V

W